T-Cell-Directed
Immunointervention

FRONTIERS IN PHARMACOLOGY & THERAPEUTICS

FRONTIERS IN PHARMACOLOGY & THERAPEUTICS

T-Cell-Directed Immunointervention

edited by

Jean-François Bach
Immunologie Clinique, Hôpital Necker
Unité de Recherches de L'INSERM U25, Paris France

OXFORD

BLACKWELL SCIENTIFIC PUBLICATIONS

LONDON EDINBURGH BOSTON

MELBOURNE PARIS BERLIN VIENNA

© 1993 by
Blackwell Scientific Publications
Editorial Offices:
Osney Mead, Oxford OX2 0EL
25 John Street, London WC1N 2BL
23 Ainslie Place, Edinburgh EH3 6AJ
238 Main Street, Cambridge
   Massachusetts 02142, USA
54 University Street, Carlton
   Victoria 3053, Australia

Other Editorial Offices:
Librairie Arnette SA
2, rue Casimir-Delavigne
75006 Paris
France

Blackwell Wissenschafts-Verlag
Meinekestrasse 4
D-1000 Berlin 15
Germany

Blackwell MZV
Feldgasse 13
A-1238 Wien
Austria

First published 1993

Set by QBF Ltd, Wiltshire
Printed and bound in Great Britain
by Hartnolls Ltd, Bodmin, Cornwall

DISTRIBUTORS

Marston Book Services Ltd
PO Box 87
Oxford OX2 0DT
(*Orders*: Tel: 0865 791155
        Fax: 0865 791927
        Telex: 837515)

USA
Blackwell Scientific Publications, Inc.
238 Main Street
Cambridge, MA 02142
(*Orders*: Tel: 800 759-6102
        617 876-7000)

Canada
Times Mirror Professional Publishing Ltd
130 Flaska Drive
Markham, Ontario L6G 1B8
(*Orders*: Tel: 800 268-4178
        416 470-6739)

Australia
Blackwell Scientific Publications
Pty Ltd
54 University Street
Carlton, Victoria 3053
(*Orders*: Tel: 03 347-5552)

A catalogue record for this title
is available from the British Library

ISBN 0-632-03105-0

Library of Congress
Cataloging in Publication Data

T-cell-directed immunointervention / edited by
Jean-François Bach.
    p cm. — (Frontiers in pharmacology &
therapeutics)
    Includes bibliographical references and
index.
    ISBN 0-632-03105-0
    1. Immunosuppressive agents. 2. T cells—
Effect of drugs on.
    I. Bach, Jean-François. II. Series.
    [DNLM: 1. Immunity, Cellular. 2.
Immunosuppressive Agents—pharmacology.
3. Receptors, Antigen, T-Cell—drug
effects. 4. T-Lymphocytes—drug effects.
5. T-Lymphocytes—immunology. QW 920
T111]
    RM373.T14 1993
    616.07'9—dc20

Contents

v

Part 3: Anti-T cell monoclonal antibodies

Part 4: Other approaches

Contributors

Hans Acha-Orbea *Ludwig Institute for Cancer Research, Lausanne Branch, 1066 Epalinges, Switzerland*

Jean-François Bach *INSERM U25, Hôpital Necker, 161 rue de Sèvres, 75743 Paris, France*

Christian Boitard *INSERM U25 and Departement d'Immunologie Clinique, Hôpital Necker, 161 rue de Sèvres, 75743 Paris, France*

Lucienne Chatenoud *INSERM U25, Hôpital Necker, 161 rue de Sèvres, 75743 Paris, France*

Irun R. Cohen *Department of Cell Biology, Weizmann Institute of Science, Rehovot 76100, Israel*

Frank Emmrich *Max Planck Society, Clinical Research Units for Rheumatology, University of Erlangen-Nurnberg, Schwabachanlage 10, 8520 Erlangen, Germany*

Gilles Feutren *Clinical Research/Immunology, Sandoz Pharma Ltd, CH-4002 Basle, Switzerland*

John Fung *Division of Transplantation, Department of Surgery, University of Pittsburgh, Pittsburgh, PA 15213, USA*

Angela Granelli-Piperno *Laboratory of Cellular Physiology and Immunology, The Rockefeller University, 1230 York Avenue, New York, NY 10021, USA*

Barry D. Kahan *Division of Immunology and Organ Transplantation, Department of Surgery, The University of Texas Medical School at Houston, 6431 Fannin, Houston, TX 77030, USA*

Vicki Rubin Kelley *Department of Medicine, Brigham and Women's Hospital, Harvard Medical School, Boston, MA 02115, USA*

Paul A. Keown *Departments of Medicine and Pathology, Vancouver General Hospital, University of British Columbia and the British Columbia Transplant Society, Vancouver, BC, Canada*

Anders Lindholm *Department of Transplantation Surgery, Huddinge Hospital, Karolinska Institute, Huddinge, Sweden*

Hugh O. McDevitt *Departments of Microbiology and Immunology, and Medicine, Stanford University School of Medicine, Stanford, California, USA*

Felix Mor *Department of Medicine 'B' Beilinson Medical Center, Petah Tiqva and The Department of Cell Biology, The Weizmann Institute of Science, Rehovot, Israel*

John R. Murphy *Department of Medicine, University Hospital, Boston University Medical Center, Boston, MA 02118, USA*

Jonathan B. Rothbard *Immunologic Pharmaceutical Corporation, Palo Alto, California, USA*

Thomas E. Starzl *Pittsburgh Transplantation Institute, University of Pittsburgh, Pittsburgh, PA 15213, USA*

Terry B. Strom *Department of Medicine, Beth Israel Hospital, Harvard Medical School, Boston, MA 02215, USA*

Angus W. Thomson *Pittsburgh Transplantation Institute, University of Pittsburgh, Pittsburgh, PA 15213, USA*

Jacky Woo *Pittsburgh Transplantation Institute, University of Pittsburgh, Pittsburgh, PA 15213, USA*

Thasia G. Woodworth *Seragen Inc., Hopkinton, MA 01748, USA*

List of abbreviations

AA	Adjuvant arthritis
ab	Antibody
ADPR	Adenosine diphosphoribosylation
ALG	Antilymphocyte globulin
APC	Antigen-presenting cell
ARRE	Antigen receptor response element
ATG	Antithymocyte globulin
AUC	Area through a dosing interval
bp	Base pair
BUN	Blood urea nitrogen
CaM	Calmodulin
CD	Cluster of differentiation
CDR	Complementarily determining region
CFA	Complete Freund's adjuvant
CNA	Calcineurin A
CNB	Calcineurin B
CNS	Central nervous system
Con A	Concanavalin A
CsA	Cyclosporin A/cyclosporin
CSF	Colony-stimulating factor
CTCL	Cutaneous T-cell lymphoma
CTL	Cytotoxic T lymphocytes
Cy	Cyclophosphamide
DAG	Diacylglycerol
DNP-KLH	Dinitrophenol-keyhole limpet haemocyanin
DT	Diphtheria toxin
DTH	Delayed-type hypersensitivity
EAE	Experimental autoimmune/allergic encephalomyelitis
EAN	Experimental allergic neuritis
EAT	Experimental autoimmune/allergic thyroiditis
EAU	Experimental autoimmune uveoretinitis
EBV	Epstein–Barr virus
EF	Elongation factor

ELISA	Enzyme-linked immunosorbant assay
EMIT	Enzyme multiplied immunoassay technique
ESR	Erythrocyte sedimentation rate
FKBP	FK 506-binding protein
FPIA	Fluorescence polarization immunoassay
FSGS	Focal segmental glomerulosclerosis
GM-CSF	Granulocyte monocyte colony stimulating factor
GVHD	Graft-versus-host disease
GVHR	Graft-versus-host reaction
HDL	High density lipoprotein
HIV	Human immunodeficiency virus
HLA	Human leukocyte antigen
HPLC	High performance liquid chromatography
HSV	Herpes simplex virus
IC	Inhibitory concentration
IDDM	Insulin-dependent diabetes mellitus
IFN	Interferon
Ig	Immunoglobulin
IL	Interleukin
IL-2R	Interleukin-2 receptor
IP3	Inositol-1,4,5-triphosphate
Ir	Immune response
i.v.	Intravenous
KLH	Keyhole limpet haemocyanin
LAK	Lymphokine activated killer
LDL	Low density lipoprotein
LFA-3	Lymphocyte function associated antigen-3
LPS	Lipopolysaccharide
MBP	Myelin-basic protein
MCF	Macrophage chemotactic factor
MCN	Minimal change nephropathy
MeBmt	4-Butenyl-4-methyl-threonine
MG	Myasthenia gravis
MHC	Major histocompatibility complex
MIF	Migration inhibition factor
MIR	Mixed lymphocyte reaction
MoAb	Monoclonal antibodies
MS	Multiple sclerosis
NAD	Nicotinamide adenine nucleotide
NF	Nuclear factor
NFAT	Nuclear factor for activated T cells
NFIL-2A	Nuclear factor (protein) involved in the activation of T cells
NF-KB	Nuclear factor (protein) involved in the activation of B lymphocytes

NK	Natural killer
NMR	Nuclear magnetic resonance
NOD	Non-obese diabetic
NS	Nephrotic syndrome
PBMC	Peripheral blood mononuclear cells
PCR	Polymerase chain reaction
PEA	*Pseudomonas* exotoxin A
PFC	Plaque-forming cell
PG	Prostaglandin
PGD_2	Prostaglandin D_2
PHA	Phytohaemagglutinin
PIF	Procoagulant-inducing factor
PKC	Protein kinase C
PLC	Phospholipase C
PLP	Proteolipid protein
PMA	Phorbol myristate acetate
PPIase	Peptidyl prolyl *cis-trans* isomerase
PTLD	Post-transplant lymphoproliferative disease
RA	Rheumatoid arthritis
RFLP	Restriction fragment length polymorphism
RIA	Radioimmunoassay
SAC	*Staphylococcus aureus* Cowan
SGOT	Serum glutamic-oxaloacetic transaminase
SGPT	Serum glutamic-pyrovic transaminase
SLE	Systemic lupus erythematosus
SRBC	Sheep red blood cells
STL	Suppressor T lymphocytes
T BIL	Total bilirubin
Tc	Cytotoxic T lymphocytes
TCR	T-cell receptor
TfR	Transferrin receptor
T_H	T helper
TI	Thymic-independent
TK	Tyrosine kinase
TNF	Tumour necrosis factor
TNP-PAA	2,4,6-Trinitrophenyl-polyacrylimade
Ts	Suppresor T lymphocytes
VLDLP	Very low density lipoproteins
VSV	Vesticular stomatitis virus

Introduction

Most undesirable immune responses involve T cells at the regulatory and/
or effector level together with B cells and mononuclear phagocytes. It
appears, however, that T cells form privileged targets for immunointervention relative to B cells (that are difficult to damp down) and to macrophages (alteration of which carries a high risk of facilitating opportunistic
bacterial infections).

A major limitation of immunosuppressive therapy has been the
difficulty of hitting T cells selectively. Azathioprine and cyclophosphamide
act on B cells as well as T cells, while corticosteroids affect both monocyte
and macrophage functions. The situation has now evolved and it appears
possible to alter or kill T cells without affecting other lymphoid or
phagocytic cells. The aim of this book is to review the main therapeutic
approaches involving T cell-specific immunointervention.

Four privileged target receptor molecules

T cells use a limited number of receptors to recognize antigens, differentiate and exert their effector functions. These receptors have logically been
selected as potential targets to generate powerful immunosuppressive
agents.

Immunophillins play an essential intermediary role in the transcription
of major lymphokines. Interestingly, it is through studies of the mode of
action of immunosuppressive drugs identified by systematic screening that
their existence was discovered. They are cytosolic receptors to which
cyclosporins, FK506 and rapamycin bind. Immunophillins are not T cell-
specific (which explains some side-effects on organs that also express
immunophillins, notably the kidneys) but their full expression is apparently more central to the function of T cells than other cell types.

The *T-cell receptor/CD3 complex* is only expressed on T cells. It is an
ideal target, which can be hit directly (using monoclonal antibodies
specific for any of its fragments (Vβ, idiotypes, constant part, CD3, etc.) or
indirectly through an action on one of its ligands (antigen peptide or
major histocompatibility complex molecules that present the peptide to
the T-cell receptor).

The *interleukin 2 receptor* (IL-2R), a T-cell growth factor, plays a central role in T-cell differentiation. IL-2R can be targeted by monoclonal antibodies. It is unfortunate that the antibodies used so far, that recognize one of the two chains (p55 or p75), show only moderate affinity for the receptor which is insufficient in case of high-level IL-2R expression or intense IL-2 production. It will be interesting to evaluate the immunosuppressive effect of bispecific (anti-p55 + anti-p75) antibodies and mixtures of the two specificities. Alternatively, IL-2-toxin conjugates, which bind with high affinity to the whole heterodimer receptor, may be of value.

The *CD4 molecule* is an adhesion molecule endowed with co-receptor-like signalling capacity. Anti-CD4 monoclonal antibodies have proved remarkably efficacious in suppressing the immune response, possibly because of the particular importance of signals sent to T cells via the CD4 molecule. Immunosuppression induced by monoclonals may depend not only on their T-cell subset selectivity, that protects other T-cell subsets (notably CD8 cells), but also on the delivery of negative signals to CD4 cells.

Search for antigen-specific T-cell-directed immunosuppression

Some of the T-cell-selective therapeutic agents just mentioned show no antigen specificity and do not induce antigen-specific unresponsiveness (tolerance). This is notably the case of cyclosporin, FK 506 and anti-IL-2 receptor monoclonal antibodies. Other agents that are not antigen-specific either may facilitate the induction of tolerance. This is the case of anti-CD4 monoclonal antibodies and, to a lesser extent, anti-CD3 monoclonal antibodies. Other agents, although not strictly antigen-specific, induce T-cell suppression that is related to certain antigens. This is particularly the case of anti-$V\beta$ antibodies and idiotypic manipulation (T-cell vaccination). It is becoming more and more apparent that some immune responses directed against well-defined antigens involve restricted $V\alpha$ and $V\beta$ T-cell receptor fragments as well as restricted idiotypes. The antigen specificity is far from absolute but $V\beta$- or idiotype-directed immunointervention only affects immune responses directed against a limited array of antigens. The situation is similar with anti-MHC class II monoclonal antibodies, that are specific for immune responses controlled by the class II gene in question. Peptide therapy aiming at blocking the interaction between the MHC molecule and the antigen peptides can be placed at the same level of specificity. Ideally one would like to use autoantigen peptides to induce antigen-specific tolerance, but there are few settings in which the auto-antigen has been chemically defined in terms of its primary structure (e.g. acetylcholine receptor in myasthenia gravis), and even then only modest results have been achieved.

It is important to realize that most available immunosuppressive agents do not strongly affect secondary responses and immunologic memory. This is notably the case of chemicals such as cyclosporin and FK 506 whose action is quantitatively overwhelmed by the events taking place in secondary immune responses. This is probably why agents such as cyclosporin and anti-CD4 antibodies do not particularly promote opportunistic infections, that are usually due to pathogens that have already been encountered by the immune system.

Therapeutic strategy

Immunosuppressive agents can be classified under three headings.

The first category is represented by agents whose action is strictly dose-dependent (e.g. cyclosporin in its effect on lymphokine synthesis). They are essentially used to prevent the onset of undesirable immune responses or to maintain a state of moderate T-cell-directed immunosuppression. These agents, which also include FK 506 and anti-IL-2R monoclonal antibodies, are no longer efficacious in the case of hyperacute immune responses such as overt organ rejection episodes and acute exacerbations of autoimmune diseases.

The second category includes agents that are capable of mitigating these intense responses, either because they can be given at very high single doses (e.g. steroids) or because their impact is not reduced by the level of activation of the target cell (CD3 or CD4 molecules, TCR). This is typically the case of anti-CD3 and anti-CD4 antibodies that can be used in the treatment of established rejection or acute phases of autoimmune diseases.

The third category comprises agents which allow tolerance induction. It is so far essentially limited to anti-CD4 and perhaps anti-CD3 monoclonal antibodies. Only these agents will prove capable of exerting long-term effects persisting after the cessation of treatment. These considerations, together with the notion of reversibility of action (observed with most immunosuppressive agents but not with depleting anti-CD4 monoclonal antibodies), form the basis for therapeutic strategies in clinical practice. The goal is to exert sufficient immunosuppression with acceptable toxicity (the less severe the patient's condition, the less toxicity is acceptable). Inappropriate or insufficiently controlled associations of efficacious doses of several T-cell-selective immunosuppressants (e.g. cyclosporin + antilymphocyte antibodies) or high doses of one of these agents can lead to overimmunosuppression facilitating the occurrence of lymphomas and viral infections (EBV, CMV, Coxsackie, etc.). Major overimmunosuppression such as that induced, for example, by high doses of cyclosporin or OKT3 for more than 3–4 weeks, will inevitably have such very harmful consequences; hence the need to use moderate doses of these strong immunosuppressors and to carry out careful pharmacological and clinical monitoring. Direct drug side-effects (e.g. cyclosporin- or FK 506-induced nephrotoxicity) are less immediately preoccupying inasmuch as they can largely be avoided by combinations of low doses of several agents such as those used in organ transplantation (double or triple therapy) and could probably be used in autoimmune diseases. We have now reached a stage where profound immunosuppression can be induced without major direct side-effects. Consequently, the problem is not so much that of finding 'more active' agents but that of developing more selective agents that will promote antigen-specific unresponsiveness without altering anti-viral defenses.

Jean-François Bach

Part 1
Cyclosporin

Chapter 1
Cellular mode of action of cyclosporin A

Angela Granelli-Piperno

Introduction

Since the discovery and pioneering studies in 1976 by J. F. Borel at Sandoz (Borel *et al.*, 1976), the immunosuppressive drug cyclosporin A (CsA) has attracted the attention of many clinical and basic scientists. CsA is a lipophilic, neutral cyclic undecapeptide (molecular weight 1203; Fig. 1.1) isolated from the fungus *Tolypocladium inflatum*. Experiments conducted both *in vivo* and *in vitro*, have established that CsA is the first immunosuppressive agent discovered that has a selective effect on lymphoid cells, especially in T cells. This accounts for the successful use of CsA to prevent allograft rejection and graft-versus-host disease. More recently, CsA has also been used in several trials to treat a number of autoimmune diseases that are suspected to be T-cell-mediated, including juvenile diabetes, psoriasis and autoimmune uveitis (Bach, 1988).

A large body of evidence has attempted to pin-point the site of action of CsA. The emerging consensus is that CsA acts at an early step of T-cell activation by inhibiting specifically a set of lymphokine genes at the transcriptional level.

This chapter focuses on the effect of CsA at the level of T lymphocytes. Thus a brief review of T-lymphocyte activation is pertinent in order to gain insight to the mode of action of CsA.

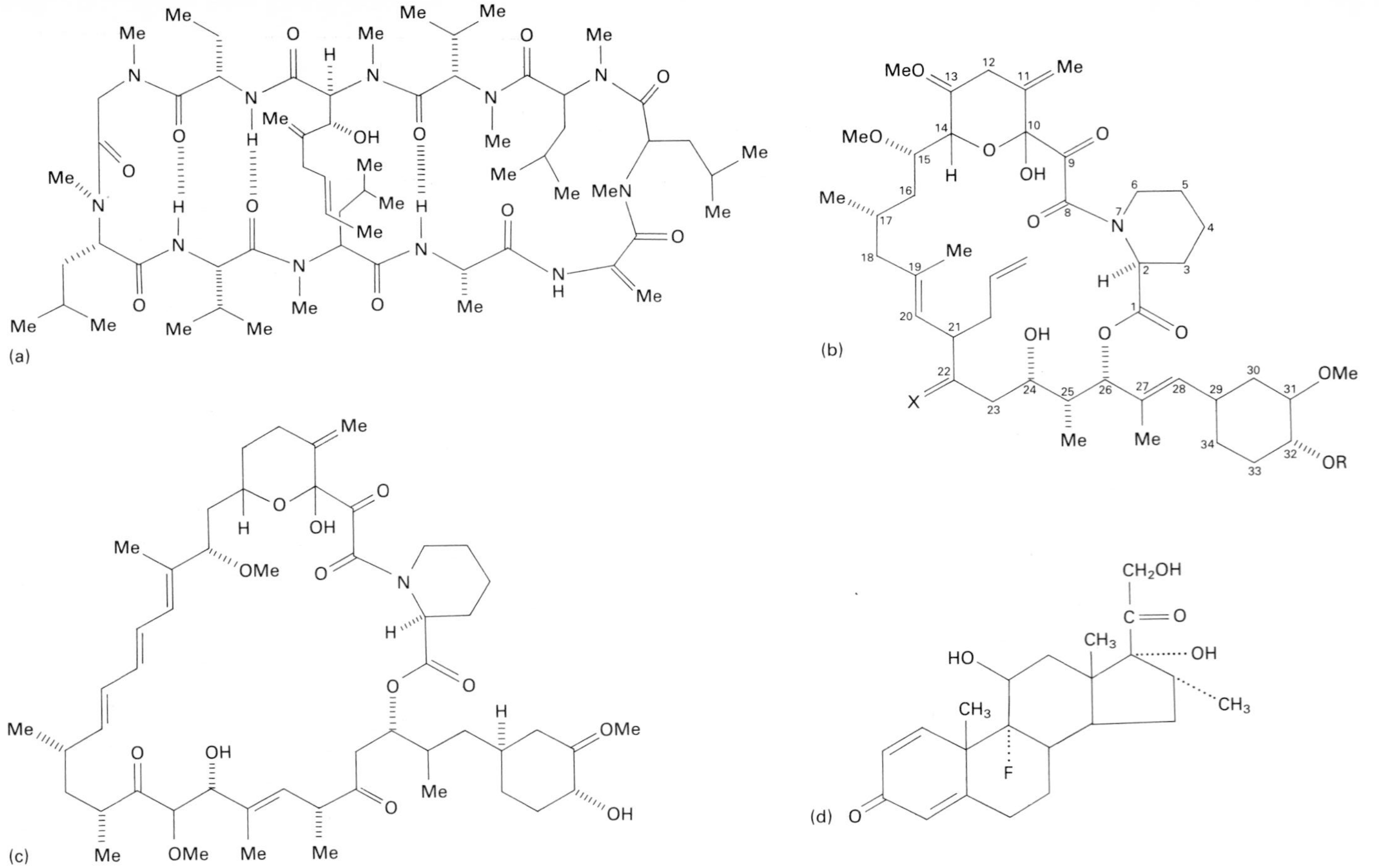

Fig. 1.1. Structure of immunosuppressants: (a) cyclosporin A; (b) FK 506; (c) rapamycin; (d) dexamethasone.

Activation of T lymphocytes

T-cell surface activation molecules

Physiological activation of T lymphocytes requires that the T-cell receptor (TCR) for antigen recognizes the major histocompatibility complex (MHC) molecules bearing antigenic fragments or the recently described superantigens (Mls, bacterial toxins), on the antigen-presenting cells (APC). Non-physiological activation of resting T cells is mediated by a diverse group of monoclonal antibodies (MoAbs) that recognize T-cell surface receptors. This includes MoAb to the TCR and to the cluster differentiation (CD) CD3 polypeptides (Samelson *et al.*, 1983). The latter are associated with the TCR and are likely to play a major role as the signal transducing units of the T-cell antigen receptor. Other MoAbs to T-cell surface antigens, e.g. certain anti-CD2 and anti-CD28 mab, can also activate T cells (Meuer *et al.*, 1984; Hara *et al.*, 1985; Martin *et al.*, 1986). Additional non-physiological stimuli for T cells include several plant lectins (phytohaemagglutinin, PHA; concanavalin A, con A), calcium ionophores and oxidizing agents (periodate and neuraminidase/galactose oxidase). A feature of all these stimuli is that a 'second signal', either phorbol myristate acetate (PMA) or antigen-presenting cells, is needed to induce T-cell proliferation. Truneh *et al.* (1985) and Hara and Fu (1985) first reported that treatment of resting T cells with phorbol esters and PHA or calcium ionophore leads to proliferation, and these two agents were subsequently found to be able to substitute for the signal delivered by antigen to T cells. Figure 1.2 shows a diagram of the events that may participate in T-cell activation.

Phosphatidylinositol turnover and Ca^{2+} rises

The membrane events initiated when antigen/MHC complexes bind to the T-cell-antigen receptor are similar to those initiated by many hormones, neurotransmitters, some grown factors, and other biologically active substances. Inositol phospholipids are hydrolysed and intracellular stores of Ca^{2+} are mobilized (Imboden & Stobo, 1985). Two second messengers, inositol triphosphate and diacylglycerol, the physiological protein kinase C (PKC) activator, are also generated (Weiss & Imboden, 1987). The effects of phorbol esters are likely to be due to direct PKC activation, while those mediated by Ca^{2+} ionophores and PHA are probably mediated by other kinases.

Protein phosphorylation in T lymphocytes

Increased phosphorylation of several proteins is observed in T lympho-cytes stimulated with mitogens (Chaplin *et al.*, 1980). Antigen engagement

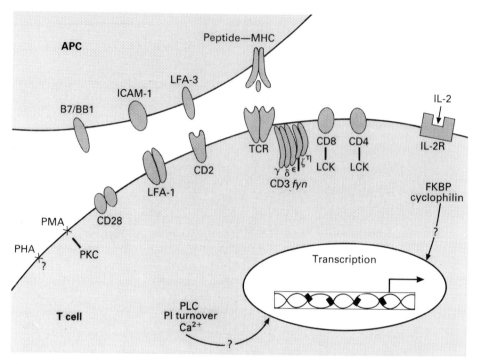

Fig. 1.2. Diagram of the cell surface molecules involved in the interaction between antigen-presenting cell (APC) and T cell and of the intracellular events following the contact between APC and T cell. Phospholypase C (PLC), phospholipids inositol (PI) turnover and Ca^{2+} are second messengers transmitting signals initiated at the antigen T-cell receptor (TCR). Cyclophilin and FKBP are cytosolic receptors for CsA and FK 506.

of the TCR results in the activation of at least two kinase pathways. One is the PKC pathway. The CD3-γ, -δ and -ϵ chains are phosphorylated on serine residues (Cantrell *et al.*, 1985, 1987). This phosphorylation can be mimicked by the addition of phorbol ester, presumably via PKC activation. Another suggested target for PKC-mediated phosphorylation in T cells is *raf*-1, which appears to participate in signal transduction from the cytoplasm to the nucleus (Morrison *et al.*, 1988; Siegel *et al.*, 1989). A second pathway is the tyrosine kinase pathway. Several phosphotyrosine kinases are expressed in T lymphocytes. A T-cell-restricted member of the *src* family of tyrosine kinases is the *lck* proto-oncogene product p56[lck]. *lck* is especially abundant in CD4[+] and CD8[+] cells and recently was found to be non-covalently associated with the cytoplasmic domains of either CD4 or CD8 molecule (Veillette *et al.*, 1988; Barber *et al.*, 1989), providing a mechanism by which the T-cell receptor and *lck* could be indirectly coupled. Thus it has been suggested that p56[lck] plays an important role in

T-cell activation (Marth *et al.*, 1987, 1989). T lymphocytes also possess the tyrosine kinases encoded by the *fyn* and the *yes* proto-oncogenes (Eiseman & Bolen, 1990); but unlike *lck*, *fyn* and *yes* are found in a variety of other tissues. However, it has been demonstrated that the *fyn* present in T cells derives from a uniquely spliced form of the gene (Cooke & Perlmutter, 1989). Some data indicate that *fyn* may also be associated with the TCR (Samelson *et al.*, 1990). Little or nothing is known about the function of *yes* protein and of the other tyrosine protein kinases that are present in T lymphocytes.

Activation of T-cell genes

The biochemical events following second messenger formation and the transduction of activation signals to the nucleus, thereby stimulating gene transcription, are poorly understood. T cells, after contact with antigen presenting cells or stimulation by mitogens, undergo morphological changes at *c*. 12 h, initiate DNA synthesis after *c*. 24 h, and then differentiate further as more and more genes are activated over several days. Dozens of distinct genes are *de novo* induced upon T-cell stimulation (Crabtree, 1989). These novel genes have distinct patterns of regulation and expression. Some encode proteins involved in cell cycle progression (c-*fos*, c-*myc*, c-*myb*) and are common to many cell types, others encode for regulatory proteins (kinases), and others are unique to T lymphocytes and encode for lymphokines whose functions are to modulate cells of the immune system as well as other cell types. Lymphokine gene expression, like T-cell proliferation, requires the synergistic action of two signals. One is provided by antigen plus MHC gene products, or lectins or antibodies with specificity for the TCR and associated molecules (CD2, CD3, CD28). The other signal is provided by accessory cells or PMA. Combinations of two signals are needed to induce interleukin (IL-2, IL-3, IL-4, IL-6), interferon (IFNγ), tumour necrosis factor (TNFα), lymphotoxin (TNF β) and granulocyte monocyte-colony-stimulating factor (GM-CSF) (Wiskocil *et al.*, 1985; Granelli-Piperno *et al.*, 1986; Thompson *et al.*, 1989). In contrast, either PHA or PMA alone induces several non-lymphokine genes, such as those for the proto-oncogenes c-*fos* and c-*myc* and p55 IL-2R (Granelli-Piperno *et al.*, 1986). Lymphokine mRNAs also are induced *de novo* in mice. Injection into the footpad of lectin, αCD3, or antigen on APC induces both IL-2 and IFNγ transcripts (Granelli-Piperno, 1990; Kasaian & Biron, 1990). Expression of IL-2 and IFNγ is more rapid then the expression of p55 IL-2R. This suggests that T cells can begin producing their differentiated products before becoming fully competent for cell growth.

In situ hybridization is useful for quantitating at the single cell level the amount of transcripts expressed. Under non-physiological T-cell stimulation, 20% of the cells contain lymphokine transcripts for a short time at the peak of the response. In contrast p55 IL-2R mRNA is present for much longer periods and in 30–50% of the cells (Granelli-Piperno, 1988). Under physiological T-cell stimulation, only 1–3% of the cells express IL-2 mRNA (Granelli-Piperno, 1988). The IL-2 produced by the activated cells influences the production of other lymphokines, but not itself. In resting T cells, IFNγ mRNA is induced by IL-2. In T blasts, IL-2 upregulates the expression of other lymphokines, e.g. IFNγ, IL-4, as well as other genes: c-fos, c-myc, c-myb, and p55 IL-2R. IL-2 seems also to be the major stimulus for the cytotoxic T-lymphocyte (CTL) genes: serine esterases and perforin (Liu et al., 1989).

Lymphokine genes are expressed transiently and the expression is tightly regulated both at the transcriptional and post-transcriptional levels. In the past years enormous progress has been made in elucidating transcription regulation. Induction of lymphokine genes require de novo protein synthesis (Weiss et al., 1987, Shaw et al., 1988). Lymphokine genes, like other transiently expressed genes, including the proto-onco-genes c-myc and c-fos, contain AU-rich sequences in their 3′ untranslated regions which by an unknown mechanism destabilize the mRNA in the cytoplasm (Shaw & Kamen, 1986). Stimulation via anti-CD28 seems to enhance the stability of several lymphokine genes (Lindsten et al., 1989); and it may be through this mechanism that the CD28 pathway appears more resistant to CsA (see below). The mechanism and the sequences involved in this process have not yet been described. Nevertheless the primary control of lymphokine gene expression occurs at the level of the promoter or enhancer regions of lymphokine genes.

Lymphokine transcriptional activating factors

Given the 'two signal' requirement for the stimulation of lymphokine gene expression, it is perhaps not surprising that the regulation of lymphokine transcription has proved difficult to unravel. IL-2 is the lymphokine that has been studied in greatest details. The IL-2 enhancer lies at −326 to −52 base pair (bp) upstream from the transcription initiation site (Fujita et al., 1983; Fujita et al., 1986; Durand et al., 1987; Williams et al., 1988). By transient transfection into the human T-cell Jurkat with wild type or deletion mutants, it was found that at least five types of promoter elements may be necessary for full inducibility of the IL-2 gene (Fujita et al., 1983; Durand et al., 1987; Shaw et al., 1988; Emmel et al., 1989). The nuclear factors binding to these sites have been identified on the basis of DNAse protection and subsequently electrophoretic mobility shift assays (Fig. 1.3). An AP-1 binding site is present at positions −151 to −145 of the human IL-2 enhancer. The AP-1 site is recognized by the transcription

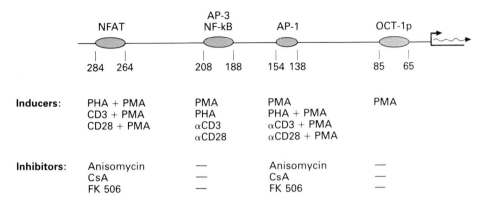

Fig. 1.3. Inducers and inhibitors of nuclear proteins isolated from stimulated primary T cells that bind to DNA motifs within the regulatory region of the IL-2 gene.

factor AP-1 (Angel *et al.*, 1987; Lee *et al.*, 1987; Chiu *et al.*, 1988), which has been recently shown to be encoded by the proto-oncogene c-*jun* (Curran & Franza, 1988). c-*jun* can associate with c-*fos* protein, and the complex augments transcription in several systems (Curran & Franza, 1988; Abate *et al.*, 1990). Primary T cells require two signals, PHA/PMA, CD3/PMA, or CD28/PMA for the optimal induction of factors that bind to the AP-1 site (Granelli-Piperno & Nolan, 1991). Therefore the two signal requirements for optimal induction of IL-2 may be exerted at the level of c-*jun* and c-*fos* transcription factors. Moreover, since AP-1 sites were defined in phorbol ester-inducible genes (Lee *et al.*, 1987), the AP-1 site in the IL-2 promoter may participate in the co-stimulatory function of PMA.

An NF-kB binding site is found at positions −188 to −208. Initially found only in nuclear extracts of B cells (Lenardo & Baltimore, 1989), it has more recently been shown that NF-kB is involved in the inducible transcription of a variety of genes including human immunodeficiency virus (HIV-1), p55 IL-2R (Bohnlein *et al.*, 1988; Kawakami *et al.*, 1988) and many lymphokine genes: TNFα (Collar *et al.*, 1990); GM-CSF (Schreck & Baeuerle, 1990); and IL-6 (Shimizu *et al.*, 1990). Recent studies have described how the nuclear localization and function of NF-kB depends on phosphorylation events, including an inhibitor that is complexed to NF-kB in the resting state (Ghosh & Baltimore, 1990). In primary T cells NF-kB can be optimally induced by a single stimulus like PHA, PMA, or CD3 (Granelli-Piperno & Nolan, 1991).

An AP-3 binding site at positions −185 to −200 lies within the non-coding strand of the NF-kB site. AP-3 is a phorbol ester inducible factor that is present also in other PMA induced genes (Chiu *et al.*, 1987). Like

NF-kB it is optimally induced in primary T cells by either PHA, PMA and CD3 (Granelli-Piperno & Nolan, 1991).

OCT-1 sites, which are found in many promoters such as those for immunoglobulin (Ig) and histone genes (Fletcher *et al.*, 1987; LaBella *et al.*, 1988) are located at position -63 to -93 (OCT-1 proximal) and at -240 to -250 (OCT-1 distal) (Kamps *et al.*, 1990). In primary T cells OCT-1p is PMA inducible (Granelli-Piperno & Nolan, 1991), while in Jurkat cells the two OCT-1 factors are constitutively expressed (Kamps *et al.*, 1990).

Positions -265 to -185 in the IL-2 enhancer represent a principal candidate for regulating the tissue specificity of the IL-2 gene (Crabtree, 1989). To this site binds a factor(s) called nuclear factor of activated T cells (NFAT), found to date only in activated Jurkat cells (Shaw *et al.*, 1988) and in activated primary T cells (Verweij *et al.*, 1990; Granelli-Piperno & Nolan, 1991). Similar to IL-2 production, the induction of NFAT requires: (i) protein synthesis; (ii) the synergistic effects of two stimuli PHA/PMA, CD3/PMA, or CD28/PMA; and (iii) a CsA sensitive step (see below). This suggests an important role for NFAT in activating the IL-2 gene. Analysis using internal deletion, or multiple copies of the NFAT site linked to a minimal promoter, indicates that the NFAT site is capable of responding to signals from the antigen receptor (Shaw *et al.*, 1988). Of interest is the report that an NFAT binding site is also present in the HIV-1 LTR (Shaw *et al.*, 1988).

The coordinate induction of several lymphokine genes, such as IL-2 and IFNγ, following T-cell stimulation, and their sensitivity to CsA (see below), suggests the existence of common regulatory elements. Unfortunately little is known about transcriptional regulation of IFNγ or other lymphokine genes so it is not known if these genes have sites comparable to NFAT. The emerging hypothesis for the activation of the IL-2 gene, using the Jurkat cell line as a model system, is that all the above sites must be occupied for full inducibility. However, the situation may differ in primary T cells. What is evident however is that IL-2 gene expression in primary T cells correlates with the induction of both NFAT and AP-1.

Immunosuppressants for T-cell activation

CsA and other immunosuppressants

In vivo and *in vitro* studies have described several agents that inhibit lymphocyte activation. However, these agents called immunosuppressants manifest different spectra of action. The prototype is CsA. Its effectiveness has been attributed to its action on T lymphocytes. There CsA effects an early event by inhibiting transcription of a variety of lymphokine genes (see below).

The recently discovered macrolide, isolated from *Streptomyces tsuku-baensis*, FK 506 also has proved to be a potent T-cell-restricted immuno-suppressant both *in vivo* and *in vitro* (Sawada *et al.*, 1987; Yoshimura *et al.*, 1989). FK 506, although structurally different from CsA (Fig. 1.1), inhibits T-cell activation by mechanisms that are similar to those of CsA but FK 506 is 10–100 times more potent (Tocci *et al.*, 1989).

Rapamycin (Fig. 1.1), is structurally related to FK 506 but inhibits T-cell activation with a mechanism that is different from FK 506 and CsA. Rapamycin, despite its structural similarity to FK 506, has no effect on the production of IL-2 but inhibits the response of T cells to IL-2 (Bierer *et al.*, 1990). Remarkably these two drugs interfere with each other's action in a variety of functional assays (Dumont *et al.*, 1990a, 1990b; Bierer *et al.*, 1990) raising the possibility that both act by means of a common receptor site. However, rapamycin does not interfere with the biological action of CsA (Dumont *et al.*, 1990a); whereas FK 506 and CsA synergize both *in vivo* and *in vitro* (Zeevi *et al.*, 1987).

Lastly, dexamethasone, a synthetic glucocorticosteroid hormone, is a potent inhibitor of T-lymphocyte proliferation induced by antigens and mitogens (Gillis *et al.*, 1979). This agent binds to specific intracellular receptors in target tissues and blocks lymphokine gene expression (Arya *et al.*, 1984). The action of dexamethasone is not specific for lymphokine genes; the drug affects the synthesis of other genes both in T cells and in antigen-presenting cells (Reed *et al.*, 1986; Kern *et al.*, 1988).

CsA: effects on T cells

The precise mechanism of CsA inhibition is not understood, perhaps due to our limited knowledge of the T-lymphocyte activation pathways. However, in the last 2 years enormous progress has been made toward this goal. To mediate its inhibitory effects, CsA can act at several points during the cascade of events involved in T-cell activation.

It has been well established that CsA has minimal or no effects on the occupancy of the antigen-specific T-cell-antigen receptor, or on the accessory molecules that mediate non-physiological activation (CD3, CD2, CD28). CsA does not seem to interfere with the generation of second messengers: activation of phospholipase C, protein kinase C (Schleuning *et al.*, 1988), and mobilization of Ca^{2+} (Manger *et al.*, 1986; Schleuning *et al.*, 1988). For the latter event there is however no general agreement. Ca^{2+} mobilization in response to CD3 was found to be insensitive to CsA (Wiskocil *et al.*, 1985), but in other settings it was found that the pathways causing measurable rises in intracellular Ca^{2+} were sensitive to CsA (Lin *et al.*, 1991). However, only subsets of Ca^{2+}-regulated signalling pathways seem affected by CsA since the Ca^{2+}-regulated expression of c-*fos* mRNA is not inhibited by the drug (Granelli-Piperno *et al.*, 1986; Mattila *et al.*, 1990).

Whether phosphorylation events are blocked by CsA remain unanswered. Significant unknowns regarding signal transduction and the physiologically relevant substrates have hindered a clear understanding of how the activation of the two kinase pathways results in lymphocyte activation. Expression of v-*src* in a murine T-cell hybridoma results in constitutive phosphorylation of the TCR-ζ chain. Interestingly, IL-2 production in the v-*src* expressing cells was blocked by CsA at doses that inhibit TCR-mediated IL-2 production (O'Shea *et al.*, 1991). *lck* and *fyn* gene products seem to be associated directly or indirectly with the TCR. Phosphorylation and mRNA expression of these products are modulated following T-cell stimulation. Since these coincide with the induction of IL-2, it has been postulated that *lck* is involved in lymphokine production (Marth *et al.*, 1987). However, these events were not affected by CsA (Granelli-Piperno, 1992) indicating that the drug exerts its action more distally. Inhibition of *lck* phosphorylation by CsA has been reported (Furue *et al.*, 1990). An effect was evident after 24 h of stimulation, a time at which IL-2 transcripts were already fully expressed. The function of *lck* and *fyn* may be more related to cell cycle progression than to lymphokine expression in primary T cells. Moreover TCR/CD3 activation did not alter the phosphorylation state of RAF-1 in T cells, whereas engagement of IL-2R resulted in a rapid increase in the phosphorylation state of a subpopulation of RAF-1 molecules progressively increasing throughout the G1 phase (Zmuidzinas *et al.*, 1991).

A precise characterization of the phosphorylated molecules involved in the early events of T-cell activation will be needed in order to assess the effects of CsA in these events.

There is general agreement that CsA inhibits expression of IL-2 and a number of other lymphokines at the transcriptional level (Table 1.1) in response to physiological and non-physiological stimuli both *in vivo* (Granelli-Piperno, 1990) and *in vitro* (Granelli-Piperno, *et al.*, 1986). A similar effect has been shown to occur in FK 506-treated cultures (Tocci *et al.*, 1989). It is worth noting that some pathways of activation (e.g. TCR/CD3) are exquisitely sensitive to low concentrations of CsA (0.1–0.3 μg/ml) or FK 506 (0.01–0.1 μg/ml), whereas others are less sensitive (e.g. CD3 and CD28 with high concentrations of PMA). Moreover a specific set of lymphokines (e.g. IL-2, IFNγ and IL-4) are blocked by CsA, whereas other lymphokines (e.g. GM-CSF, IL-6) or other genes (e.g. c-*fos*, heat shock protein, p55 IL-2R) are not (Granelli-Piperno *et al.*, 1986; Granelli-Piperno, unpublished data). CsA has similar effects on gene expression in CD8 and CD4 T-cell subsets (Granelli-Piperno *et al.*, 1986).

A good correlation exists between immunosuppression and lymphokine expression, in that the non-immunosuppressive analogue of CsA, CSH, or the less potent analogue, CSF, did not or only partially inhibited IL-2mRNA (Granelli-Piperno *et al.*, 1986; Granelli-Piperno *et al.*, 1988).

Table 1.1. Summary of effects of CsA on specific mRNA expression

	T cells (% inhibit.)	Monocytes (% inhibit.)
Proto-oncogenes		
myc	45	0
fos	0	0
lck	10	ND
fyn	10	NT
yes	50	NT
Cytokines		
IL-1	ND	0
IL-2	100	ND
IL-4	100	ND
IL-6	5	0
GM-CSF	10	0
IFNγ	100	ND
Others		
IL-2R	5	ND
HSP-70	0	0
γIP-10	ND	0
HLA-DR	NT	0
Actin	0	0
Plasminogen activator	ND	0
Perforin	25	NT
Serine esterase	20	NT

inhibit., inhibition; ND, not detected; NT, not tested.

T cells stimulated in the presence of CsA not only express high and low affinity IL-2R, but these receptors are functional since they respond to low doses of exogenously added IL-2. The reported reduction of IL-2R by CsA may be secondary to IL-2 inhibition, indeed it has been shown that IL-2 upregulates transcription of its own receptor (Depper *et al.*, 1985). In accordance with this, the reported inhibition of MHC class II on monocytes after CsA treatment, could be the result of the inhibition of IFNγ, a factor well known to induce MHC class II expression (Steeg *et al.*, 1982; Collins *et al.*, 1984).

At least one of the effects of CsA on lymphokine transcription is at the level of factors binding to regulatory sequences located in the lymphokine genes. Several factors bind to the IL-2 enhancer, and it has been shown that CsA inhibits the activation of specific nuclear factors (Emmel *et al.*, 1989; Granelli-Piperno *et al.*, 1990; Randak *et al.*, 1990). Studies of primary T cells have documented that both CsA and FK 506 markedly inhibit the activation of factors binding to the AP-1 and NFAT sites

(Granelli-Piperno *et al.*, 1990; Granelli-Piperno & Nolan, 1991; see Fig. 1.3). Since these two factors require protein synthesis and two signals for optimal induction, just as with IL-2 gene expression, they may represent targets for these immunosuppressants (Granelli-Piperno *et al.*, 1990).

CsA: effects on non-T cells

Although research on this immunosuppressant has focused on T lympho-cytes, several reports indicate that CsA may inhibit a number of cellular functions in other cell types. While CsA inhibits B-cell response to T-cell-independent antigens (e.g. dinitrophenyl-Ficoll), to polyclonal anti-immunoglobulin or ionomycin plus PMA (Bijsterbosch & Klaus, 1986), the drug fails to inhibit lipopolysaccharide (LPS) responses (Bijsterbosch & Klaus, 1986). It has been hypothesized that CsA, as in T cells, blocks calcium-dependent signalling pathways in B cells (Bijsterbosch & Klaus, 1986).

CsA has moderate and only indirect effects on accessory cells. CsA does not interfere with antigen presentation or lectin stimulation. The expression of genes induced in monocytes under different conditions is not altered by CsA (Table 1.1) (Granelli-Piperno & Keane, 1988; Granelli-Piperno *et al.*, 1988). Most likely, the effect of CsA on monocytes is an indirect effect due to the lack of circulating cytokines that regulate their function. The paucity of the effects of CsA on monocytes cannot be attributed to uptake phenomenon, since the uptake of ^{3}H CsA is similar both in T cells and accessory cells.

The observation that CsA inhibits receptor-mediated exocytosis in both T cells (Trenn *et al.*, 1989) and mast cells (Hultsch *et al.*, 1990) demonstrates that CsA has alternative functions in other cell types. The inhibition of mediators released by mast cells occurs without affecting phosphatidylinositol hydrolysis or rises in Ca^{2+} (Hultsch *et al.*, 1990).

CsA has profound effects on thymocyte development. CsA interferes with the development of mature TCR α/β single positive cells and additionally blocks the deletion of potentially autoreactive T-cell clones that mature in the presence of CsA (Gao *et al.*, 1988; Shi *et al.*, 1989). In the absence of clonal deletion, potentially autoreactive T cells could develop (Gao *et al.*, 1988; Jenkins *et al.*, 1988). The effects on thymocytes, however, may occur via the same mechanism that is involved in the inhibition of signalling in mature T cells.

Targets for CsA

A large body of evidence indicates that CsA exerts its inhibitory action distal to the known early membrane-associated events, but proximal to the transcription factors involved in gene activation.

Specific receptors for CsA in T cells were described in early 1980 (Donatsch *et al.*, 1980) and more recently by Cacalano *et al.* (1992). However, CsA, being very hydrophobic, appears to bind to the plasma membrane via non-specific hydrophobic interactions.

The hypothesis that calmodulin, a mediator of certain Ca^{2+}-dependent processes, might represent a target of CsA action (Colombani *et al.*, 1985) was questioned for several reasons. The most important being that active and inactive analogues of CsA bind calmodulin equally (LeGrue *et al.*, 1986). The discovery of cyclophilin, a cytoplasmic CsA-binding protein has been of major interest (Handschumacher *et al.*, 1984). Radiolabelled CsA has been used to identify and purify this predominantly cytoplasmic CsA-binding protein. Cyclophilin is an abundant and ubiquitous protein of 17 kD with a basic isoelectric point (pI 9.3) (Harding *et al.*, 1986). Cyclophilin is widely distributed and found in both prokaryotic and eukaryotic organisms where it represents more than 0.1% of total cellular proteins (Handschumacher *et al.*, 1984). The correlation between the affinity of CsA and its analogues for cyclophilin *in vitro* and the immunosuppressive potencies *in vivo* (Quesniaux *et al.*, 1987) prompted researchers to postulate that CsA mediates its effect through cyclophilin. Two groups have reported that cyclophilin is identical to peptidyl proline *cis-trans* isomerase, a protein that plays a role in protein folding (Fischer *et al.*, 1989; Takahashi *et al.*, 1989). The enzymatic activity of the cyclophilin (rotamase activity) is apparently inhibited by CsA (Harding *et al.*, 1989). The nina A gene in *Drosophila* and a gene in yeast are homologous to cyclophilin and possess isomerase activity (Montell & Rubin, 1988; Shieh *et al.*, 1989). However, recent findings, indicate that the isomerase/rotamase activity of cyclophilin may not explain immunosuppression (Schreiber, 1991; Sigal *et al.*, 1991). Much higher concentrations of the drug are required to inhibit the rotamase activity of this binding protein.

A great deal of interest was generated when it was found that FK 506 binds and blocks the activity of FK-binding-protein (FKBP) that also possesses peptidyl-proline *cis-trans* isomerase activity (Harding *et al.*, 1989; Siekierka *et al.*, 1989). Human FKBP is a 12-kD enzyme and like cyclophilin is a basic cytosolic protein (pI 8.9). FK 506 inhibits the rotamase activity of FKBP but not cyclophilin; and vice versa CsA inhibits the rotamase activity of cyclophilin but not that of FKBP (Rosen *et al.*, 1990). Rapamycin, an analogue of FK 506, blocks the rotamase activity of FKBP but, notably, does not block IL-2 gene expression (Bierer *et al.*, 1990). These results indicate that distinct immunophilins are responsible for mediating the actions of CsA and FK 506, and a common immunophilin may be responsible for mediating the action of both FK 506 and rapamycin.

Although the immunophilins, cyclophilin A and FKBP, are well characterized CsA and FK 506 cytosolic receptors, other members of these families exist (Fischer *et al.*, 1989; Harding *et al.*, 1989; Sierkierka *et al.*, 1989; Takahashi *et al.*, 1989; Friedman & Weissman, 1991; Jin *et al.*, 1991; Price *et al.*, 1991) and are currently being investigated for their effects in T cells. The biological characteristics of immunophilins are summarized in Table 1.2.

The structural chemistry of the immunophilins can give some clues of how the drugs might work. X-ray crystallography and nuclear magnetic resonance (NMR) spectroscopy reveal a hydrophobic drug-binding pocket which not only retains the drug in a particular orientation but also changes the shape of the drug upon binding. The immunosuppressants can be visualized as possessing two domains: one important for binding to immunophilins (binding domain) and one essential for biological action (effector domain) (Schreiber, 1991).

An attractive area of research is to investigate the physiological role of immunophilins in the absence of the drug. Indeed the presence of cyclophilin and FKBP in high concentration and in many organisms suggests that these cytosolic proteins, possessing rotamase activity, may have general cellular functions.

Conclusion and perspectives

The transcription of specific genes is inhibited in T cells by CsA and FK 506. This means that CsA must interfere with precise, specific pathways of activation that are restricted to the induction of these particular genes. It is unclear and difficult to reconcile how a protein as ubiquitous as cyclophilin could mediate such a selective effect. One can speculate that CsA

Table 1.2. Biological characteristics of immunophilins

	Cyclophilin A	FKBP
M.W.	17 000	11 800
Kd	5–200 nM	0.2–0.8 nM
Isolectric point (pl)	9.1–9.3	8.9–9.2
Distribution	Ubiquitous	Ubiquitous
Abundance	0.1–1%	0.1–1%
Activity	Rotamase	Rotamase
Bind to	Cyclosporin A	FK 506
		Rapamycin
Isoforms	Cylophilin A[1,2]	FKBP 12[5,6]
	Cyclophilin B[3]	FKBP 13[7]
	Cyclophilin C[4]	

References: 1, Fischer *et al.*, 1989; 2, Takahashi *et al.*, 1989; 3, Price, *et al.*, 1991; 4, Friedman & Weissman, 1991; 5, Sierkierka *et al.*, 1989; 6, Harding *et al.*, 1989; 7, Jin *et al.*, 1991.

influences directly or indirectly the transcriptional machinery of the sensitive genes (e.g. IL-2, IFNγ). With respect to the factors shown to participate in the transcription of the IL-2 gene, NFAT has the requisite that corresponds to the induction of IL-2 expression in primary T cells. Induction of NFAT requires protein synthesis, as does the induction of IL-2 mRNA; requires two signals, e.g. anti-CD3, anti-CD28, or lectin plus PMA; is sensitive to CsA and FK 506; and seems restricted to T cells. Of the other control sites monitored, only AP-1 meets many of the above criteria, the exception being that the AP-1 site and activity (c-*fos*:c-*jun*) is found in many cell types, although there is a tremendous variability in the nucleotide sequences of AP-1 binding sites.

CsA could interfere directly with the binding of NFAT to its DNA cognate, or CsA could somehow reduce the activity of the transducing kinase(s) that couples induced Ca^{2+} signals to the phosphorylation and activation of NFAT. As described for other substrates, more than one kinase could regulate NFAT phosphorylation, NFAT being a target of multiple signal transduction. NFAT has not yet been characterized; and because multiple NFAT binding proteins may exist, it is difficult to evaluate how CsA influences NFAT activity. Therefore it will be necessary to have well characterized molecules to explore their functions.

On the other hand, the similarity between the immunosuppressant FK 506 and CsA with respect to the cytoplasmic binding proteins is intriguing. These binding proteins, FKBP and cyclophilin, have identical enzymatic activities (peptidyl proline *cis-trans*-isomerases), and this has prompted the idea that these receptors or an isomerization about peptidyl proline might actively participate in the mechanism of immunosuppression. Although CsA and FK 506 bind and inhibit the activity of cyclophilin and FKBP, inhibition requires much higher concentrations than are apparently needed to bring about immunosuppression. The drugs may mediate inhibition by mechanisms that are not directly associated with the inhibition of the enzymatic activities of their cytosolic receptors. This hypothesis is strengthened by the results obtained by Sigal *et al.* (1991) using several analogues of CsA. Their work shows a very weak correlation between immunosuppression and inhibition of the enzymatic activity of cyclophilin, questioning the direct role of cyclophilin in mediating CsA immunosuppressive activity. Likewise, both FK 506 and rapamycin inhibit the rotamase activity of FKBP, but the drugs inhibit distinct pathways of activation in T cells. Therefore it seems that the inhibition of the enzymatic activity of FKBP isomerase activity by FK 506 is not sufficient to mediate its immunosuppressive action.

Studies in lower eukaryotes have made use of CsA-resistant mutants (lacking cyclophilin or having a mutated cyclophilin that prevented binding) and suggest that the cyclophilin–CsA complex, but not CsA itself is responsible for the toxic effects (Tropschug *et al.*, 1989). Similarly, small

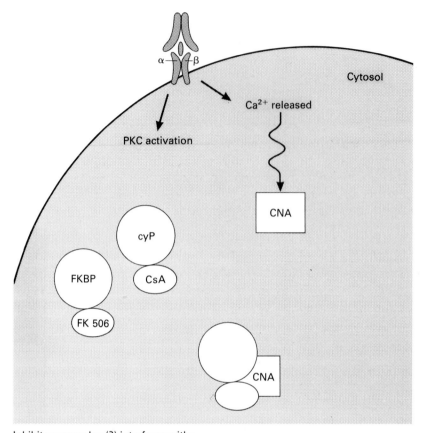

Inhibitory complex (?) interferes with:

Ca^{2+} signal transduction
phosphorylation of target proteins: NFAT, AP-1
translocation of cytoplasmic components

Fig. 1.4. Proposed model of inhibitory action of CsA and FK 506. Binding of antigens to the T-cell receptor complex stimulate activation of protein kinase C (PKC) and intracellular release of calcium ions (Ca^{2+}). Calcium activates the phosphatase calcineurin (CNA). CsA and FK 506 bind to their receptors cyclophilin (cyP) and FKBP. Both drug–receptor complexes may interfere with Ca^{2+} signal transduction, phosphorylation of target proteins.

amounts of the complexes between cyclophilin and CsA may mediate the effect of CsA on some T-cell-restricted sites. Recently, Fesik *et al.* (1990) have shown that CsA adopts a new conformation when bound to its target binding protein. The immunosuppressants bound to their cytosolic receptors may form complexes that possess specificity to interfere with proteins (kinases, transcription factors) important in signal transduction in T lymphocytes. Indeed Liu *et al.* (1991) have recently reported that the complexes cyclophilin–CsA and FKBP–FK 506, but not cyclophilin or FK 506 by themselves, competitively bind to and inhibit the Ca^{2+} and calmodulin-dependent phosphatase calcineurin. These results suggest that calcineurin may be involved in a common step associated with T-cell receptor signalling pathways and that cyclophilin and FKBP mediate the actions of CsA and FK 506 respectively by forming drug-dependent complexes with calcineurin and altering the activity of calcineurin (Fig. 1.4).

It is to be expected that while scientists unravel the mechanism of action of CsA and FK 506, they will further illuminate the mechanism of T-cell signalling and the induction of T-cell-specific gene expression.

Many questions remain unanswered concerning the mechanism of action of these immunosuppressants at the cellular level. However, progress has been made in the past year towards the identification of the target factors that participate in this event.

Acknowledgements

The author is grateful to past and present colleagues and to Dr Ralph Steinman for his critical review of the manuscript. The study was supported by NIH grants GM37643 and AI24775.

References

Abate, C., Luk, D., Gentz, R., Rauscher, F. J. III & Curran, T. (1990). Expression and purification of the leucine zipper and DNA-binding domains of *Fos* and *Jun*: both *fos* and *jun* contact DNA directly. *Proceedings of the National Academy of Sciences of the USA* **87**, 1032–1036.

Angel, P., Imagawa, M., M., Chiu, R., Stein, B., Imbra, R. J., Rahmsdorf, H. J., Jonat, C., Herrlich, P & Karin, M. (1987). Phorbol ester-inducible genes contain a common *cis* element recognized by a TPA-modulated *trans*-acting factor. *Cell* **49**, 729–739

Arya, S. K., Wong-Staal, F. & Gallo, R. C. (1984). Dexamethasone-mediated inhibition of human T cell growth factor and interferon messenger RNA. *Journal of Immunology* **133**, 273–276.

Bach, J. F. (1988). Cyclosporine in autoimmunity. *Transplantation Proceedings* **20**, 379–389.

Barber, E. K., Dasgupta, J. D., Schlossman, S. F., Trevillyan, J. M. & Rudd, C. E. (1989). The CD4 and CD8 antigens are coupled to a protein-tyrosine kinase (p56lck) that phosphorylates the CD3 complex. *Proceedings of the National Academy of Sciences USA* **86**, 3277–3281.

Bierer, B. E., Mattila, P. S., Standaert, R. F., Herzenberg, L. A., Burakoff, S. J., Crabtree, G. & Schreiber, S. L. (1990). Two distinct signal transmission pathways in T lymphocytes are inhibited by complexes formed between an immunophilin and either FK506 or rapamycin. *Proceedings of the National Academy of Sciences USA* **87**, 9231–9235.

Bijsterbosch, M. K. & Klaus, G. G. B. (1986). Concanavalin A induces Ca^{2+} mobilization, but only minimal inositol phospholipid breakdown in mouse B cells. *Journal of Immunology* **137**, 1294.

Bohnlein, E., Lowenthal, J. W., Siekevitz, M., Ballard, D. W., Franza, B. R. & Greene, W. C. (1988). The same inducible nuclear proteins regulates mitogen activation of both the interleukin-2 receptor-alpha gene and type 1 HIV. *Cell* **53**, 827–836.

Borel, J. F., Feurer, C., Guber, H. U. & Stahelin, H. (1976). Biological effects of cyclosporin A: a new antilymphocyte agent. *Agents Actions* **6**, 468.

Cacalano, N. A., Chen, B.-X., Cleveland, W. L. & Erlanger, B. F. (1991). Evidence for functional receptor for cyclosporin A (CSA) on the surface of T cells. *PNAJ* **89**, 4353.

Cantrell, D., Davies, A. A., Londel, M., Feldman, M. & Crumpton, M. J. (1987). Association of phosphorylation of the T3 antigen with immune activation of T lymphocytes. *Nature* **325**, 540.

Cantrell, D. A., Davies, A. A. & Crumpton, M. J. (1985). Activators of protein kinase C down-regulate and phosphorylate the T3/T-cell antigen receptor complex of human T lymphocytes. *Proceedings of the National Academy of Sciences USA* **82**, 8158.

Chaplin, D. D., Wedner, H. J. & Parker, C. W. (1980). Protein phosphorylation in human peripheral blood lymphocytes. Mitogen-induced increases in protein phosphorylation in intact lymphocytes. *Journal of Immunology* **124**, 2390–2398.

Chiu, R., Imagawa, M., Imbra, R. J., Bockoven, J. R. & Karin, M. (1987). Multiple *cis*- and *trans*-acting elements mediate the transcriptional response to phorbol esters. *Nature* **329**, 648–651.

Chiu, R., Boyle, W. J., Meek, J., Smeal, T., Hunter, T. & Karin, M. (1988). The c-*fos* protein interacts with c-*jun*/AP-1 to stimulate transcription of AP-1 responsive genes. *Cell* **54**, 541–552.

Collar, M. A., Baeuerle, P. & Vassalli, P. (1990). Regulation of tumor necrosis factor alpha transcription in macrophages: involvement of four kB-like motifs and of constitutive and inducible forms of NF-kB. *Molecular and Cellular Biology* **10**, 1498–1506.

Collins, T., Korman, A. J., Wake, C. T., Bass, J. M., Kappes, D. J., Fiers, W., Ault, K. A., Gimbrone, M. A., Strominger, J. L. & Pober, J. S. (1984). Immune interferon activates multiple class II major histocompatibility complex genes and the associated invariant chain gene in human endothelial cells and dermal fibroblasts. *Proceedings of the National Academy of Sciences USA* **81**, 4917–4921.

Colombani, P. M., Robb, A. & Hess, A. D. (1985). Cyclosporin A binding to calmodulin: a possible site of action on T lymphocytes. *Science* **228**, 337–339.

Cooke, M. P. & Perlmutter, R. M. (1989). Expression of a novel form of the *fyn* proto-oncogene in hematopoietic cells. *New Biology* **1**, 66–74.

Crabtree, G. R. (1989). Contingent genetic regulatory events in T lymphocyte activation. *Science* **243**, 355–361.

Curran, T. & Franza Jr., B. R. (1988). Fos and Jun: the AP-1 connection. *Cell* **55**, 395–397.

Depper, J. M., Leonard, W. J., Drogule, C., Kronke, M., Waldmann, T. A. & Greene, W. C. (1985). Interleukin 2 (IL-2) augments transcription of the IL-2 receptor gene. *Proceedings of the National Academy of Sciences USA* **82**, 4230.

Donatsch, B. R. P., Gotz, U. & Tschopp, M. (1980). Cyclosporin receptor in mouse lymphocytes. *Immunology* **41**, 913–919.

Dumont, F. J., Melino, M. R., Staruch, M. J., Koprak, S. L., Fischer, P. A. & Sigal, N. H. (1990a). The immunosuppressive macrolides FK-506 and rapamycin act as reciprocal antagonists in murine T-cells 1. *Journal of Immunology* **144**, 1418–1424.

Dumont, F. J., Staruch, M. J., Koprak, S. L., Melino, M. R. & Sigal, N. H. (1990b). Distinct mechanisms of suppression of murine T cell activation by the related macrolides FK-506 and rapamycin. *Journal of Immunology* **144**, 251–258.

Durand, D. B., Bush, M. R., Morgan, J. G., Weiss, A. & Crabtree, G. R. (1987). A 275 base pair fragment at the 5′ end of the interleukin-2 gene enhances expression from a heterologous promoter in response to signals from the T cell antigen receptor. *Journal of Experimental Medicine* **165**, 395–407.

Eiseman, E. & Bolen, J. B. (1990). *src*-Related tyrosine protein kinases as signaling components in hematopoietic cells. *Cancer Cells* **2**, 303–310.

Emmel, E. A., Verweij, C. L., Durand, D. B., Higgins, K. M., Lacy, E. & Crabtree, G. R.

(1989). Cyclosporin A specifically inhibits function of nuclear proteins involved in T cell activation. *Science* **246**, 1617–1620.

Fesik, S. W., Gampe, R. T., Holzman, J. T. F., Egan, D. A., Edalji, R., Luly, J. R., Simmer, R., Heflrich, R., Kishore, V. & Rich, D. H. (1990). Isotope-edited NMR studies show cyclosporin A has a *trans* 9,10 amide bond when bound to cyclophilin. *Science* **250**, 1406–1409.

Fischer, G., Wittmann-Liebold, B., Lang, K., Kiefhaber, T. & Schmid, F. X. (1989). Cyclophilin and peptidyl-prolyl *cis-trans* isomerase are probably identical proteins. *Nature* **337**, 476–478.

Fletcher, C., Heintz, N. & Roeder, R. G. (1987). Purification and characterization of OTF-1, a transcription factor regulating cell cycle expression of a human histone H2b gene. *Cell* **51**, 773–781.

Friedman, J. & Weissman, I. (1991). Two cytoplasmic candidates for immunophilin action are revealed by affinity for a new cyclophilin: one in the presence and one in the absence of CsA. *Cell* **66**, 799–806.

Fujita, T., Takoaka, C., Matsui, H. & Taniguchi, T. (1983). Structure of the human interleukin 2 gene. *Proceedings of the National Academy of Sciences USA* **80**, 7437–7441.

Fujita, T., Shibuya, H., Ohashi, T., Yamanishi, K. & Taniguchi, T. (1986). Regulation of human interleukin-2 region functional DNA sequences in the 5′ flanking region for the gene expression in activated T lymphocytes. *Cell* **46**, 401–407.

Furue, M., Katz, S. I., Kawakami, Y. & Kawakami, T. (1990). Coordinate expression of *src* family protooncogenes in T cell activation and its modulation by cyclosporine. *Journal of Immunology* **144**, 736–739.

Gao, E-K., Lo, D., Cheney, R., Kanagawa, O. & Sprent, J. (1988). Abnormal differentiation of thymocytes in mice treated with cyclosporin A. *Nature* **336**, 176–179.

Ghosh, S. & Baltimore, D. (1990). Activation *in vitro* of NF-kB by phosphorylation of its inhibitor IkB. *Nature* **344**, 678–682.

Gillis, S., Crabtree, G. R. & Smith, K. A. (1979). Glucocorticoid-induced inhibition of T cell growth factor production. I. The effect on mitogen induced lymphocyte proliferation. *Journal of Immunology* **123**, 1624–1631.

Granelli-Piperno, A. (1988). *In situ* hybridization for interleukin 2 and interleukin 2 receptor mRNA in T cells activated in the presence or absence of cyclosporin A. *Journal of Experimental Medicine* **168**, 1649–1658.

Granelli-Piperno, A. (1990). Lymphokine gene expression *in vivo* is inhibited by cyclosporin A. *Journal of Experimental Medicine* **171**, 533–544.

Granelli-Piperno, A. (1992). SRC-related proto-oncogenes and transcription factors in primary human T cells: modulation by cyclosporin A and FK-50. *Journal of Autoimmunity* **5**, 145–158.

Granelli-Piperno, A., Andrus, L. & Steinman, R. M. (1986). Lymphokine and nonlymphokine mRNA levels in stimulated human T cells: kinetics, mitogen requirements, and effects of cyclosporin A. *Journal of Experimental Medicine* **163**, 922–937.

Granelli-Piperno, A. & Keane, M. (1988). Effects of cyclosporin A on T lymphocytes and accessory cells from human blood. *Transplantation Proceedings* **20**, 136–142.

Granelli-Piperno, A., Keane, M. & Steinman, R. M. (1988). Evidence that cyclosporin inhibits cell-mediated immunity primarily at the level of the T lymphocyte rather than the accessory cell. *Transplantation* **46**, 53S–60S.

Granelli-Piperno, A. & Nolan, P. (1991). Nuclear transcription factors that bind to elements of the IL-2 promoter: induction requirements in primary human T cells. *Journal of Immunology* **147**, 2734–2739.

Granelli-Piperno, A. Nolan, P., Inaba, K. & Steinman, R. M. (1990). The effect of immunosuppressive agents on the induction of nuclear factors that bind to sites on the interleukin 2 promoter. *Journal of Experimental Medicine* **172**, 1869–1872.

Handschumacher, R. E., Harding, M. W., Rice, J. & Drugge, R. J. (1984). Cyclophilin: a specific cytosolic binding protein for cyclosporin A. *Science* **226**, 544–546.

Hara, T., & Fu, S. M. (1985). Human T cell activation. I. Monocyte-independent activation and proliferation induced by anti-T3 monoclonal antibodies in the presence of tumor promoter 12-*O*-tetradecanoyl phorbol-13-acetate. *Journal of Experimental Medicine* **161**, 641–656.

Hara, T., Fu, S. M. & Hansen, J. A. (1985). Human T cell activation. II. A new activation pathway used by a major T cell population via a disulfide-bonded dimer of a 44 kilodalton polypeptide (9.3 antigen) *Journal of Experimental Medicine* **161**, 1513–1524.

Harding, M. W., Handschumacher, R. E. & Speicher, D. W. (1986). Isolation and amino acid sequence of cyclophilin. *Journal of Biological Chemistry* **261**, 8547.

Harding, M. W., Galat, A., Uehling, D. E. & Schreiber, S. L. (1989). A receptor for the immunosuppressant FK506 is a *cis-trans* peptidyl-prolyl isomerase. *Nature* **341**, 758–760.

Hultsch, T., Rodriguez, J. L., Kaliner, M. A. & Hohman, R. J. (1990). Cyclosporin A inhibits degranulation of rat basophilic leukemia cells and human basophils. *Journal of Immunology* **144**, 2659–2664.

Imboden, J. B. & Stobo, J. D. (1985). Transmembrane signalling by the T-cell-antigen receptor: perturbation of the T3–antigen receptor complex generates inositol phosphates and releases calcium ions from intracellular stores. *Journal of Experimental Medicine* **161**, 466.

Jenkins, M. K., Schwartz, R. H. & Pardoll, D. M. (1988). Effects of cyclosporine A on T cell development and clonal deletion. *Science* **241**, 1655–1658.

Jin, Y.-J., Albers, M. W., Lane, W. S., Bierer, B. E., Schreiber, S. L. & Burakoff, S. J. (1991). Molecular cloning of a membrane-associated human FK506- and rapamycin-binding protein, FKBP-13. *Proceedings of the National Academy of Sciences USA* **88**, 6677–6681.

Kamps, M. P., Corcoran, L., LeBowitz, J. H. & Baltimore, D. (1990). The promoter of the human interleukin-2 gene contains two octamer-binding sites and is partially activated by the expression of Oct-2. *Molecular and Cellular Biology* **10**, 5464–5472.

Kasaian, M. T. & Biron, C. A. (1990). Cyclosporin A inhibition of interleukin 2 gene expression, but not natural killer cell proliferation, after interferon induction *in vivo*. *Journal of Experimental Medicine* **171**, 745–762.

Kawakami, K., Scheidereit, C. & Roeder, R. G. (1988). Identification and purification of a human immunoglobulin-enhancer-binding protein (NFkB) that activates transcription from a human immunodeficiency virus type 1 promoter *in vitro*. *Proceedings of the National Academy of Sciences USA* **85**, 4700–4704.

Kern, J. A., Lamb, R. J., Reed, J. C., Daniele, R. P. & Nowell, P. C. (1988). Dexamethasone inhibition of interleukin 1 beta production by human monocytes. *Journal of Clinical Investigation* **81**, 237–244.

LaBella, F., Sive, H. L., Roeder, R. G. & Heintz, N. (1988). Cell-cycle regulation of a human histone H2b gene is mediated by the H2b subtype-specific consensus element. *Genes Development* **2**, 32–39.

Lee, W., Mitchell, P. & Tjian, R. (1987). Purified transcription factor AP-1 interacts with TPA-inducible enhancer elements. *Cell* **49**, 741–752.

LeGrue, S. J., Turner, R., Weisbrodt, N. & Dedman, J. R. (1986). Does the binding of cyclosporin to calmodulin result in immunosuppression? *Science* **234**, 68–71.

Lenardo, M. J. & Baltimore, D. (1989). NF-kB: a pleiotropic mediator of inducible and tissue-specific gene control. *Cell* **58**, 227–229.

Lin, C. S., Boltz, R. C., Siekierka, J. J. & Sigal, N. H. (1991). FK-506 and cyclosporin A inhibit highly similar signal transduction pathways in human T lymphocytes. *Cellular Immunology* **133**, 269-284.

Lindsten, T., June, C. H., Ledbetter, J. A., Stella, G. & Thompson, C. B. (1989). Regulation of lymphokine messenger RNA stability by a surface-mediated T cell activation pathway. *Science* **244**, 339-342.

Liu, C. C., Rafii, S., Granelli-Piperno, A., Trapani, J. A. & Young, J. D-E. (1989). Perforin and serine esterase gene expression in stimulated human T cells. *Journal of Experimental Medicine* **170**, 2105-2118.

Liu, J., Farmer, J. D., Lane, W. S., Friedman, J., Weissman, I. & Schreiber, S. L. (1991). Calcineurin is a common target of cyclophilin-cyclosporin A and FKBP-FK506 complexes. *Cell* **66**, 807-815.

Manger, B., Hardy, K. J., Weiss, A. & Stobo, J. D. (1986). Differential effect of cyclosporin A on activation signaling in human T cell lines. *Journal of Clinical Investigation* **77**, 1501-1506.

Marth, J. D., Lewis, D. B., Wilson, C. B., Gearn, M. E., Krebs, E. G. & Perlmutter, R. M. (1987). Regulation of pp56 *lck* during T cell activation: functional implications for the *src*-like protein tyrosine kinases. *EMBO Journal* **6**, 2727-2734.

Marth, J. D., Lewis, D. B., Cooke, M. P., Mellins, E. D., Gearn, M. E., Samelson, L. E., Wilson, C. B., Miller, A. D. & Perlmutter, R. M. (1989). Lymphocyte activation provokes modification of a lymphocyte-specific protein tyrosine kinase (p56 *lck*) *Journal of Immunology* **143**, 2430-2437.

Martin, P. J., Ledbetter, J. A., Morishita, Y., June, C. H., Beatty, P. G. & Hansen, J. A. (1986). A 44 kilodalton cell surface homodimer regulates interleukin 2 production by activated human T lymphocytes. *Journal of Immunology* **136**, 3282-3287.

Mattila, P. S., Ullman, K. S., Fiering, S., Emmel, E. A., McCutcheon, M., Crabtree, G. R. & Herzenberg, L. A. (1990). The actions of cyclosporin A and FK506 suggest a novel step in the activation of T lymphocytes. *EMBO Journal* **9**, 4425-4433.

Meuer, S. C., Hussey, R. E., Fabbi, M., Fox, D., Acuto, O., Fitzgerald, K. A., Hodgdon, J. C., Protentis, J. P., Schlossman, S. F. & Reinherz, E. L. (1984). An alternative pathway of T-cell activation: a functional role for the 50 kd T11 sheep erythrocyte receptor protein. *Cell* **36**, 897-906.

Montrell, C. & Rubin, G. M. (1988). The drosophila ninaC locus encodes two photoreceptor cell specific proteins with domains homologous to protein kinases and the myosin heavy chain head. *Cell* **52**, 757-772.

Morrison, D. K., Kaplan, D. R., Rapp, U. & Roberts, T. M. (1988). Signal transduction from membrane to cytoplasm: growth factors and membrane-bound oncogene products increase *raf*-1 phosphorylation and associated protein kinase activity. *Proceedings of the National Academy of Sciences USA* **85**, 8855-8858.

O'Shea, J. J., Ashwell, J. D., Bailey, T. L., Cross, S. L., Samelson, L. E. & Klausner, R. D. (1991). Expression of v-*src* in a murine T-cell hybridoma results in constitutive T-cell receptor phosphorylation and interleukin 2 production. *Proceedings of the National Academy of Sciences USA* **88**, 1741-1745.

Price, E., Zydowsky, L., Jin, M., Baker, C., McKeon, F. & Walsh, C. (1991). Human cyclophilin B: a second cyclophilin gene encodes a peptidyl-prolyl isomerase with a signal sequence. *Proceedings of the National Academy of Sciences USA* **88**, 1903-1907.

Quesniaux, V. F. J., Schreier, M. H., Wenger, R. M., Hiestand, P. C., Harding, M. W. & Van Regenmortel, M. H. V. (1987). Cyclophilin binds to the region of cyclosporine involved in its immunosuppressive activity. *European Journal of Immunology* **17**, 1359-1365.

Randak, C., Brabletz, T., Hergenrother, M., Sobotta, I., & Sefling, E. (1990). Cyclosporin A suppresses the expression of the interleukin 2 gene by inhibiting the binding of lymphocyte-specific factors to the IL-2 enhancer. *EMBO Journal* **9**, 2529–2536.

Reed, J. C., Abidi, A. H., Alpers, J. D., Hoover, R. G., Robb, R. J. & Nowell, P. C. (1986). Effect of cyclosporin A and dexamethasone on interleukin 2 receptor gene expression. *Journal of Immunology* **137**, 150–154.

Rosen, M. K., Standaert, R. F., Galat, A., Nakasuka, M. & Schreiber, S. L. (1990). Inhibition of FKBP rotamase activity by immunosuppressant FK506: twisted amide surrogate. *Science* **248**, 863–866.

Samelson, L. E., Germain, R. N. & Schwartz, R. H. (1983). Monoclonal antibodies against the antigen receptor on a cloned T-cell hybrid. *Proceedings of the National Academy of Sciences USA* **80**, 6972–6976.

Samelson, L. E., Phillips, A. F., Luong, E. T. & Klausner, R. D. (1990). Association of the *fyn* protine-tyrosine kinase with the T-cell antigen receptor. *Proceedings of the National Academy of Sciences USA* **87**, 4358–4362.

Sawada, S., Suzuki, G., Kawase, Y. & Takaku, F. (1987). Novel immunosuppressive agent, FK506 *in vitro* effects on the cloned T cell activation. *Journal of Immunology* **139**, 1797–1803.

Schleuning, M., Duggan, A. & Reem, G.-H. (1988). Cyclosporin does not inhibit the early transducing lipids generated by the activated human thymocytes. *Transplantation Proceedings* **20**, 63–68.

Schreck, R. & Baeuerle, P. A. (1990). Nf-kB as inducible activator of the granulocyte-macrophage colony-stimulating factor gene. *Molecular and Cellular Biology* **10**, 1281–1286.

Schreiber, S. L. (1991). Chemistry and biology of the immunophilins and their immunosuppressive ligands. *Science* **251**, 283–287.

Shaw, G. & Kamen, R. (1986). A conserved AU sequence from the 3' untranslated region of GM-CSF mRNA mediates selective mRNA degradation. *Cell* **46**, 659–667.

Shaw, J. P., Utz, P. J., Durand, D. B., Toole, J. J. Emmel, E. A. & Crabtree, G. R. (1988). Identification of a putative regulator of early T cell activation genes. *Science* **241**, 202–205.

Shi, Y., Sahai, B. M. & Green, D. R. (1989). Cyclosporin A inhibits activation-induced cell death in T-cell hybridomas and thymocytes. *Nature* **339**, 625–626.

Shieh, B.-H., Stamnes, M. A., Seavello, S., Harris, G. L. & Zuker, C. S. (1989). The ninaA gene required for visual transduction in *Drosphila* encodes a homologue of cyclosporin A-binding protein. *Nature* **338**, 67–70.

Shimizu, H., Mitomo, K., Watanabe, T., Okamoto, S. & Yamamoto, K-I. (1990). Involvement of an NF-kB-like transcription factor in the activation of the interleukin-6 gene by inflammatory lymphokines. *Molecular and Cellular Biology* **10**, 561–568.

Siegel, J. N., Klausner, R. D., Rapp, U. R. & Samelson, L. E. (1989). Rapid changes in phosphorylation of c-*raf* following T cell activation. *FASEB Journal* **3**, A518.

Sierkierka, J. J., Hung, S. H. Y., Poe, M., Lin, C. S. & Sigal, N. H. (1989). A cytosolic binding protein for the immunosuppressant FK506 has peptidyl-prolyl isomerase activity but is distinct from cyclophilin. *Nature* **341**, 755–757.

Sigal, N. H., Dumont, F., Durette, P., Siekierka, J. J., Peterson, L., Rich, D. H., Dunlap, B. E., Staruch, M. J., Melino, M. R., Koprak, S. L., Williams, D., Witzel, B. & Pisano, J. M. (1991). Is cyclophilin involved in the immunosuppressive and nephrotoxic mechanisms of action of cyclosporin A. *Journal of Experimental Medicine* **173**, 619–629.

Steeg, P. S., Moore, R. N., Johnson, H. M. & Oppenheim, J. J. (1982). Regulation of murine macrophage Ia antigen expression by a lymphokine with immune interferon activity. *Journal of Experimental Medicine* **165**, 1780–1793.

Takahashi, N., Hayano, T. & Suzuki, M. (1989). Peptidyl-prolyl *cis-trans* isomerase is the cyclosporin A-binding protein cyclophilin. *Nature* **337**, 473–475,

Thompson, C. B., Lindsten, T., Ledbetter, J. A., Kunkel, S. L., Young, H. A., Emerson, S. G., Leiden, J. M. & June, C. H. (1989). CD28 activation pathway regulates the production of multiple T cell-derived lymphokines/cytokines. *Proceedings of the National Academy of Sciences USA* **86**, 1333–1337.

Tocci, M. J., Matkovick, D. A., Collier, K. A., Kwok, P., Dumont, F., Lin, S., Degudicibus, S., Siekierka, J. J., Chin, J. & Hutchinson, N. I. (1989). The immunosuppressant FK506 selectively inhibits expression of early T cell activation genes. *Journal of Immunology* **143**, 718–726.

Trenn, G., Taffs, R., Hohman, R., Kincaid, R., Shevach, E. M. & Sitkovsky, M. (1989). Biochemical characterization of the inhibitory effect of CsA on cytolytic T lymphocyte effector functions. *Journal of Immunology* **142**, 3796–3802.

Tropschug, M., Barthelmess, I. B. & Neupert, W. (1989). Sensitivity to cyclosporin A is mediated by cyclophilin in *Neurospora crassa* and *Saccharomyces cerevisiae*. *Nature* **342**, 953–955.

Truneh, A., Albert, F., Goldstein, P. & Schmitt-Verhulst, A. M. (1985). Early steps of lymphocyte activation bypassed by synergy between calcium ionophores and phorbol ester. *Nature* **313**, 318–320.

Veillette, A., Bookman, M. A., Horak, E. M. & Bolen, J. B. (1988). The CD4 and CD8 T cell surface antigens are associated with the internal membrane tyrosine-protein kinase p56 *lck*. *Cell* **55**, 301–308.

Verweij, C. L., Guidos, C. & Crabtree, G. R. (1990). Cell type specificity and activation requirements for NFAT-1 (nuclear factor of activated T-cells) transcriptional activity determined by a new method using transgenic mice to assay transcriptional activity of an individual nuclear factor. *Journal of Biological Chemistry* **265**, 15788–15795.

Weiss, A. & Imboden, J. B. (1987). Cell surface molecules and early events involved in human T lymphocyte activation. *Annual Review of Immunology* **41**, 1–38.

Weiss, A., Shields, R., Newtown, M., Manger, B. & Imboden, J. (1981). Ligand–receptor interactions required for commitment to the activation of the interleukin 2 gene. *Journal of Immunology* **138**, 2169–2176.

Williams, T. M., Eisenberg, L., Burlein, J. E., Norris, C. A., Pancer, S., Yao, D., Burger, S., Kamoun, M. & Kant, J. A. (1988). Two regions within the human IL-2 gene promoter are important for inducible IL-2 expression. *Journal of Immunology* **141**, 662–666.

Wiskocil, R., Weiss, A., Imboden, J., Kamin-Lewis, R. & Stobo, J. (1985). Activation of a human T cell line: a two-stimulus requirement in the pretranslational events involved in the coordinate expression of interleukin 2 and gamma-interferon genes. *Journal of Immunology* **134**, 1599–1603.

Yoshimura, N., Matsui, S., Hamashima, T. & Okada, T. (1989). Effect of a new immunosuppressive agent, FK506 on human lymphocyte responses *in vitro*. *Transplantation* **47**, 356–359.

Zeevi, A., Duquesnoy, R., Eiras, G., Rabinowich, H., Todo, S., Makowka, L. & Starzl, T. E. (1987). Immunosuppressive effect of FK-506 on *in vitro* lymphocyte alloactivation: synergism with cyclosporine A. *Transplantation Proceedings* **19**, 40–44.

Zmuidzinas, A., Mamon, H. J., Roberts, T. M. & Smith, K. A. (1991). Interleukin-2-triggered *raf*-1 expression, phosphorylation, and associated kinase activity increase through G1 and S in CD3-stimulated primary human T cells. *Molecular Cellular Biology* **11**, 2794–2803.

Chapter 2
Immunological effects of cyclosporin A

Angus W. Thomson

Introduction

Cyclosporin A (CsA) is important, clinically, as an immunosuppressive agent in the fields of transplantation and autoimmunity. It is also, however, an invaluable tool for research immunologists who wish to probe: (i) molecular mechanisms underlying signal transduction and gene activation within lymphocytes and mast cells; (ii) mechanisms underlying the induction of tolerance or autoimmunity in experimental animals; (iii) and the roles of T lymphocytes and their cytokine products in cell-mediated immunity, including allograft rejection.

The potential of CsA as a clinical immunosuppressant was readily apparent from the first description of the properties of the drug by J.-F. Borel *et al.* (1976). Unlike the principal drugs used as anti-rejection therapy before the advent of CsA, the anti-metabolites (azathioprine and cyclophosphamide) and corticosteroids, CsA was shown to exhibit a selective and reversible, non-cytotoxic inhibitory effect on early events in T (CD4$^+$) lymphocyte activation and proliferation and to be non-toxic to the bone marrow. In the ensuing 15 years, as a result of its capacity to prolong graft survival safely, CsA has been accepted universally as the first choice immunosuppressive drug to prevent the rejection of a variety of organ allografts, predominantly kidney and also those organs (heart, liver, and heart–lung), with respect to which graft and patient survival had been especially poor before the introduction of CsA (Kahan, 1988, 1989). More recently, the clinical efficacy of CsA has been demonstrated in a variety of autoimmune disorders, including psoriasis, uveitis, type 1 insulin-dependent diabetes, rheumatoid arthritis, Crohn's disease and nephrotic syndrome (von Graffenried *et al.*, 1989). Using CsA, significant improvement in a higher proportion of patients with autoimmune conditions of presumed T-cell aetiology can be achieved than previously observed using cytotoxic agents or corticosteroids.

In parallel with these clinical developments, exhaustive laboratory studies have been conducted to elucidate the precise subcellular events in T cells following recognition of antigen which are affected by CsA. The functions of leukocytes other than T cells in the presence of CsA, in particular B lymphocytes, macrophages, other accessory cells and mast cells have also come under careful scrutiny. The results of these investigations have indicated very clearly that T cell subsets (CD4, T_{H1}, T_{H2}, CD8) are not all affected equally by CsA. In murine systems, for example, low doses of CsA can result in selective loss of CD4-mediated T_H function, whereas high doses abrogate both CD4- and CD8-mediated T_H function as well as T-effector-cell function. Murine $CD8^+$ T_H-cell function appears particularly sensitive to CsA suppression *in vivo* (Auchincloss & Winn, 1989). Certain B-cell functions (e.g. in mice) may be inhibited directly by CsA. Moreover, cytokine-dependent activities of B cells, macrophages and other leukocytes are affected indirectly by CsA, as a result of its capacity to block the production of a variety of cytokines by activated $CD4^+$ cells.

Compared with a very large number of *in vitro* studies, there are much fewer *in vivo* studies which have investigated the mechanism of action of CsA. Numerous investigations have, nevertheless, been performed to define the influence and mode of action of CsA on classical models of humoral and cell-mediated immunity. These include analyses of antibody production, delayed-type hypersensitivity, anti-allograft responses, and both graft-versus-host and autoimmune reactions in various species, including man. Comprehensive reviews of the influence of CsA on T-lymphocyte function, cell-mediated immunity, allograft rejection and autoimmunity have been published (White, 1982; Borel, 1986; Schindler, 1985; Kahan, 1988; Borel, 1989; Di Padova, 1989; Ryffel, 1989; Thomson, 1989). The purpose of this chapter is to provide the reader with an updated overview of the immunological effects of CsA, based largely on work with experimental models *in vitro* and *in vivo*. Other chapters in this volume are concerned with effects of CsA in transplantation and autoimmunity and these topics will not be covered in this chapter. The most significant recent developments which will be presented have improved our understanding of the subcellular molecular action of CsA. These findings will be dealt with first. A survey of the influence of CsA on T cell and non-T cell components on the immune system will follow and the effects on CsA on T-cell function *in vivo* will then be discussed. Where topics have been extensively reviewed in the recent literature, the reader is referred in the text to the appropriate publication as a source of references.

Effects on T-cell activation via different pathways

The principal target of the inhibitory action of CsA on the immune system is the T lymphocyte. During induction of an immune response, antigen processed by antigen-presenting cells (APC) and presented on the surface of these cells in the context of major histocompatibility complex (MHC) gene products is recognized by T-cell receptors (TCR) on $CD4^+$ or $CD8^+$ T helper (T_H) cells. Human T_H cell–APC interactions exhibit differential sensitivity to CsA *in vitro*, the most sensitive being the $CD4^+$ T_H-self–APC, followed by the $CD8^+$ T_H-allo–APC and the $CD4^+$ T-allo–APC interaction (Clerici & Shearer, 1990). This T_H cell–APC interaction, together with secondary signals resulting from interaction between CD2 on T cells and lymphocyte function associated antigen-3 (LFA-3) in the membrane of APC, leads to activation of the T cells and to synthesis both by APC and T_H cells of numerous cytokines (interleukins 1-10, interferon (IFN)γ, tumour necrosis factor (TNF)α/β, colony stimulating factors (CSFs), etc.) which have multiple, regulatory effects on cell activation, differentiation and proliferation. These effects include the autocrine stimulation of T_H cells and the differentiation and maturation of cytotoxic and suppressor T lymphocytes (Tc and Ts), B cells and natural killer (NK) cells.

The influence of CsA on the *in vitro* activation of T lymphocytes by antigen (including alloantigen) and a wide variety of mitogenic ligands, including monoclonal antibodies directed against the TCR/CD3 complex or CD2, antilymphocyte serum, phytomitogens, ionophores and phorbol esters has been investigated in detail (reviewed by Di Padova, 1989; Thomson & Duncan, 1989). The most studied stimuli are these inducing activation via the TCR/CD3 structure in the presence of accessory signals, as they mimic physiological responses. Notably, however, at different concentrations, CsA may exhibit disparate effects on T-cell subsets or clones, on different stages of activation in the same subset and on different modes of cell activation. In contrast to its potent inhibitory effects on resting T cells, CsA is much less effective in suppressing activated T lymphocytes. Furthermore, to achieve its effect on mitogen-stimulated cells, it must be added during the first few hours of culture; if removed during this period, inhibition is reversed. More 'physiological', primary mixed lymphocyte reactions (MLR) however, are inhibited by CsA, even if the drug is added up to 96 h after start of cultures.

Evidence based on experiments using ligands which recognize the

TCR and associated structures indicates that CsA does not affect activation signal recognition at the level of the TCR. Thus, binding of anti-idiotypic TCR antibody by cloned murine T cells, or binding of anti-CD3 antibodies (which recognize the invariant part of the TCR) by mouse lymphocytes is unaffected by CsA.

Stimuli which induce T-cell activation independent of the TCR/CD3 complex are of value in delineating the activation pathways affected by CsA. The CD2 pathway, through ligands such as lymphocyte associated antigen-3 (LFA-3), can activate T cells in a non-antigen-specific manner. Stimulation via CD2 in the presence of CsA shows similar sensitivity to activation via CD3 (Bloemena et al., 1989; Bierer et al., 1991). In contrast, however, the pathway activated by CD28 plus phorbol myristate acetate (PMA), which is independent of the TCR/CD3 complex and accessory cells, is resistant to CsA. Proliferation induced by anti-CD3 in the presence of CsA-resistant stimuli, such as CD28 or PMA, shows reduced sensitivity to the drug.

Phytohaemagglutinin (PHA) induces accessory cell-dependent T-cell proliferation via multiple activation pathways which have distinct lymphokine requirements. A small proportion of PHA-stimulated human T cells and a greater incidence of mouse T lymphocytes (c. 50%) are resistant to inhibition by CsA, indicating the existence of a subset of T cells which can undergo IL-2-independent proliferation. Further understanding of the mechanism of CsA resistance may help elucidate IL-2-independent T-cell activation in vivo (see below) and may also provide insight into both experimental and clinical situations in which CsA fails to control specific immune responses. Combination of the phorbol ester PMA with the calcium ionophore ionomycin induces proliferation in T cells which is almost completely inhibited by CsA and although IL-2R (α chain) mRNA is detectable, the response is not restored by addition of exogenous IL-2. This provides further evidence that the inhibitory effects of CsA are primarily directed against the early phase of T-lymphocyte activation.

Effects on CTL generation and CTL clones

Generation of cytotoxic T cells

Administration of CsA to mice during the period of sensitization to alloantigens (spleen cells) inhibits the in vitro expression of T-cell-mediated cytotoxicity. Even high doses of CsA, however, do not affect already generated cytotoxic T cells. In CsA-treated renal allografted animals, there are reductions in CD8[+] lymphocytes within the graft and substantial reductions in donor-specific cytotoxicity (Bradley et al., 1985).

The requirements for stimulating MLR, —an in vitro correlate of anti-allograft reactions, differ from those of mitogen-stimulated cultures. After allogeneic stimulation, the majority of IL-2-producing cells are $CD4^+$, whereas following antigen or mitogen activation, both $CD4^+$ and $CD8^+$ cells proliferate and secrete IL-2. Allorecognition results in the generation and IL-2 driven clonal expansion of $CD8^+$ cytotoxic T lymphocytes (CTL) that recognize and kill the target cells. CsA inhibits several steps in this process, including lymphokine secretion by $CD4^+$ T_H cells and the induction of competence in CTL. CsA may block maturation of CTL by inhibiting the induction of IL-2 and several other cytokines, including IFNγ and CSF. In CsA-suppressed human MLRs, precursors of CTL can accumulate (Hooton *et al.*, 1990). Other events, including progression of CTL and the activation of Ts cells are insensitive to CsA. It appears that an IL-4-dependent, CsA-resistant signal pathway may allow CTL differentiation in the absence of significant cell proliferation (Bubeck *et al.*, 1989). Exogenous rIL-2 is capable of reversing inhibition of CTL generation at low but not high concentrations of CsA, which must be present within the first 24 h of culture to prevent activation of CTL precursors. Although it is recognized that CsA prevents the generation of CTL in the MLR, considerable controversy exists in the literature about the effects of CsA on the effector phases of CTL function. CsA inhibits the Ca^{2+}-dependent, but not the Ca^{2+}-independent, pathway of target cell lysis. It partially reduces induction of mRNAs for perforin and serine esterase by IL-2 or PMA/mitogen in $CD8^+$ human T cells (Liu *et al.*, 1989). In addition, CsA profoundly inhibits granule exocytosis induced by antigen, anti-TCR monoclonal antibody, or the combination of PMA and ionophore (Trenn *et al.*, 1989). The inhibitory effects of CsA are not mediated by the triggering of cAMP-dependent protein kinase and are not due to inhibition of binding of calmodulin (CaM) to CaM-binding proteins. Moreover, concentrations of CsA that inhibit exocytosis in T cells produce a profound effect on IgE receptor-mediated exocytosis in rat basophils, yet do not inhibit receptor-mediated phosphatidylinositol hydrolysis. Therefore, one of the activities of CsA may be to inhibit a step common to Ca^{2+}-dependent exocytosis in secretory cells of the immunological system.

The inhibitory effect of CsA on MLR and CTL may be explained by induction of $CD8^+$ Ts cells, which is dependent on the presence of $CD4^+$ T_H cells and requires IL-2. High concentrations of CsA, however, inhibit Ts induction. It is not clear whether the Ts induced in the presence of CsA act on T_H cells or on CTL precursors to limit the generation of cytotoxicity in MLR.

Extensive studies have been conducted of the proliferative responses of $CD4^+$ T_H or $CD8^+$ CTL clones in the presence of CsA. Proliferation of alloantigen stimulated T_H clones is very sensitive to CsA and is partially restored by exogenous IL-2 at low CsA concentrations. Similarly, the proliferative response of antigen-dependent IL-2-dependent CTL clones is

CsA sensitive. On the other hand, conventional antigen-independent, IL-2-dependent, alloreactive CTL are CsA-resistant. Taken together, the data concerning a variety of T cell clones, activated using diverse stimuli, indicate that CsA suppresses activation mediated through the TCR/CD3 complex (resting cells) but is less effective in inhibiting growth stimulated via the IL-2R pathway.

The production of lymphokines by cloned T_H or CTL is very sensitive to inhibition by CsA and maximal inhibition is dependent on the presence of CsA at the initiation of cultures. The cytolytic activity *per se* of these cells, however, is not inhibited directly by CsA although the drug does interfere with maturation of lytic action. Cytolytic activity, mediated by antigen-independent, IL-2-dependent CTL is insensitive to CsA, whereas lymphocytotoxicity mediated by antigen-dependent, IL-2-dependent CTL and by antigen-dependent T-cell hybridomas may be affected by the drug.

Molecular action of CsA

Essential to comprehension of the postulated molecular action of CsA is an understanding of the subcellular molecular events which lead eventually, to cytokine gene activation within stimulated T cells. What follows is a description of these events, which are as yet imprecisely defined, together with an indication of where CsA is thought to act.

Signal transduction in T cells

Stimulation of T lymphocytes through binding of the TCR to the corresponding MHC-associated antigen, alloantigen or T-cell mitogen, elicits complicated biochemical changes in the cytosol that eventually lead to changes in activity in the nucleus. Priming of T cells by stimulation through the TCR/CD3 complex results in an increase in activity of membrane-bound phospholipase C, which is coupled to TCR/CD3 through a G-protein. This results in the generation of diacylglycerol (DAG) and inositol-1,4,5-triphosphate (IP3) from phosphatidylinositol-4, 5-bisphosphate. The increase in DAG, in turn, activates the phosphorylation activity of protein kinase C (PKC), and IP3 causes the liberation of Ca^{2+} ions from intracellular Ca^{2+} sources. Phosphorylation of IP3 to inositol-1,3,4,5-tetrakisphosphate allows the opening of the undefined membrane channel for influx of extracelluar Ca^{2+}, and thus results in an increase in cytosolic Ca^{2+}. These increases in PKC phosphorylation activity and cytosolic Ca^{2+} are regarded as secondary signals that, by acting on undefined targets, generate a tertiary signal that passes the message from the cytoplasm through the nuclear envelope to the nucleus (Crabtree, 1989). These signal transduction pathways are illustrated in Fig. 2.1, which also shows the proposed sites of action of CsA.

The nature of the tertiary signals is unclear, but recent findings suggest that certain proteins, known as nuclear factors (NF) may be the missing link in this activation network. These nuclear factors may be present in resting lymphocytes, such as NFIL-2A in T cells and NF-KB in B lymphocytes. Others, however, are absent in resting T cells, but their generation soon occurs once lymphocytes are activated, e.g. the T-cell-specific nuclear factor NFAT-1. Apart from the development of the concept of nuclear factors, a novel class of enzymes known as peptidyl prolyl *cis-trans* isomerases (PPIases) has recently emerged as an important entity in the control of signal transduction. The cytosolic, cyclosporin-binding protein cyclophilin is a PPIase. PPIases catalyse the *cis-trans* isomerization of prolyl residues, which are known to be important in the folding of peptides or proteins to their native conformation. These

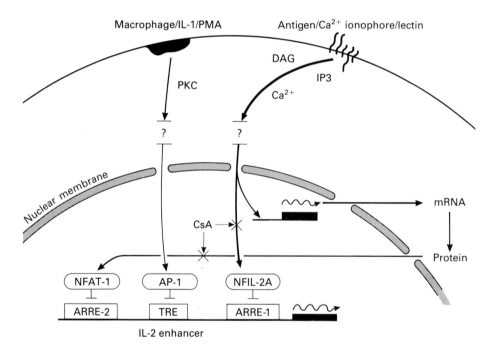

Fig. 2.1. A model of the pathways involved in activation of the interleukin (IL)-2 gene in the Jurkat human T-cell line by either IL-1 and PMA or antigen and lectin/ionophore. The relative contribution of each pathway to the activation of the IL-2 gene is indicated by the thickness of each arrow and is estimated from the effects of deletion of the responses element from the intact enhancer in transfection studies. The gene activated to produce the NFAT-1 complex may not encode the DNA binding activity but may only contribute to the formation of the complex. The proposed sites of action of cyclosporin A are indicated by crosses. DAG (diacylglycerol), Ca^{2+}, IP3 (inositol-1,4,5-trisphosphate) and PKC (protein kinase C) are postulated to be second messengers in transmitting signals initiated at the antigen receptor. TRE is the PMA response element (figure reproduced with permission from Crabtree, 1989).

enzymes may modify signal transduction by interfering with the *trans*-acting factor or by affecting the *cis*-acting gene segment, either directly or indirectly through undefined, specific physiological substrates.

Expression of the IL-2 gene is regulated by five transcriptional segments in the enhancer lying between -548 and $+39$ base pairs 5′ to the transcription initiation site of the gene. Two enhancer sequences, -285 to -255 and -93 to -63, activate a linked promoter in response to the signal generated from the antigen receptor. These two regions are bound by two distinct nuclear factors to protect them from DNase I digestion. The nuclear factor NFIL-2A, present in both activated and non-activated T cells, binds to the regulatory site identified in the IL-2 enhancer between base pairs -93 and -63. This sequence is referred to as antigen receptor response element 1 (ARRE-1), since it can be activated only through the TCR and not by PMA (Fig. 2.1). The promoter of the IL-2 gene is then activated by the sequence protected from DNase I digestion once an activation signal is elicited in the TCR. The constitutive activity of the IL-2 promoter, when the NFIL-2A binding activity is disrupted by mutation, implies a negative signal of this NFIL-2A protein in resting T cells. Thus, NFIL-2A provides a dual function, suppressing IL-2 gene expression in resting T cells and promoting expression in activated T cells.

Another antigen receptor response element (ARRE-2) present between base pairs -285 and -255 of the IL-2 enhancer is protected from DNase by nuclear factor NFAT-1 which is expressed only in activated T cells. Evidence indicates that deletion of the NFAT-1 binding site significantly impairs activity of the IL-2 enhancer. Besides, an increase in NFAT-1 binding activity in nuclear extracts of activated T cells and the appearance of NFAT-1 precede the earliest detectable appearance of IL-2 mRNA by about 10 min. This implies that activation of the IL-2 gene is dependent on the prior activation of NFAT-1. Cooperation between NFAT-1 and NFIL-2A results in full enhancer activity, although each of them binds to a different sequence.

The role of CsA–cyclophilin complexes

The cytosolic PPIase cyclophilin (MW 17 737 Da), one of the recently discovered family of immunosuppressant drug-binding 'immunophilins' (Schreiber, 1991) is now believed to play an essential role in the molecular action of CsA. Messenger RNA specific for cyclophilin is found in every tissue. The PPIase activity of cyclophilin is strongly and specifically inhibited by CsA. The inhibition of PPIase activity, however, is insufficient to explain the immunosuppressive action of CsA (Sigal *et al.*, 1991), which is now envisaged as a pro-drug (Schreiber & Crabtree, 1992). Recent evidence strongly suggests that the immunosuppressive effects of CsA are mediated by the CsA–cyclophilin complex. This complex has been shown to bind specifically to three polypeptides — CaM and the two subunits of the enzyme calcineurin (a Ca^{2+}-activated, serine-threonine protein phosphatase). The interaction of cyclophilin appears to be with calcineurin. This drug–immunophilin complex has been shown to block the phosphatase activity of calcineurin (Liu *et al.*, 1991). Thus calcineurin appears to be the target of the CsA–cyclophilin complex (Schreiber & Crabtree, 1992). A further set of key observations relates to the nuclear factor NFAT. Granelli-Piperno *et al.* (1990) showed that CsA inhibited binding of NFAT to the IL-2 transcriptional element. Further insight has come from the work of Flanagan *et al.* (1991), who have shown that the drug–immunophilin complex blocks Ca^{2+}-dependent translocation of the pre-existing, cytoplasmic component of NFAT to the nucleus. The nuclear component of NFAT is transcriptionally inactive in all cells other than activated T lymphocytes (see above) and is induced by signals from the TCR. Its appearance is not blocked by CsA. It appears that CsA blocks dephosphorylation of the cytoplasmic component of NFAT which is required for its translocation to the nucleus. In the absence of both nuclear and cytoplasmic components, binding of NFAT to DNA and transcriptional activation of the IL-2 gene is suppressed.

Cytokine production and receptor expression

CsA inhibits not only the transcription of IL-2 but also the synthesis *in vitro* of a broad spectrum of other cytokines and proto-oncogenes (including c-*myc*, c-*fos* and *sra* family genes) after T-cell activation (reviewed by Ryffel, 1989). These observations were recently extended by the demonstration that CsA inhibits alloantigen-induced T-cell cytokine gene expression *in vivo* (Granelli-Piperno, 1990). A list of cytokines and the influence of CsA is shown in Table 2.1. Whilst production of IL-1α and β by monocytes and synthesis of granulocyte-monocyte-colony-stimulating factor (GM-CSF) are CsA-resistant, the synthesis of IL-2–IL-6, TNF and IFNγ is inhibited by CsA. There is evidence that CsA does not inhibit transcription of the IL-7 gene (Motta *et al.*, 1991). The drug has no effect on constitutive cytokine synthesis.

Inhibition of cytokine receptor expression generally occurs at concentrations of CsA higher than those required to block cytokine secretion. CsA inhibits both low (p55) and intermediate (p75) affinity IL-2R expression, as shown by ^{125}I-IL-2 equilibrium binding studies on anti-CD3-stimulated human T cells (Foxwell *et al.*, 1990). The effect on receptor expression may be due either to a direct effect, or to absence of the respective ligand, such as IL-2, which is known to upregulate expression of its own receptor. Indeed rIL-2 reverses CsA inhibition of IL-2R expression. CsA does not inhibit IL-1R. The effect of the drug on IL-2R expression has been more controversial and may depend on the method of

Table 2.1. Effects of CsA on cytokine production

Cytokine	Cellular source	Activity	CsA sensitivity
IL-1α	Monocytes	Pleiotropic effect on T lymphocytes and fibroblasts (cytokine release, growth)	−
IL-1β	Monocytes		−
IL-2	T cells	Proliferation of activated T cells	+
IL-3	Monocytes, T cells	Proliferation of haemopoietic multipotential stem cells	+
IL-4	T cells	Proliferation of T cells	+
IL-5	T cells	Differentiation of eosinophils	+
IL-6	T cells, monocytes, fibroblasts	Pleiotropic effects, production of acute phase proteins by hepatocytes, MHC class I expression on fibroblasts	+
IL-7	Bone marrow stromal cells	Haemopoietic factor; and B- and T-cell-growth factor	−
IFNγ[1]	T cells	Expression of MHC class II on endothelial cells and fibroblasts; antimicrobial and tumoricidal activity	+
TFNα[2]	HL-60		+
TNFβ	Peripheral blood		+
GM-CSF	Macrophage cell line	Haemopoietic growth factors	−
G-CSF	Human bladder	Haemopoietic growth factors	?
M-CSF	Human urine	Haemopoietic growth factors	?

[1]IFNγ, interferon-γ; [2]TNF, tumour necrosis factor.

analysis and the stimulant used. Thus the appearance of IL-2R on anti-CD3 stimulated T cells may be inhibited by CsA whilst plant lectin (PHA or concanavalin A (Con A))-induced receptor expression is more resistant. CsA inhibits anti-CD3-induced upregulation of IL-4R on human blood mononuclear cells as well as expression of high affinity binding sites (Foxwell *et al.*, 1990). However upregulation of IL-4R by IL-2 or its own ligand on activated IL-4R$^+$ T cells is CsA-resistant.

The immunosuppressive efficacy of CsA may be due, at least in part, to indirect effects of the drug on non-T cell components of the immune system, resulting from the inhibition of cytokine production. Thus, inhibition of IL-1, IL-2, IL-4-6, TNFα/β or INFγ production can affect B-cell responses. There is also evidence, however, that at least *in vitro*, CsA can inhibit directly certain B-cell activities. Moreover, it has been reported that some functions of mononuclear phagocytes and other accessory cells may be affected directly by CsA. Recent data have also shown that CsA blocks mediator release from activated mast cells *in vitro*. As with T-cell responses, these reports must be interpreted with due consideration to the CsA concentration used, the nature of the antigen or other stimulus, and the physiological relevance of the experimental system.

B lymphocytes

There is considerable evidence that, in both the mouse and man, CsA can directly inhibit the activation of B lymphocytes and that the biochemical mechanism is similar to that in T cells. Drug sensitivity is determined both by the nature of the stimulus and by the mechanism of cell activation. Thus, with respect to murine B cells, CsA blocks Ca^{2+}-dependent signals downstream of phosphatidyl inositol biphosphate hydrolysis. Typically, proliferative responses to anti-immunoglobulin (Ig) (which are dependent on Ca^{2+} mobilization) are exquisitely sensitive to inhibition by CsA ($IC_{50} < 10$ ng/ml), whilst lipopolysaccharide (LPS)-stimulated B-cell proliferation (Ca^{2+}-independent) is only affected at much higher drug concentrations (Table 2.2). This is well illustrated by the recent work of Wicker *et al.* (1990), who demonstrated a differential inhibitory action of CsA on anti-IgM and LPS-induced human B-cell responses. In combination with submitogenic concentrations of anti-Ig, IL-4 induces B cell DNA synthesis, which is highly sensitive to CsA. The stimulation of B-cell growth and the induction of antibody production by IL-5 are susceptible to low concentrations of CsA ($IC_{50} < 10$ ng/ml). Other cell activators which do not cause cell proliferation but induce a marked increase in cell surface membrane MHC antigen expression can also be classified as either

Table 2.2. Influence of CsA on murine B cells

Stimulus	Ca^{2+} mobilization	Sensitivity to CsA
Anti-IgM	+ + +	High
Con A	+ +	High
Ca^{2+} ionophore	+ + +	High
LPS[1]	−	Low
PMA	−	Low
IL-4	−	Low
IL-5	−	High
Ca^{2+} ionophore plus PMA[2]	+ + +	High
IL-4 plus anti-IgM	+ +	High

[1]LPS, *E. coli* lipopolysaccharide; [2]PMA, phorbol myristate acetate.

CsA-sensitive (e.g. Ca^{2+} ionophore or Con A) or CsA-insensitive (IL-4 or PMA).

In mice, specific primary IgM and IgG antibody responses to thymic-dependent antigens, e.g. dinitrophenol-keyhole limpet haemocyanin (DNP-KLH) are suppressed by CsA, whilst secondary responses are not (Klaus, 1988). With respect to primary antibody responses to thymic-independent (TI)-antigens *in vivo*, there appear to be those B cells responsive to TI-1 antigens (e.g. DNP-LPS) which are CsA-resistant (even at 300 mg/kg) and those B cells responsive to TI-2 antigens (e.g. DNP-Ficoll or DNP-dextran) which are very sensitive to CsA (50 mg/kg).

Results from studies with human lymphocytes also indicate that CsA can have *direct* effects on B cells. Thus *Staphylococcus aureus* Cowan (SAC) or anti-μ-induced human B-cell proliferation, which is T-cell independent, is suppressed by CsA. As in the mouse, stimulation of human B cells by agents that interact with surface Ig receptors is CsA-sensitive. On the other hand, activation by Epstein-Barr virus (EBV) is resistant. Thus, in both species, the nature of the B-cell stimulus markedly affects drug sensitivity. Recent studies by Renz et al. (1990) concerned with IL-4 induced human IgE production, show that pre-treatment of B cells with CsA fails to inhibit their responsiveness to IL-4 in the presence of normal T cells, whereas pre-treatment of T cells abrogates the IgE response. These observations clearly illustrate the indirect effects of CsA on B-cell responses and the insensitivity of IL-4-induced antibody production to the drug.

Mononuclear phagocytes

Early work which examined the influence of CsA on macrophage functions other than antigen presentation, such as phagocytic (*in vitro* or *in vivo*) or migratory activity and LPS-induced, monokine (IL-1) production indicated that these were insensitive to drug concentrations which markedly affect T-cell functions. Expression of IL-6 mRNA by stimulated monocytes is not inhibited by CsA. Moreover, the responses of macrophages to various cytokines *in vitro* were shown to be unaffected by CsA (Thomson et al., 1983). The various properties of mononuclear phagocytes and the influence of CsA are summarized in Table 2.3. Although CsA does not affect antigen uptake and catabolism, oxidative burst (phorbol ester-induced superoxide production may be an exception) or bactericidal activity, it has been found to enhance elimination of intracellular *Leishmania major* parasites by mouse macrophages (Chiara et al., 1989). In this instance, it appears that CsA may reduce the resistance of the intracellular parasites against leishmanicidal oxidative macrophage products (Bogdan et al., 1989).

Examination of the capacity of CsA to impair the antigen-presenting

Table 2.3. Influence of CsA on macrophage functions

Chemotactic migration	Unchanged or decreased
Phagocytosis	Unchanged
Secretion	
· Lysozyme	Unchanged
PG	Increased
Thromboplastin	Variable
Monokine production	
IL-1	Unchanged or reduced
IL-6	Unchanged
TNFα	Unchanged
Responses to cytokines	
e.g. MIF, IFNγ, MCF, PIF	Unchanged
Superoxide release	Unchanged or reduced
MHC antigen expression	Unchanged or reduced

PG, prostaglandin; MIF, migration inhibition factor; MCF, macrophage chemotactic factor; PIF, procoagulant inducing factor.

role of macrophages and other APC has focused on the regulation of cell surface MHC antigen expression. There are numerous reports (summarized in Table 2.4) that CsA either fails to inhibit HLA-DR or Ia antigen expression on human monocytes or rodent APCs respectively, or that the drug blocks MHC class II antigen expression on mononuclear phagocytes, epithelial or endothelial cells. Either indirect (via inhibition of IFNγ

Table 2.4. Inhibition of MHC antigen expression by CsA

Cell	Response
Not affected	
Human monocyte	Mitogen-induced HLA-DR mRNA expression
Human monocyte	Basal/IFN-γ induced HLA-DR expression
Rat lymphocytes	Ia expression on graft infiltrating cells
Murine macrophage	Ia antigen expression
Retinal pigment epithelial cells	Ia antigen expression
Inhibited	
Human monocyte	HLA-DR expression in MLR
Murine renal epithelium	Basal and GVHD/IFNγ-induced Ia expression
Vascular endothelium (canine kidney)	MHC class II expression

production) or possibly, direct mechanisms may be responsible, with the balance of evidence in favour of failure of CsA to inhibit MHC antigen expression directly at concentrations which suppress lymphokine production.

The effect of CsA on the function of APCs has been evaluated extensively, using different read-out assays, such as antigen-specific T-cell (including T-cell line) proliferation, IL-2 release by T-cell hybridomas, proliferative responses to mitogens and mixed lymphocyte reactions (Table 2.5). The literature of this topic has been reviewed in detail by Di Padova (1989). Many factors affect interpretation of the data, including, in particular, the possibility of drug 'carry-over' to the indicator system and as stated by the latter author, a unitary interpretation of these findings is not possible. Nevertheless, by blocking cytokine secretion and subsequent MHC expression on various cells, CsA may alter (allo) antigen presentation in the affected organ and regional lymphoid tissue, resulting in impairment of sensitization to the (allo) antigens.

Table 2.5. Effects on CsA on antigen presentation

APC	Species	Antigen	Read-out
Monocytes	Man	Tetanus toxoid	T-cell proliferation
Irradiated peripheral blood mononuclear cells	Man	Purified protein derivative	T-cell proliferation
Irradiated monocytes	Man	Tetanus toxoid	Lymphocyte proliferation
		Diphtheria toxoid	Lymphocyte proliferation
		Cytomegalovirus	Lymphocyte proliferation
		Allogeneic MLR	Lymphocyte proliferation
Langerhans' cells	Mouse	Con A	T-cell proliferation
Peritoneal cells	Mouse	*L. monocytogenes*	Proliferation of T-cell line
B-lymphoma line	Mouse	Hen egg white lysozyme	IL-2 production by T-cell hybridoma
Peritoneal macrophages	Mouse	*L. monocytogenes*	IL-2 production by peritoneal T cell
Irradiated spleen cells	Mouse	Thyroglobulin	Proliferation of T-cell line
Peritoneal macrophages	Mouse		IL-2 production by T-cell hybridoma
Veiled cells	Rabbit	Con A	T-cell proliferation

Neutrophils

No interference by CsA with chemotaxis, arachidonic acid release and metabolism, oxidative burst or microbicidal activity by neutrophils has been reported.

Mast cells and basophils

Whilst it is well recognized that CsA interferes with Ca^{2+} signalling within lymphocytes, there is now also evidence that inhibition of extracellular Ca^{2+} uptake by CsA may relate directly to the inhibition of mast cell activation by the drug. It has been shown recently that physiologically-relevant concentrations of CsA inhibit histamine release from rat mast cells induced by three unrelated secretagogues — compound 48–80, calcium ionophore A23187 and Con A + phosphatidylserine (Draberova, 1990). It has also been reported that CsA rapidly and irreversibly inhibits the release of preformed (histamine) and *de novo* synthesized mediators (prostaglandin D_2 (PGD_2)) from activated human lung mast cells *in vitro*. Thus, as shown by Triggiani *et al.* (1989), CsA (0.03—3 µg/ml) inhibited histamine and PGD_2 release from anti-IgE treated cells. Since CsA is active when added after anti-IgE challenge, inhibition is likely to be at a level post-mRNA transcription, unlike the pre-transcriptional action of CsA on lymphocyte activation. CsA inhibits IgE receptor-mediated exocytosis in rat basophils (Trenn *et al.*, 1989) and also rapidly inhibits histamine release from human peripheral blood basophils challenged with anti-IgE. Significantly, if added from 1–10 min during the reaction, CsA inhibits the *ongoing* release of histamine caused by anti-IgE and by the ionophore A23187 (Cirillo *et al.*, 1990).

Treatment of either normal rats or animals with an expanded jejunal mast cell population (due to graft-versus-host reaction or helminth infection) with CsA leads to depletion of the mucosal mast cells and to reduced secretion of mast cell granule specific protease (Cummins *et al.*, 1988). These observed effects of CsA on mucosal mast cells are entirely in line with its capacity to inhibit T-cell-mediated regulatory stimuli to mast cell proliferation (IL-3) and/or migration and to inhibit T-cell promoted mediator secretion. Taken together, these observations suggest that CsA may be suitable for the treatment of severe allergic diseases in man, such as severe steroid-resistant, bronchial asthma.

Eosinophils

It has long been recognized that eosinophilia is T-cell dependent although, under normal circumstances, T-cell mediated immunity is not accompanied by enhanced eosinophil production. Pre-treatment of mice or rats with high-dose cyclophosphamide (Cy), however, induces eosinophilia in response to T-dependent antigens, such as KLH and ovalbumin. This effect has been attributed to elimination of (T) suppressor cells and to removal of the normal restraints on cytokine (IL-5)-driven eosinophil production. In this model, CsA is highly effective in inhibiting eosinophilia (Thomson *et al.*, 1986) and, thus, may be of value in the treatment of those clinical conditions where eosinophils play a central role, including the hypereosinophilic syndrome.

NK cells and LAK cells

Most studies show that CsA does not influence directly either human or rodent NK or lymphokine activated killer (LAK) cell activities. CsA does not influence the increase in NK cell activity induced by IFNγ (Kasaian & Biron, 1990) or IL-2, although an indirect effect of CsA on NK or LAK activities mediated via suppression of cytokine secretion by CD4$^+$ T cells is possible. Very recently, however, augmentation of the generation of NK cells (number and function) by CsA has been demonstrated in CsA-treated, bone marrow transplanted mice (Kosugi & Shearer, 1991). These results are the first demonstration of a positive effect of CsA on NK cell generation and may provide insight into the role of cytokines that regulate NK cell proliferation and differentiation. In CsA-treated renal transplant patients, marked increases in NK cell activity have been observed during rejection (Verslius *et al.*, 1988). On the other hand, a reduction in NK cell activity has been observed following conversion from CsA to azathioprine.

Conclusions based on *in vitro* studies

CsA is a potent inhibitor of Ca^{2+} dependent, TCR-directed CD4$^+$ T$_H$ cell activation and suppresses both the expression of cytokine mRNA message and protein secretion. Most of the effects of CsA on the immune system, such as inhibition of T-cell proliferation, generation of cytotoxic T cells and inhibition of T-dependent antibody production, are a direct consequence of inhibition of cytokine production. CsA may, however, *directly* inhibit certain B cell functions, most significantly proliferation, depending on the nature of the stimulus and the signalling pathway used. There is also evidence that certain accessory cell functions, including antigen processing, may be affected by CsA, although cautious interpretation of the data is essential. Recently, it has been shown that CsA inhibits release of preformed and *de novo* synthesized mediators from activated mast cells, whilst the upregulated production of eosinophils in experimental models can be markedly suppressed by CsA. Taken together, these well established and more recently identified properties of the drug extend the range of its potential clinical applications.

Effects of CsA on lymphoid tissue

In laboratory rodents, CsA induces rapid atrophy of the thymic medulla, associated with loss of the medullary but not cortical epithelium. Accompanying the medullary atrophy are decreases in numbers of mature, medullary thymocytes, as defined by the mutually exclusive expression of CD4 or CD8 antigens, and in the amount of MHC class II antigen expression evident within the medulla, especially the Hassall's corpuscles. In contrast, the cortical thymocytes show no apparent alterations in thymocyte or MHC class II antigen expression. Following CsA withdrawal in young adult rats, there is full recovery of medullary components within 3 weeks. These observations have important implications with regard to the influence of CsA on cell-mediated immunity. In specific terms, they indicate that there is temporary loss of thymic hormones and self-MHC class II antigen expression on medullary stromal cells necessary for the generation of T_H and self-antigen recognition. Loss of self-MHC antigen expression within the thymus may also contribute to the induction of syngeneic graft-versus-host disease observed in rats following irradiation, syngeneic bone marrow transplantation and a short course of CsA (see below). Medullary regeneration in lethally irradiated mice reconstituted with syngeneic bone marrow is also inhibited if CsA is given at the time of grafting. Thus CsA appears to impair development of prothymocytes (pre-T cells) from common stem cells in the marrow.

Marked reductions in T lymphocytes within periarteriolar sheaths and marginal zones of the spleen, whilst the splenic red pulp and thymic cortex remained relatively unaffected, have been observed in normal rodents given high doses of CsA and in cardiac allografted rats with lower doses of immunosuppressant. This selective depletion of T_H and T_C areas lends credence to the view that CsA may 'spare' the $T_{C/S}$ compartment *in vivo* and, indeed, flow cytometric analysis of spleen cells of CsA-treated rats reveals significant reductions in absolute numbers of $CD4^+$ cells and in the $CD4^+:CD8^+$ ratio. The reductions in overall bone marrow cellularity induced by high doses of CsA in rats is consistent with 'subclinical marrow depression' which has been reported in transplant patients receiving CsA.

Antibody production (animal models)

The powerful inhibitory action of CsA on antibody production was first demonstrated with respect to haemagglutinin titres in mice or rhesus monkeys immunized with sheep erythrocytes. These studies also showed that the immunosuppressive effect was rapidly reversible. Thus, even high doses of CsA given to mice up to 1 day before immunization were ineffective in suppressing hemagglutinating antibody levels. Strong inhibitory effects on the production of the primary and secondary splenic antibody (IgM and IgG) plaque-forming cell (PFC) response were also demonstrated, especially when CsA was given just before (day -1), at the same time, or shortly after (day $+1$) immunization. The secondary PFC response was less readily suppressed than the primary. CsA was also shown to depress primary humoral responses to other thymic-dependent antigens, including human serum albumin and pneumococcus type 3 in rabbits. Secondary responses were again more difficult to suppress. At least in the mouse, this appears to be due to the emergence of CsA-resistant, primed T_H cells after priming with antigen.

Formation of IgM antibodies to the thymus-independent antigen LPS in normal or congenitally athymic nude mice is not inhibited by CsA, suggesting that the drug does not affect antibody production by B cells directly. Use of two types of thymic-independent antigens (TI1 and TI2) in mice has revealed the importance of the nature of the antigen in determining whether antibody responses are inhibited by CsA. Thus, as discussed above under 'B cells', primary B cell (IgM) responses to TI1 antigens (e.g. DNP-LPS) are CsA-resistant, whereas antibody production (IgM or IgG) to TI2 antigens (e.g. DNP-Ficoll) is extremely sensitive to the drug. At the level of B cell memory activation, it was found that those lymphocytes activated by TI1 antigens were resistant to CsA, whereas those activated by TI2 cells were not. The behaviour of the memory cells thus conforms to the pattern of their respective (TI1 or TI2) precursors.

In addition to suppressing IgM and IgG responses, CsA also inhibits primary IgE production (e.g. to ovalbumin in rats); differential effects on primary and secondary IgE responses in experimental animals have, however, been reported and depend on the dosage and timing of drug administration in relation to immunization. The observation that administration of CsA along with antigen augments IgE responses in mice has been attributed to a change in the balance of isotope-specific immunoregulatory T_H and Ts cells (Chen *et al.*, 1989).

Reversible inhibition of alloantibody production following skin grafting has been demonstrated in CsA-treated rats. In the same species, CsA can prevent the alloantibody response to blood transfusion and suppress on-going alloantibody production. This effect has been ascribed to development of anti-idiotypic antibodies. In multiparous rats previously sensitized to paternal alloantigens, CsA prevents primary humoral responses produced by blood transfusion, but does not abrogate established responsiveness resulting from previous pregnancies. Contrary to results obtained with various other antigens, CsA does not appear to affect secondary alloantibody responses in the rat.

With respect to viral antigens, the influence of CsA on antibody responses to vesicular stomatitis virus (VSV), influenza A and herpes simplex virus (HSV) have been examined in mice. In one study, CsA had no effect on the primary, T-cell-independent IgM response to VSV, but completely suppressed the switch to primary IgG anti-VSV antibodies. Thereafter, the IgG response was refractory to CsA and secondary, IgG responses were highly resistant to the drug. In a separate investigation, interference with the switch from IgM to IgG was also demonstrated in influenza A-infected mice. Other studies have failed to show an inhibitory effect of CsA on antibody production in response to HSV or influenza A infection in mice.

The effect of CsA on the production of autoantibodies in various experimental autoimmune disease models has been reviewed. Amongst the many reports, inhibition by the drug of anti-acetylcholine receptor antibodies in experimental myasthenia gravis, circulating anti-S antigen in experimental autoimmune uveitis, and anti-thyroglobulin antibodies in experimental autoimmune thyroiditis has been demonstrated in the context of prevention or therapy of the disease. In NZB/WF_1 hybrid mice, however, which spontaneously develop lupus disease, preventive treatment with CsA was found to reduce levels of anti-ds DNA autoantibodies but not anti-ss DNA, anti-erythrocyte or anti-IgG autoantibodies.

Cell-mediated immunity

Well documented effects of CsA on T cells *in vivo* which are consistent with its immunosuppressive properties are summarized in Table 2.6.

Delayed-type hypersensitivity

In keeping with its selective inhibitory action on T-cell functions, CsA is highly effective in inhibiting delayed-type hypersensitivity (DTH) reactions and the generation of cytotoxic T lymphocytes in experimental models. CsA suppresses the induction of primary DTH skin reactions in mice to the contact sensitizing agents oxazalone and dinitrofluorobenzene

Table 2.6. Effects of CsA on T cells *in vivo* consistent with its immunosuppressive properties

Interference with thymocyte maturation
Reductions in T-dependent areas of spleen
Reductions in CD4:CD8 ratio
Reduction in expression of T-cell-activation markers (e.g. IL-2R)
Generation of suppressor cells
Reduced lymphoproliferative and lymphokine-secreting capacity
Inhibition of cytotoxic T-cell generation
Capacity to transfer transplantation tolerance adoptively (rat)
Interference with cell migration

or to alloantigens in a dose-dependent manner. It also inhibits DTH reactions when withheld until the time of challenge and suppresses secondary responses whether or not the primary response has been suppressed. Adoptive cell transfer experiments have shown that T cells from immunized, CsA-treated donors fail to transfer DTH to naive recipients; conversely, DTH responses are blocked in recipient mice treated with CsA. CsA will also suppress DTH induced in mouse footpads by injection of cloned T_H lymphocytes, but does not inhibit footpad swelling caused by local cytokine injection. This latter observation is consistent with failure of CsA to inhibit responses of T cells or macrophages to preformed cytokines *in vitro*. Inhibition of contact sensitivity reactions by CsA in mice can be reversed by simultaneous treatment with IL-2 but not IFNγ.

DTH reactions to viruses, such as HSV or influenza in mice are also suppressed by CsA. Interestingly, however, it appears that MHC class II restricted T_{DTH} cells are generated in CsA-treated, influenza-inoculated animals, since T cells from CsA-treated donors can transfer DTH to naive recipients.

In guinea pigs, CsA given daily between immunization and skin testing, or withheld until the time of challenge, markedly impairs DTH reactions to antigens such as tuberculin or ovalbumin. A short course of the drug following immunization also suppresses contact sensitivity to dinitrochlorobenzene (DNCB). Applied topically, to the test site, CsA is also effective in inhibiting contact sensitivity skin reactions to DNCB or dinitrofluorobenzene (DNFB) in sensitized animals when applied at the time of epicutaneous antigen challenge.

It is evident that CsA inhibits both the induction and effector phases of DTH reactions in experimental animals or man, including patients immunized with KLH and tetanus toxoid. As with other immunosuppressive agents, these effects of CsA are dependent on the temporal relationship between drug and antigen administration. Under certain experimental conditions, e.g. when CsA is given to animals for only a short period after immunization, or before an otherwise tolerogenic dose of antigen, augmentation of DTH which is transferable by spleen cells can be observed.

Ex vivo and *in vitro* studies have shown clearly that the efficacy of CsA in suppressing DTH reactions is due to inhibition of the antigen-specific release of cytokines from sensitized T cells, including mediators such as macrophage inhibition factor and chemotactic and procoagulant-inducing factors. There is also evidence, however, that, in certain DTH models, CsA may spare or even promote the induction of Ts cells. Thus, CD8$^+$ spleen cells from mice immunized with alloantigens and CsA suppressed the transfer of DTH by sensitized cells in an MHC-restricted and antigen-specific manner. In contrast, there are reports that CsA given during sensitization may prevent the induction of Ts cells by high dose contact sensitizer in mice. As demonstrated by cell transfer experiments, short courses of CsA following immunization may also impair the induction of antigen-specific Ts in guinea pigs. These discrepant observations on Ts cell activities in distinct *in vivo* experimental models make it difficult to construct a unifying concept of the influence of CsA on these regulatory cells in DTH reactions.

Interestingly, chronic treatment of mice with CsA before and after infection with murine AIDS-inducing leukaemia viruses protects against development of the disease which is dependent on the presence of CD4[+] T cells and B cells (Cerny *et al.*, 1991).

Graft-versus-host reactivity

CsA is effective in inhibiting local and systemic graft-versus-host reactions. Administration of the drug to F1 hybrid rats from the time of subcutaneous injection of parental spleen cells into the hind footpad suppresses the local graft-versus-host reaction (GVHR). The GVRH within the draining popliteal lymph node is maximal at 7 days. A delay in treatment until day 4 after sensitization renders CsA ineffective. It has also been shown that *in vitro* treatment of parental spleen cells with CsA prior to injection into F1 hybrids markedly reduces the local GVHR. Analysis of the early events in the local GVHR by Kroczek *et al.* (1987) has shown that CsA has little effect on alloantigen-induced increases in cell size, IL-2R[+] cells or on the induction of cell proliferation or cytolytic activity. These and more recent studies on T cell priming to alloantigen *in vivo* (Pereira *et al.*, 1990) indicate that IL-2-independent pathways can play a major role in the expression of cell-mediated immunity.

Syngeneic graft-versus-host disease

When CsA is used prophylactically against graft-versus-host diseases (GVHD) after allogeneic bone marrow transplantation (BMT) GVHD has been shown to develop upon withdrawal of CsA treatment. Interestingly, on cessation of CsA treatment after syngeneic BMT, a disease similar to GVHD develops in rats. This syndrome has been termed syngeneic GVHD and is an exception to the prevailing concept that histocompatibility differences are required for GVHD. Syngeneic GVHD has been adoptively transferred into irradiated recipients, but not normal animals, indicating that normal animals may maintain a tolerance mechanism that inhibits the expansion of autoreactive T cells generated during CsA treatment. Both CD4[+] and CD8[+] splenic T cells are required for the adoptive transfer of active disease (Hess *et al.*, 1990). Although the induction of syngeneic GVHD has been reproducible in the rat, data concerning this disease in mice have been controversial. Two groups have demonstrated the development of a syngeneic GVHD-like disease in mice following CsA treatment of syngeneic mouse radiation chimeras, whereas others have been unable to induce this syndrome in mice. Syngeneic GVHD in mice appears to be age-dependent and strain-specific. These factors may account for some of the differences concerning the use of mice in this model.

The mechanism(s) by which syngeneic GVHD develops in CsA-treated syngeneic or autologous rodent radiation chimeras is not understood. CsA has been shown to mediate the destruction of thymic medullary components (discussed above) and/or prevent tolerance induction after syngeneic BMT. These findings have been shown to be manifested by alterations in thymocyte maturation when CsA was administered both *in vivo* and *in vitro*. Jenkins *et al.* (1988) and Gao *et al.* (1989) have shown that autoreactive T cells bearing self-reactive TCR (Vβ 17a$^+$ and Vβ 11$^+$, respectively) develop in I-E$^+$ mice after syngeneic or autologous BMT and CsA treatment. It has therefore been postulated that such autoreactive T cells generated as a result of CsA-mediated inhibition of clonal deletion could be responsible for the development of syngeneic GVHD in rodents. In a recent study, however, Bryson *et al.* (1991) found that in mouse syngeneic radiation chimeras, development of CsA-induced autoreactive T cells as assessed by Vβ TCR expression showed strain variation that did not correlate with the induction of syngeneic GVHD. One suggested mechanism by which CsA might interfere with clonal deletion and acquisition of self-tolerance *in vivo*, is by downregulating the expression of class II MHC molecules on APC in the thymus. An alternative mechanism of action of CsA is by direct interference with the intracellular deletional process. Thus, CsA may interfere with activation-induced thymocyte death (apoptosis) (Shi *et al.*, 1989) by blocking activation of a gene and/or biochemical pathway directly involved in programmed cell death, following activation via the TCR. The effect of CsA on apoptosis both *in vitro* and *in vivo* may provide important clues to the mechanism of programmed cell death.

Acknowledgements

The author is grateful to Ms Shelly Conklin and Ms Bonnie Lemster for help in the preparation of the manuscript.

References

Auchincloss, H. & Winn, H. J. (1989). Murine CD8$^+$ T cell helper function is particularly sensitive to cyclosporine suppression *in vivo*. *Journal of Immunology* **143**, 3940–3943.

Bierer, B. E., Schreiber, S. L. & Burakoff, S. J. (1991). The effect of the immunosuppressant FK-506 on alternate pathways of T cell activation. *European Journal of Immunology* **21**, 439–445.

Bloemena, E., Van Oers, R. H., Weinreich, S., Stilma-Meinesz, A. P., Schellekens, P. T. & Van Lier, R. A. (1989). The influence of cyclosporin A on the alternative pathways of human T cell activation *in vitro*. *European Journal of Immunology* **19**, 943–946.

Bogdan, C., Streck, H., Rollinghoff & Solbach, W. (1989). Cyclosporin A enhances elimination of intracellular *L. major* parasites by murine macrophages. *Clinical Experimental Immunology* **75**, 141–146.

Borel, J. F. (1986). *Ciclosporin. Prog. Allergy*, No. **38**. Karger, Basel.

Borel, B. F. (1989). Pharmacology of cyclosporine. Pharmacological effects on immune function: *in vivo* studies. *Pharmacological Reviews* **41**, 304–372.

Borel, J.-F., Feurer, C., Gubler, H. V. & Stahelin, H. (1976). Biological effects of cyclosporin A: a new antilymphocytic agent. *Agents Actions* **6**, 468–475.

Bradley, J. A., Mason, D. W. & Morris, P. J. (1985). Evidence that rat renal allografts are rejected by cytotoxic T cells and not by nonspecific effector. *Transplantation* **39**, 169–175.

Bryson, J. S., Caywood, B. E. & Kaplan, A. M. (1991). Relationship of cyclosporine A-mediated inhibition of clonal deletion and development of syngeneic graft-versus-host disease. *Journal of Immunology* **147**, 391–397.

Bubeck, R., Meithke, T., Heeg, K. & Wagner, H. (1989). Synergy between interleukin 4 and interleukin 2 conveys resistance to cyclosporin A during primary *in vitro* activation of murine CD8 cytotoxic T cell precursors. *European Journal of Immunology* **19**, 624–630.

Cerny, A., Merino, R., Makino, M., Waldvogel, F. A., Morse, H. C. & Izui, S. (1991). Protective effect of cyclosporin A on immune abnormalities observed in the murine acquired immunodeficiency syndrome. *European Journal of Immunology* **21**, 1747–1450.

Chen, S.-S., Stanescu, G., Magalski, A. E. & Qian, Y.-Y. (1989). Cyclosporin A is an adjuvant in murine IgE antibody responses. *Journal of Immunology* **142**, 4225–4232.

Chiara, M. D., Bedoya, F. & Sobrino, F. (1989). Cyclosporin A inhibits phorbol ester-induced activation of superoxide production in resident mouse peritoneal macrophages. *Biochemical Journal* **264**, 21–26.

Cirillo, R., Triggiani, M., Siri, L., Ciccarelli, A., Pettit, G. R., Condorelli, M. & Marone, G. (1990). Cyclosporin A rapidly inhibits mediator release from human basophils presumably by interacting with cyclophilin. *Journal of Immunology* **144**, 3891–3897.

Clerici, M. & Shearer, G. M. (1990). Differential sensitivity of human T helper cell pathways by *in vitro* exposure to cyclosporin A. *Journal of Immunology* **144**, 2480–2485.

Crabtree, G. R. (1989). Contingent genetic regulatory events in T lymphocyte activation. *Science* **243**, 355–361.

Cummins, A. G., Munro, G. H. & Ferguson, A. (1988). Effect of cyclosporin A on rat mucosal mast cells and the associated protease RMCPII. *Clinical Experimental Immunology* **72**, 136–140.

Di Padova, F. E. (1989). Pharmacology of cyclosporine. V. Pharmacological effects on immune function: *in vitro* studies. *Pharmacological Reviews* **41**, 373–405.

Draberova, L. (1990). Cyclosporin A inhibits rat mast cell activation. *European Journal of Immunology* **20**, 1469–1473.

Flanagan, W. M., Corthesy, B., Bram, R. J. & Crabtree, G. R. (1991). Nuclear association of a T-cell transcription factor blocked by FK 506 and cyclosporin A. *Nature* **352**, 803–807.

Foxwell, B. M., Simon, J., Herrero, J. J., Taylor, D., Woerly, G., Cantrell, D. & Ryffel, B.

(1990). Anti-CD3 antibody-induced expression of both p55 and p75 chains of the high affinity interleukin-2 receptor. *Immunology* **69**, 104–109.

Foxwell, B. M., Woerly, G. & Ryffel, B. (1990). Inhibition of interleukin-4 receptor expression on human lymphoid cells by cyclosporin. *European Journal of Immunology* **20**, 1185–1188.

Gao, E., Lo, D., Cheney, R., Kanagawa, O. & Sprent, J. (1989). Abnormal differentiation of thymocytes in mice treated with cyclosporin A. *Nature* **336**, 176–.

Granelli-Piperno, A. (1990). Lymphokine gene expression *in vivo* is inhibited by cyclosporin A. *Journal of Experimental Medicine* **171**, 533–544.

Granelli-Piperno, A., Nolan, P., Inaba, K. & Steinman, R. M. (1990). The effect of immunosuppressive agents on the induction of nuclear factors that bind to sites on the interleukin-2 promoter. *Journal of Experimental Medicine* **172**, 1869–1872.

Hess, A. D., Fischer, A. C. & Beschorner, W. E. (1990). Effector mechanisms in cyclosporin A-induced syngeneic graft-versus-host disease. Role of CD4[+] and CD8[+] T lymphocyte subsets. *Journal of Immunology* **145**, 526–533.

Hooton, J. W. L., Miller, C. L., Helgason, C. D., Bleackley, R. C., Gillis, S. & Paetkau, V. (1990). Development of precytotoxic T cells in cyclosporine-suppressed mixed lymphocyte reactions. *Journal of Immunology* **144**, 816–823.

Jenkins, M. K., Schwartz, R. H. & Pardoll, D. M. (1988). Effects of cyclosporine A on T cell development and clonal selection. *Science* **241**, 1655.

Kahan, B. D. (ed.) (1988). *Cyclosporine. Therapeutic Use in Transplantation*. Grune and Stratton, Orlando.

Kahan, B. D. (1989). Cyclosporine. *New England Journal of Medicine* **321**, 1725–1728.

Kasaian, M. T. & Biron, C. A. (1990). Cyclosporin A inhibition of interleukin 2 gene expression, but not natural killer proliferation, after interferon induction *in vivo*. *Journal of Experimental Medicine* **171**, 745–762.

Klaus, G. G. B. (1988). Cyclosporine-sensitive and cyclosporine-insensitive modes of B cell stimulation. *Transplantation* **46**, 11S–14S.

Kosugi, A. & Shearer, G. M. (1991). Effect of cyclosporin A on lymphopoiesis. III. Augmentation of the generation of natural killer cells in bone marrow transplanted mice treated with cyclosporin A. *Journal of Immunology* **146**, 1416–1421.

Kroczek, R. A., Black, C. D. V., Barbet, J. & Shevach, E. M. (1987). Mechanism of action of cyclosporin A *in vivo*. I. Cyclosporin A fails to inhibit T lymphocyte activation in response to alloantigens. *Journal of Immunology* **139**, 3597–3603.

Liu, C. C., Rafii, S., Granelli-Piperno, A., Trapani, J. A. & Young, J. D. (1989). Perforin and serine esterase gene expression in stimulated human T cells. Kinetics, mitogen requirements and effects of cyclosporin A. *Journal of Experimental Medicine* **170**, 2105–2108.

Liu, J., Farmer, J. D., Lane, W. S., Friedman, J., Weissman, I. & Schreiber, S. L. (1991). Calcineurin is a common target of cyclophilin–cyclosporin A and FKBP–FK506 complexes. *Cell* **66**, 807–815.

Motta, I., Colle, J. H., Shidani, B. & Truffa-Bachi, P. (1991). Interleukin-2/interleukin 4-independent T helper cell generation during an *in vitro* antigenic stimulation of mouse spleen cells in the presence of cyclosporin A. *European Journal of Immunology* **21**, 551–557.

Pereira, G. M. B., Miller, J. F. & Shevach, E. M. (1990). Mechanism of action of cyclosporine A *in vivo*. II. T cell priming *in vivo* to alloantigen can be mediated by an IL-2-independent cyclosporine A-resistant pathway. *Journal of Immunology* **144**, 2109–2116.

Renz, H., Mazer, B. D. & Gelfand, E. W. (1990). Differential inhibition of T and B cell function of IL-4-dependent IgE production by cyclosporin A and methylprednisolone. *Journal of Immunology* **145**, 3541–3646.

Ryffel, B. (1989). Pharmacology of cyclosporine (Sandimmun) VI. Cellular activation: regulation of intracellular events by cyclosporine. *Pharmacological Reviews* **41**, 407–422.

Schindler, R. (ed.) (1985). *Ciclosporin in Autoimmune Diseases*. Springer-Verlag, Berlin.

Schreiber, S. L. (1991). Chemistry and biology of the immunophilins and their immunosuppressive ligands. *Science* **251**, 283–287.

Schreiber, S. L. & Crabtree, G. R. (1992). The mechanism of action of cyclosporin A and FK-506. *Immunology Today* **13**, 136–142.

Shi, Y., Sahai, B. M. & Green, D. R. (1989). Cyclosporin A inhibits activation-induced cell death in T-cell hybridomas and thymocytes. *Nature* **339**, 625–626.

Sigal, N. H., Dumont, F., Durette, P., Siekierka, J. J., Peterson, L., Rich, D. H., Dunlap, B. E., Staruch, M. J., Melino, M. R., Koprak, S. L., Williams, D., Witzel, B. & Pisano, J. M. (1991). Is cyclophilin involved in the immunosuppressive and nephrotoxic mechanism of action of cyclosporin A. *Journal of Experimental Medicine* **173**, 619–628.

Thomson, A. W. (ed.) (1989). *Cyclosporin. Mode of Action and Clinical Applications*. Kluwer Academic Publishers, London.

Thomson, A. W. & Duncan, J. I. (1989). The influence of cyclosporin A on T cell activation, cytokine gene expression and cell mediated immunity. In Thomson, A. W. (ed.) *Cyclosporin. Mode of Action and Clinical Applications*, pp. 50–81, Kluwer Academic Publishers, London.

Thomson, A. W., Milton, J. I., Aldridge, R. D., Davidson, R. J. L. & Simpson, J. G. (1986). Inhibition of drug-induced eosinophilia by cyclosporin A. *Scandinavian Journal of Immunology* **24**, 163–170.

Thomson, A. W., Moon, D. K., Geczy, C. L. & Nelson, D. S. (1983). Cyclosporin A inhibits lymphokine production but not the responses of macrophages to lymphokines. *Immunology* **48**, 291–299.

Trenn, G., Taffs, R., Hohman, R., Kincaid, R., Shevach, E. M. & Sitkovsky, M. (1989). Biochemical characterization of the inhibitory effect of CsA on cytolytic T lymphocyte effector functions. *Journal of Immunology* **142**, 3796–3802.

Triggiani, M., Cirillo, R., Lichtenstein, L. M. & Marone, G. (1989). Inhibition of histamine and prostaglandin D_2 release from human lung mast cells by ciclosporin A. *International Archives of Allergy and Applied Immunology* **88**, 253–255.

Versluis, D. J., Metselaar, H. J., Bijma, A. M., Vaessen, L. M. B., Wenting, G. J. & Weimar, W. (1988). The effect of long-term cyclosporin therapy on natural killer cell activity. *Transplantation Proceedings* **22**, 179–185.

von Graffenried, B., Friend, D., Shand, N., Scheiss, W. & Timonen, P. (1989). Cyclosporin A (Sandimmun) in autoimmune disorders. In Thomson, A. W. (ed.) *Cyclosporin. Mode of Action and Clinical Applications*, pp. 213–251. Kluwer Academic Publishers, London.

White, D. J. G. (ed.) (1982). *Cyclosporin A*. Elsevier Biomedical Press, Amsterdam.

Wicker, L. S., Boltz, R. C. Jr., Matt, V., Nichols, E. A., Peterson, L. B. & Sigal, N. H. (1990). Suppression of B cell activation by cyclosporin A, FK 506 and rapamycin. *European Journal of Immunology* **20**, 2277–2283.

Chapter 3
Pharmacokinetics, drug interactions and analytical measurement of cyclosporin

Paul A. Keown

Introduction

Cyclosporin (CsA) is a lipophilic, cyclic undecapeptide produced by the fungus *Tolypocladium inflatum Gams*, which causes a potent and selective inhibition of the transcriptional signals leading to antigen-mediated T-lymphocyte activation (Kahan, 1989). During the last decade, CsA has become the principal immunosuppressant employed in solid organ and bone marrow transplantation, and is now emerging as an important agent in the therapy of several autoimmune disorders (Keown, 1990). The clinical use of CsA, however, is complicated by its variable bioavailability, narrow therapeutic index, and complex pharmacokinetic and pharmacodynamic interactions. This chapter will review the current advances in pharmaceutical chemistry, clinical metabolism and therapeutic measurement of CsA, which have contributed to a safer and more effective use of this drug.

Molecular structure

The molecular structure and physicochemical properties of CsA are integral to its immunosuppressive action and pharmacokinetic behaviour. Ten of the eleven residues forming the cyclic structure of CsA are known aliphatic amino acids, while a novel C9 derivative of threonine, 4-butenyl-4-methyl-threonine (MeBmt) occupies position 1 in the ring (Fig. 3.1). The conformation of CsA, determined experimentally by X-ray diffraction in the solid state and by nuclear magnetic resonance in non-aqueous solution, is characterized by two structural motifs (Wenger, 1990). Residues MeBmt[1] to MeLeu[6] comprise an antiparallel β-sheet which is stabilized by three transannular hydrogen bonds, while the residues Ala[7] to MeVal[11] form a loop in which the 9-10 peptide bond is in the *cis*

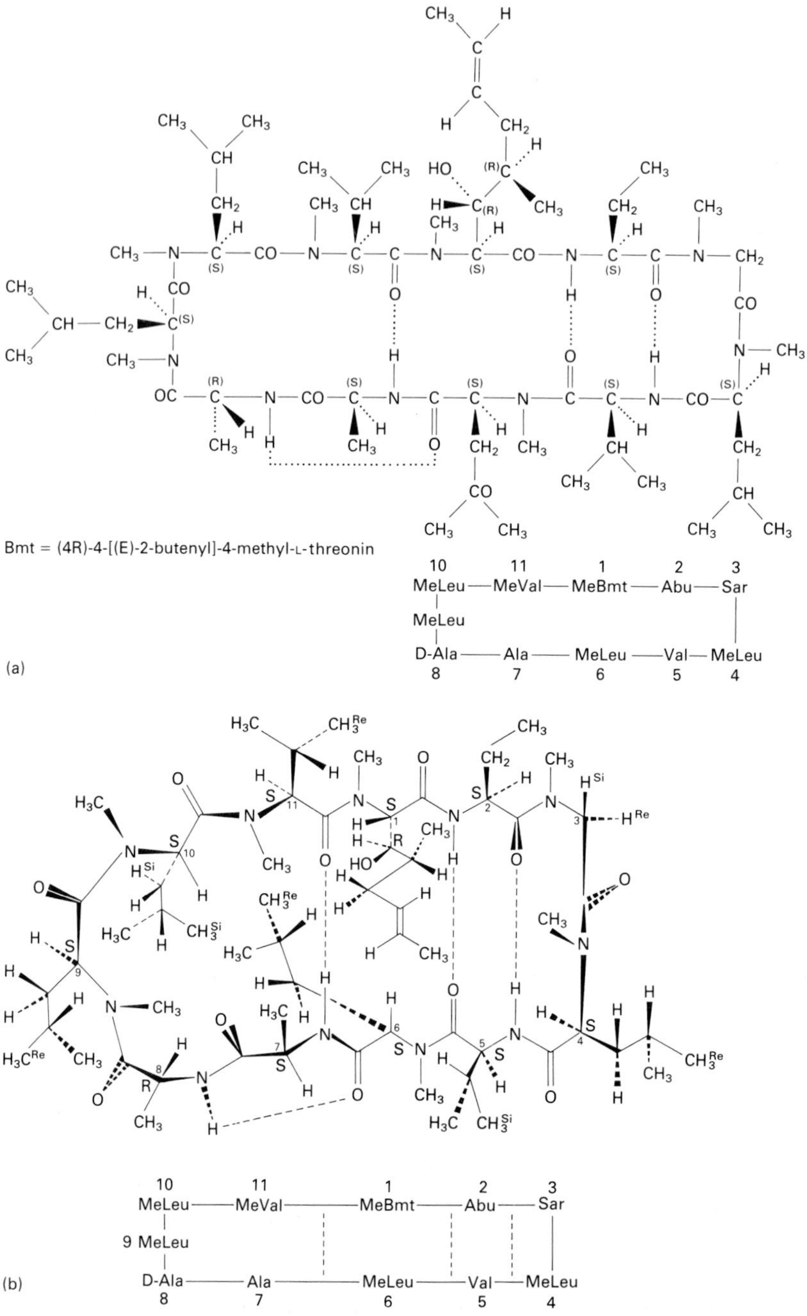

Bmt = (4R)-4-[(E)-2-butenyl]-4-methyl-ʟ-threonin

```
        10          11          1          2      3
      MeLeu ——— MeVal ——— MeBmt ——— Abu ——— Sar
        |
      MeLeu
        |
      D-Ala ——— Ala ——— MeLeu ——— Val ——— MeLeu
        8          7          6          5      4
```

(a)

```
        10          11                    1          2      3
      MeLeu ——— MeVal ———————————— MeBmt ——— Abu ——— Sar
        |
     9 MeLeu
        |
      D-Ala ——— Ala ———————————— MeLeu ——— Val ——— MeLeu
        8          7                    6          5      4
```

(b)

Fig. 3.1. (a) Structural formula of CsA showing MeBmt extended. (b) Schematic conformation showing MeBmt folded under the ply of the molecule.

position. An additional extra-annular hydrogen bond links the NH of DAla[8] to the carbonyl oxygen of MeLeu[6]. In the solid state, crystallographic studies indicate that the C9 MeBmt side chain is folded under the ply of the β-sheet (Fig. 3.1b), whereas in aprotic solvents it protrudes from the body of the molecule due to a simple rotation of 120° about the Cα–Cβ bond (Fig. 3.1a). It is now believed that this latter conformation is essential for interaction with the initial intracellular receptor, cyclophilin, via the active portion of the CsA molecule encompassing the residues 10 to 3. Modification of the three-dimensional structure within this active portion reduces receptor binding and decreases its molecular action. Recent studies indicate that binding to a second receptor, now recognized to be calcineurin, is essential for full expression of the inhibitory effect of CsA (Schreiber, 1991). Although not yet proven, it is likely that this interaction occurs through the antipodean residues 4 to 9. Molecular substitution within this region would therefore similarly impair biological effect, a consequence which is observed with the metabolites so far examined.

Pharmacokinetics

Subcutaneous, intramuscular and intraperitoneal routes of administration have been employed in experimental animals, but absorption from these sites is unreliable in man (Keown et al., 1981; Wassef et al., 1985). CsA is therefore normally administered by intravenous or oral routes, which have a relative bioavailability of approximately 3:1. Preliminary studies of topical and local administration are also underway. For intravenous use, CsA is produced commercially stabilized at a concentration of 100 mg/ml with the castor oil derivative, cremophore. It is dispensed from glass containers to avoid leaching of plasticizers, and administered by constant infusion over 24 h to minimize toxicity and provide constant blood levels at steady state, or by intermittent infusion over a period of 4–6 h. Alternative preparations utilizing liposomes or Intralipid have been evaluated in animals, and achieve a higher volume of distribution at steady state (Vd_{ss}) and a lower total body clearance (Venkataram et al., 1990). For oral use, CsA is available as a 100 mg/ml solution with olive oil vehicle or as gelatin capsules containing 25 mg or 100 mg of CsA. These two commercial forms appear to be bioequivalent (Nashan et al., 1988; Hilbrands et al., 1991), but recent studies suggest that microemulsion preparations may increase absorption (Tarr & Yalkowsky, 1989; Ritschel et al., 1990). CsA is administered orally once or twice daily in patients with normal absorption and elimination characteristics. More frequent administration may be required in children, patients with malabsorption, or those receiving concommitant interactive chemotherapy.

CsA absorption occurs predominantly in the upper gastrointestinal tract. Studies in the experimental animal (Freeman, 1991), supported by similar data in man, demonstrate that only a minor degree of CsA absorption occurs via the lymphatic system. Absorption half-life ($t_{1/2}$) is approximately 60 min after a lag time of 30–60 min, and peak concentrations (C_{max}) in blood or plasma are normally reached within 3–4 h. Uptake is incomplete, ranging from 2 to 89% of administered drug (Kahan & Grevel, 1988), with about one-third of the administered dose reaching the systemic circulation. Pharmacokinetic modelling suggests that absorption occurs via a zero-order process in which the rate of absorption is constant and independent of drug concentration at the absorption site. This is consistent with the concept of an absorption 'window' in the upper part of the small intestine and the carrier-mediated transfer of CsA across the intestinal wall (Freeman, 1991).

Absorption of CsA is influenced by numerous factors including food intake, bile flow, gastrointestinal motility and disorders of the absorptive surface (McMillan, 1989). The characteristics of CsA render it particular susceptible to alterations in absorption in the presence of food, but the magnitude and direction of this effect are individual and controversial. Food has been reported to both delay and impair (Keown et al., 1982) or, paradoxically, to increase (Honcharick, 1991) the absorption of CsA in renal transplant patients and healthy volunteers. While post-prandial alteration in hepatic blood flow is not believed to influence CsA absorption, the timing and composition of the meal in relation to dosage may be critical; the concomitant administration of a high fat load has been demonstrated to facilitate intestinal transport of CsA, increasing bioavailability in plasma from 21 to 79% (Gupta et al., 1990). It is therefore recommended that administration be standardized for each patient. Bile plays a key role in solubilizing CsA within the intestinal lumen so that mixing may occur with the aqueous phase at the absorptive surface, an effect also recently reported with vitamin E (Sokol et al., 1991). Administration of bile salts increases CsA absorption in experimental animals and in normal subjects, although whether this applies in allograft recipients remains uncertain (Ericzon et al., 1987; Lindholm et al., 1990). In contrast, biliary diversion, bile duct ligation, subtotal hepatectomy or the administration of cholestyramine impair uptake of the drug (Ericzon et al., 1987; Takaya et al., 1987). Normalization of bile flow after clamping of the T-tube post-liver transplantation results in a significant increase in both the rate and magnitude of CsA absorption, with a decrease in t_{max} from 6 to 3 h, and a simultaneous increase in bioavailability from 16 to 30% (Naoumov et al., 1989). Disorders of gastrointestinal motility or the absorptive surface represent perhaps the most important clinical problem. Delayed gastric emptying and intestinal dysmotility due to the autonomic neuropathy of diabetes mellitus lead to erratic and impaired CsA uptake. Similarly, accelerated transit accompanying acute diarrhoea, bacterial overgrowth in a blind loop or reduced absorptive area as in the short gut syndrome or sprue may all produce malabsorption of lipid-soluble substances including CsA. Metoclopramide can improve the former by decreasing gastric emptying time (Wadhwa et al., 1987), but treatment is particularly difficult in the latter group and may require correction of the underlying disorder or the use of intravenous CsA. Finally, absorption of CsA appears to be affected by the duration of therapy, and an increase in bioavailability of up to 50% has been observed in renal transplant patients during the first 3 months after transplantation (Tufveson et al., 1986). Whether this reflects an alteration in the mechanisms of CsA transport, a change in distribution and binding of CsA and metabolites, or a resolution in the enteropathy accompanying chronic renal disease is not yet established (Awni et al., 1990).

Topical application of CsA has been evaluated in the eye, skin and bowel. Ophthalmic formulations (2–4% CsA in olive oil) produce high levels of CsA in the conjunctiva, cornea, sclera and lacrimal glands, and have been demonstrated to control anterior ocular disease and to prolong the survival of corneal allografts. Transport of CsA across the anterior ocular barrier is poor, and topical application does not produce detectable levels of CsA within the aqueous or vitreous humour or other intraocular structures, except in the presence of severe uveitis when intermediate concentrations may be found in the anterior chamber (Diaz-Llopis & Menezo, 1989; BenEzra et al., 1990). Topical treatment is therefore ineffective for the treatment of intraocular inflammation, which requires the use of systemic therapy. This produces detectable levels of CsA in nearly all tissues of the inflamed eye despite the relative impenetrability of the blood–retinal barrier (BenEzra & Maftzir, 1990). No successful topical formulation of CsA for clinical use in skin disease has been produced thus far, mainly due to the lack of drug penetration. Recent studies suggest that the addition of penetration enhancers such as azone and propylene glycol permit the accumulation of immunosuppressive concentrations of CsA in the skin (Duncan et al., 1990), although this remains to be evaluated in clinical trials. Topical administration of CsA by retention enema has also been investigated for patients with inflammatory bowel disease. This route produces high distal colonic tissue concentrations after a single dose, which are comparable to those achieved by intravenous administration and up to 10-fold greater than by oral administration, without perceptible absorption (Sandborn et al., 1991). Rectal administration may ultimately prove valuable, with or without pulse intravenous CsA, for patients with severe ileitis and colitis.

Following absorption, CsA is transported in the blood bound predominantly to erythrocytes, leukocytes and plasma proteins, while between 1 and 6%, depending on the method of analysis, remains free in the plasma (Legg et al., 1988; Londholm & Henricsson, 1989). Distribution within the blood compartment is governed by a complex equilibrium which depends on drug concentration, temperature, haematocrit and lipoprotein concentration (Legg et al., 1988; Lensmeyer et al., 1989). At concentrations of 500 μg/l in whole blood, approximately 50% of CsA is bound to red cells and 10% to leukocytes, while 30–40% resides in the plasma (Lemaire & Tillement, 1982); as the CsA concentration increases further, the red cell/plasma ratio falls reflecting saturation of erythrocyte binding. Red blood cell affinity for CsA is inversely related to temperature, so that the blood-to-plasma concentration at 37° C increases by approximately 25% as the temperature declines to 22° C or less, an important consideration in therapeutic monitoring of CsA. Partitioning between the red cell and plasma is inversely related to haematocrit, and a 10% increase in packed cell volume is associated with a fall in plasma CsA concentration of around 12% (Rosano, 1985). In plasma, CsA is primarily bound to lipoproteins (and to a lesser extent chylomicrons), which exhibit non-saturable, low affinity binding and high capacity uptake for the drug (Awni et al., 1990). Distribution among individual lipoprotein classes is similar in both organ transplant recipients and healthy subjects. The greatest proportion is bound to high density lipoproteins (HDL) (33–46%), followed by low density lipoprotein (LDL) (28–35%) and very low density lipoprotein (VLDL) (6–19%) (Awni et al., 1990), in a ratio inversely reflecting the clearance rates. Elimination of CsA from the VLDL fraction is more rapid than from other biological fluids, and the systemic clearance of CsA from total plasma or VLDL fractions is more rapid than from whole blood or HLD and LDL fractions. The remaining CsA is associated with the non-lipoprotein fraction. It has been postulated that LDL serves as a carrier for CsA, facilitating delivery to the immuno-competent cell and transport to metabolic sites via the LDL receptor pathway. Although not formally established, this mechanism could explain the similarity in tissue distribution of CsA binding and LDL receptor expression, and the recognized inverse relationship between biological effect of CsA and total serum cholesterol levels (Ballantyne et al., 1989).

The distribution of CsA in vivo (Fig. 3.2) is variably described by either a bi- or tri-exponential model (Karlsson & Lindberg-Freijs, 1990). CsA accumulates readily in body fat producing a high Vd_{SS} which ranges from 2 to 8 l/kg depending on the route of administration and the analytic assay employed, and varies markedly from patient to patient (Ptachcinski et al., 1986; Kahan, 1988). CsA distributes readily across most biological membranes and accumulates primarily in the liver, followed in decreasing order by the pancreas, heart, lung, kidney, spleen, lymph nodes, and blood (Maurer et al., 1984). Diffusional resistance governs the transfer of CsA into the brain and fetus (Sangalli et al., 1990). CsA does not readily cross the blood–brain barrier, and drug concentrations are low in cerebrospinal fluid, brain and spinal cord. In the experimental animal, muscle and fat are the major sites of CsA deposition during pregnancy, while the thoracic and abdominal organs show intermediate accumulation. Little drug accumu-

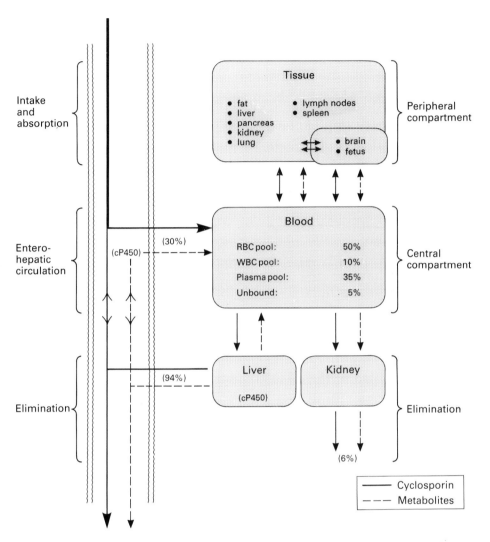

Fig. 3.2. Absorption, distribution and elimination of CsA following oral administration.

lates in the fetus, and CsA is not detectable in maternal and fetal brains or in the amniotic fluid. Placental transfer of CsA is also low in humans. *In vitro* studies using a dual perfusion technique of isolated placental lobules confirm *in vivo* measurements, and show negligible transfer for CsA from the maternal to fetal circulation, representing less than 5% of the maternal drug load (Nandakumaran & Eldeen, 1990). Significant concentrations of CsA accumulate in breast milk, and breast feeding may be contraindicated in order to protect the developing neonatal immune system (Fletchner *et al.*, 1985; Behrens *et al.*, 1989).

Metabolism of CsA occurs predominantly in the liver, and to a lesser degree in the bowel (Kolars et al., 1991), under the influence of the cytochrome P-450 III gene family (Kronbach et al., 1988). Biotransformation is initiated by oxidative attack at five main points on the molecular face opposite the cyclophilin binding site, comprising the γ-carbons of the MeLeu at positions 4, 6, and 9, the terminal methyl group of the MeBmt side chain, and the N-methyl group of Leu at position 4 (Wenger, 1990). Mathematical analysis predicts 41 mono-, di- or tri-oxidized derivatives of this process, and more than 25 metabolites have now been documented in human blood, bile and urine. All retain the cyclic oligopeptide structure, and approximately 12 of these have been further structurally identified with nuclear magnetic resonance and mass spectroscopy (Maurer & Lemair, 1986). To simplify description, a novel coding system has recently been adopted for metabolite designation which is based upon the molecular position of metabolic biotransformation (Table 3.1). In vitro studies utilizing liver microsomes show that the first oxidation products of CsA are the primary metabolites M1, M9 and M4N, produced by stepwise biotransformation beginning with a single conversion: either a region-specific hydroxylation at the n or γ positions of amino acid 1, or a demethylation at amino acid 4 (Fig. 3.3). Further oxidation of these compounds then produces a second group of metabolites which exhibit combined biotransformation, such as M19 characterized by dihydroxylation at both n and γ positions of amino acids 1 and 9, M49 which is oxidized at positions 4 and 9, or M4N9 which is oxidized at positions 4(N) and 9. Other secondary derivatives include M4N69 and M69 found in human urine, both of which are oxidized at position 6 and may represent further oxidation products of M4N9 and M9 respectively, M1AL, an aldehyde obtained by oxidation of the primary alcohol M1, and M1A, the corresponding acid first isolated as the bile acid metabolite Ma. Both of the latter may be further oxidized in positions 4, 4(N), 6 and 9, or cyclicized in position 1. Of these possibilities only M1A and M4N69 have so far been isolated and their structures elucidated (Wenger, 1990). A third conversion mechanism is intramolecular tetrahydrofuran ether formation at amino acid 1, producing M1c (Kahan et al., 1988), while the ultimate formation of linear CsA metabolites formed as γ lactones has also been predicted and at least one of these has been produced synthetically (Wenger, 1990).

In addition to the complex interpatient variations, it is now clear that the metabolism and accumulation of CsA differs quantitatively in individual tissues. While unchanged CsA represents the major component in plasma, M1 and M9 are present in high concentration in erythrocytes and other tissues. In contrast, M1 is the major component in urine, while unchanged CsA represents only 0.1% of the administered dose, and an acid derivative of M1 predominates in bile where CsA is present in only trace amounts (Lemaire et al., 1990). Although all natural and synthetic

Table 3.1. Nomenclature of CsA metabolites according to position of oxidation. Consensus document, Hawks Cay meeting on Therapeutic Drug Monitoring of Cyclosporine, 1990

New	Position of oxidation	Old
M1	$1\eta(8')$	M17
M1c	1η; 1ε-cyclized	M18
M4	4-γ	NI*
M4N	4-N-desmethylated	M21
M9	9-γ	M1
M9N	N-desmethylated in position 9	NI
M6	6-γ	NI
M19	1η, 9-γ	M8
M14	1η,4-γ	NI
M14N	1η, 4-N-desmethylated	M25
M16	1η, 6-γ	NI
M49	4-γ, 9-γ	M10
M46	4-γ, 6-γ	NI
M4N6	4-N-desmethylated, 6-γ	NI
M4N9	4-N-desmethylated, 9-γ	M13
M69	6-γ, 9-γ	M16
M1c4	1η, 1ε-cyclicized, 4-γ	NI
M1c6	1η, 1ε-cyclicized, 6-γ	NI
M1c9	1η, 1ε-cyclicized, 9-γ	M26
M4N69	4-N-desmethylated, 6-γ, 9-γ	M9
M1	1η	M17
M1AL	1η oxidized to an aldehyde	NI
M1A	1η oxidized to an acid	203-218
M1cAL	$1\eta = $ CHO, 1ε-cyclized	'biliary aldehyde'
M1cA	$1\eta = $ COOH, 1ε-cyclized	cyclic 203-218
MOX1	1ε, teta-oxirane $=$ MOX(S)1 $+$ MOX(R)1	epoxide
M1OX	1η, 1ε-teta-oxirane $=$ M1OX(S) $+$ M1OX(R)	M17-epoxide
M1TRI	1ε, 1 teta, 1η M1OX $\rightarrow$ M1TRI-hydroxy	NI
M1DI	MOX1 H_2O $\rightarrow$ M1DI; 1 teta, $1\eta =$ M1DI(6S,7R) $+$ M1DI(6R, 7S)	(dihydroxy) MeBmt[1]-CS

structural congeners with substitutions or deletions on the ring structure are demonstrably less immunosuppressive than unchanged CsA (Fahr *et al.*, 1990), it has been suggested that under certain circumstances the local accumulation of metabolites may contribute to the individual toxicity observed with this drug. However, experimental or clinical evidence to support this is scarce.

Interspecies comparisons show that the elimination of CsA is similar throughout the mammalian kingdom, with the possible exception of the dog which has an increased metabolic capacity (Sangalli *et al.*, 1988). In man, CsA elimination is determined by demographic parameters including age and sex, obesity, blood lipid levels and organ dysfunction, while the

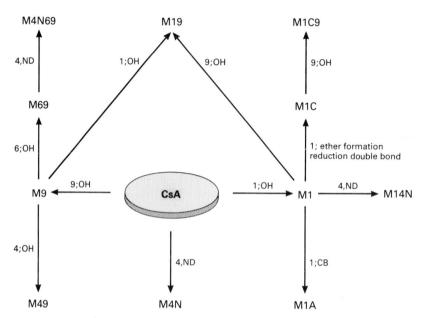

Fig. 3.3. Principal pathways for CsA biotransformation with primary and secondary metabolites.

timing of administration may exert a further minor influence. Clearance is increased by approximately 40% in children, and is correspondingly slower in older patients (Ptachcinski *et al.*, 1986). Females appear to clear CsA more slowly than males (Kahan *et al.*, 1986), reflecting partly the accumulation of the drug in body fat. The influence of obesity on the elimination of CsA is intriguing. Obese patients show higher blood levels than non-obese subjects when CsA is administered according to actual body weight, but pharmacokinetic analyses show no perceptible difference when normalized for ideal body weight and the difference in blood level is eliminated when the administered dose is adjusted for ideal body weight (Flechner *et al.*, 1989). Alterations in lipid profile markedly influence the pharmacokinetics of CsA, both by modifying distribution and by facilitating hepatic metabolism when the cleavage of lipids under the action of hepatic lipase releases free drug (Gupta & Benet, 1990). In addition, CsA increases lipoprotein concentration in both experimental animals and in man, thereby reciprocally modulating its own distribution. The plasma $t_{1/2}$ and Vd_{ss} of CsA correlate directly with fasting HDL cholesterol levels, while HDL CsA clearance correlates inversely with the serum creatinine and total bilirubin levels (Brunner *et al.*, 1990). CsA is eliminated primarily by biliary excretion, with median $t_{1/2}$ of 6–8 h. Clearance of CsA is significantly impaired in patients with liver disease and the elimination $t_{1/2}$ may be prolonged by fourfold or more. Longer dosing intervals or a substantial reduction in dose are therefore necessary in the presence of hepatic dysfunction. In contrast, renal excretion represents a minor pathway of elimination, accounting for approximately 6% of total body clearance in man (Kahan, 1989) (Fig. 3.3), and renal failure does not alter CsA clearance. Finally, the elimination of CsA has been reported to follow a circadian variation, with higher blood levels and lower clearance values after day-time dosing, although this is not well established.

Drug interactions

Pharmacokinetic interactions involving CsA occur with a broad range of drugs, including anticonvulsants, antibiotics, antimycotics, calcium channel inhibitors, adrenal steroids and other agents. Interaction may occur at the levels of drug absorption, disposition, metabolism or elimination, and may be divided into two classes which produce either an increase or a decrease in CsA concentration.

Phenytoin is the archetype of the first group of agents. This interaction, initially described following renal transplantation (Hoyer et al., 1984; Keown et al., 1984), has subsequently been widely observed in other solid organ and bone marrow transplant recipients and in normal subjects (Freeman et al., 1984; Schmidt et al., 1989). Pharmacokinetic studies in healthy subjects show that both C_{max} and area under the time/concentration curve (AUC) are reduced, without a significant change in $t_{1/2}$ or either parent drug or metabolites (Freeman et al., 1984). Phenobarbital and carbamazepine exert similar but sequentially less potent dose-related effects, while valproic acid exhibits no clinically important interaction and may be substituted in this situation (Hillebrand et al., 1987; Yee & McGuire, 1990a). Phenytoin produces a rapid decline in blood CsA concentration within several days of administration which persists throughout the duration of treatment and up to 3 weeks following drug withdrawal (Keown et al., 1984). The effect is often most dramatic in children, perhaps related to the higher intrinsic CsA clearance in this age group (Yee et al., 1988). All three drugs are potent inducers of the cytochrome P-450 enzyme system, and it is now believed that interaction occurs at two sites, producing an increase in presystemic metabolism of CsA thus reducing bioavailability, and an acceleration in hepatic metabolism of CsA which increases systemic clearance (Freeman et al., 1984; Rowland & Gupta, 1987).

Rifampicin induces a potent pharmacokinetic interaction quantitatively similar to that of phenytoin. Other antituberculous drugs may exert a less important effect, but this has not been well characterized. CsA concentrations decrease quickly after commencement of rifampicin, a consequence which may lead to acute graft rejection in renal and cardiac transplant patients (Langhoff & Madsen, 1983; Van Buren et al., 1984; Allen et al., 1985; Coward et al., 1985; Howard et al., 1985; Modry et al., 1985; Offerman et al., 1985). Pharmacokinetic studies show that rifampicin decreases the AUC, C_{max}, t_{max} and elimination $t_{1/2}$ of CsA (Yee, 1990), and an increase in CsA dosage of two- to threefold is required to compensate for this effect. Rifampicin is a known inducer of microsomal enzymes, and at least one of the cytochrome P-450 enzymes integral to the metabolism of CsA is strongly inducible by the drug.

A variety of other agents including nafcillin, octreotide and sulphonamide/trimethoprim have recently been reported to decrease CsA concentrations *in vivo* (Jones *et al.*, 1986; Landgraf *et al.*, 1987; Veremis *et al.*, 1987). Nafcillin probably accelerates CsA metabolism by inducing hepatic microsomal enzymes, although the mechanism of drug interaction is not yet fully established. The somatostatin analogue octreotide has been reported to decrease blood CsA concentrations in man following renal and pancreatic transplantation (Landgraf *et al.*, 1987; Rosenberg *et al.*, 1987), while in the experimental animal it delays t_{max} without affecting CsA trough levels, and potentiates renal and hepatic toxicity and glucose intolerance (Yale *et al.*, 1991). It has been hypothesized that octreotide decreases oral CsA absorption, possibly by inhibiting the secretion of pancreatic lipase or bile acids, or interferes with the enterohepatic recirculation of CsA. Finally, there are conflicting reports of the interaction between CsA and sulphonamide/trimethoprim (Thompson *et al.*, 1983; Jones *et al.*, 1986). Although a pharmacodynamic effect in increasing serum creatinine concentration has been well documented, the magnitude of any pharmacokinetic interaction appears to be minor and the mechanism is unknown.

Several classes of drug, including antibiotics, antifungals and calcium channel inhibitors exert an opposite but equally important pharmacokinetic effect resulting in a marked increase in CsA concentration. Erythromycin is perhaps the most potent and well recognized of the first group (Martell *et al.*, 1986), although quantitatively lesser interactions have been reported with other macrolide derivatives such as josamycin (Kreft-Jais *et al.*, 1987), ponsinomycin (Couet *et al.*, 1990), and rosithromycin (Billaud *et al.*, 1990). Interestingly, no change in CsA level has been observed during administration of spiramycin, a derivative which does not form a stable complex with the cytochrome P-450 enzyme that metabolizes CsA (Fabre *et al.*, 1988; Birmele *et al.*, 1989). The drug interaction caused by erythromycin is dose- and time-dependent, producing an increase in CsA levels within 2–14 days of treatment, and normally necessitates a reduction in CsA dose by 50% or more. Pharmacokinetic studies indicate that both the CsA AUC and C_{max} increase substantially during coadministration of erythromycin (Freeman *et al.*, 1987), although the effect on measured elimination rate is more contentious and the $t_{1/2}$ is variably reported to remain unchanged or increase slightly, though significantly, from 6.8 to 8.8 h (Freeman *et al.*, 1987; Vereestraeten *et al.*, 1987). The mechanism of interaction is complex, and appears to encompass a simultaneous increase in CsA absorption and a decrease in CsA elimination, due respectively to a reduction in gastrointestinal motility, a decrease in CsA metabolism by enteric flora, or to inhibition of intestinal and hepatic cyctochrome P-450 enzyme activity (Zara *et al.*, 1985; Watkins *et al.*, 1987; Henricsson & Lindholm, 1988). The increase in bioavailability may be quantitatively more important than the reduction in elimination, as emphasized by the fact that erythromycin produces a 13% decrease in plasma clearance of CsA with no change in $t_{1/2}$ when CsA is administered intravenously, compared with an almost threefold increase in C_{max} and a twofold rise in AUC after oral CsA administration (Gupta *et al.*, 1989). Further, erythromycin increases the AUC for the principal metabolite AM1 after oral, but not intravenous, administration of CsA.

The antifungal agent ketoconazole is a potent inhibitor of CsA metabolism in both microsomal enzymes and in the experimental animal, reducing CsA clearance from 15 to 7 ml/h with a corresponding increase in elimination $t_{1/2}$ from 4.1 to 11.2 h (Anderson & Blaschke, 1986; Henricsson & Lindholm, 1988). This effect is evident also in man, where ketoconazole has been reported to cause a pathological increase in CsA blood concentration in renal, cardiac and bone marrow transplant recipients, often producing renal dysfunction secondary to acute CsA nephrotoxicity (Yee & McGuire 1990a). Because of the magnitude of this interaction, ketoconazole has recently been employed experimentally to reduce the dose of CsA required, and hence the cost associated with maintenance immunosuppressive treatment in renal and cardiac graft recipients (Butman *et al.*, 1989; First *et al.*, 1989). Fluconazole is a potent inhibitor of phenazone metabolism in the experimental animal, but produces a quantitatively smaller increase in blood concentration when administered simultaneously with CsA (Canafax *et al.*, 1991). Whether itraconazole has a discernable influence on CsA metabolism in man remains contentious (Novakova *et al.*, 1987; Trenk *et al.*, 1987), although it does not inhibit either cytochrome P-450 enzyme activity *in vitro* or hepatic drug metabolism *in vivo* in the experimental animal (Lavrijsen *et al.*, 1987; Shaw *et al.*, 1987). The mechanism of interaction between these agents and CsA is not clearly established, but is most probably related to the concentration-dependent inhibition of microsomal enzyme activity demonstrated both *in vitro* and *in vivo*.

The influence of calcium channel inhibitors is particularly important in view of the prevalent use of these agents in the management of post-transplant cardiovascular disease. Diltiazem causes the most potent interaction, and increases the trough blood CsA concentration by up to 400% within 3–4 days of commencing treatment (McCauley *et al.*, 1989; Sabate *et al.*, 1989; Wagner *et al.*, 1989). Pharmacokinetic studies demonstrate a decrease in clearance of both CsA and its primary metabolites, with a consequent rise in C_{max} and a variable influence on elimination $t_{1/2}$ (Sabate *et al.*, 1989; Brockmoller *et al.*, 1990). A similar, though quantitatively lesser effect has been reported with verapamil (Sabate *et al.*, 1988) and with nicardipine (Cantarovich *et al.*, 1987) in recipients of heart and kidney transplants, while nifedipine or nitrendipine have no demonstrable influence on CsA pharmacokinetics (Copur *et al.*, 1989; Wagner *et al.*, 1989). These are therefore the preferred agents for use in patients receiving CsA. Interaction appears to occur predominantly at the level of CsA metabolism. Diltiazem and verapamil inhibit cytochrome P-450 enzyme activity both *in vitro* and *in vivo* in the experimental animal (Renton, 1985), and cause a dose-dependent non-competitive inhibition of CsA metabolism in liver microsomes *in vitro* (Henricsson & Lindholm, 1988; Brockmoller *et al.*, 1990). This explanation however, is clearly incomplete, as studies in human liver microsomes show that nifedipine behaves similarly to diltiazem and verapamil in inhibiting CsA metabolism (Henricsson *et al.*, 1988), and that both nifedipine and CsA are substrates for the same cytochrome P-450 enzymes (Combalbert *et al.*, 1989). The clinical consequence of this drug interaction are mitigated by the protective effects of calcium channel inhibitors which oppose the constrictor influence of CsA on the renal microvasculature (Petric *et al.*, 1992). Renal blood flow and glomerular filtration thus remain unchanged, or even increase despite a rise in CsA levels (Wagner *et al.*, 1987; Sabate *et al.*, 1989). Because of this, calcium channel inhibitors are now being widely evaluated as prophylactic therapy to simultaneously minimize CsA nephrotoxicity and control hypertension.

Drug interactions have been reported to occur with a number of other miscellaneous agents including acetazolomide, alcohol, colchicine, fluoroquinolones and non-steroidal anti-inflammatory agents (reviewed in Yee & McGuire, 1990b), although these are clinically less important and well established. Isoflurane increases CsA levels in the rodent (Gelb *et al.*, 1991), but whether this occurs in man is not yet clear. Cimeditine and ranitidine do not influence CsA concentration, but may raise serum creatinine, possibly by interfering with tubular secretion of creatinine. Oral contraceptives are weak inhibitors of cytochrome P-450 enzymes (Orme *et al.*, 1983), and have been reported to increase CsA concentration in recipients of renal and liver transplants. Estradiol inhibits CsA metabolism in human liver microsomes (Henricsson *et al.*, 1988), and the major enzyme that metabolizes CsA also catalyses 6-B hydroxylation of steroids. CsA and prednisolone are also metabolized by the same hepatic microsomal enzymes, and human liver microsomal studies show a bidirectional inhibition of CsA and corticosteroid metabolism (Yee, 1990). There are reports that administration of high-dose intravenous methylprednisolone (> 3 mg/kg/day) *in vivo* may increase CsA trough levels (Klintmalm & Sawe, 1984) but this remains controversial (Ptachcinski *et al.*, 1987) and any serious interaction is infrequent and of uncertain clinical importance.

Therapeutic monitoring

Therapeutic monitoring has become increasingly important as a guide to CsA dosage. It provides an accurate assessment of the absorption, distribution and metabolism of CsA, permits definition of, and compensation for, altered drug handling due to demographic factors or drug interactions, and facilitates the recognition of non-compliance (Kahan & Grevel, 1988). Considerations regarding therapeutic monitoring of CsA may be divided into four major areas, relating to sample selection, analytical method, quality assurance and therapeutic interpretation.

At steady state, CsA is distributed between both plasma and erythrocytes in the central blood compartment. Partitioning between these phases is temperature-dependent, erythrocyte binding increasing as the temperature falls below 37°C, so that the blood:plasma ratio increases from 1.5:3 at body temperature to 2.5:10 at room temperature (Van den Berg et al., 1985). Equilibration occurs within approximately 2 h, reaching a new steady state. The selection of serum/plasma or whole blood as valid matrices for analysis has been a controversial issue, and important advantages and disadvantages have been martialled for and against both (Anonymous, 1990). Excellent clinical correlations have been established with the serum matrix, which is assumed to be in closest equilibrium with intracellular cyclophilin receptor, but the variability of separation and the low concentrations of CsA in serum with current immunosuppression are important drawbacks. In addition, manipulation of whole blood samples is technically simple, and samples may be transported at ambient temperature without partitioning concerns. For these reasons, whole blood is now most commonly used as the matrix of choice (Shaw et al., 1990), although fluctuations in hematocrit remain a potential bias.

Measurement of CsA is currently performed predominantly by high performance liquid chromatography (HPLC) or radioimmunoassay (RIA), and a number of additional automated analytical methods are under evaluation. All permit specific measurement of the parent compound, as recommended by the international task force reports (Anonymous, 1987; Kahan et al., 1990; Shaw et al., 1990).

HPLC was the first specific method developed for analysis of CsA (Niederberger et al., 1980), and more than 60 variants of the original method have now been described. HPLC is accurate and precise, and remains the standard against which the analytical accuracy of other techniques are compared. It may be adapted to measure individual metabolites, in which case the assay is standardized using pure preparations of the metabolite in question. Most current HPLC methods use isocratic reverse-phase conditions for analysis, although some gradient methods have been reported. Extraction of CsA from the blood or plasma matrix may be performed by solvents such as ether or methyl-T-butyl ether, or by solid phase extraction systems including Sep-Pak (C18), BondElut, and CN which reduce the time and labour required. Column switching, the use of two or more columns in series to purify, separate, and quantify CsA is less widely employed, although meets many of the needs for efficiency and automation. The advantage of this approach is that all of the analyte in the sample is deposited onto the analytical column, and sample preparation is thus minimized (Gmur *et al.*, 1985). The conditions for analytical separation and the columns employed vary widely according to the method reported. Chromatography is normally performed at an elevated temperature (73–75°C), which speeds up interconversion and yields a sharp single peak. Accuracy can be further improved by the use of a more polar stationary phase (C1 or CN versus C18, which can also be operated at a slightly lower temperature. Despite its specificity, HPLC has a number of important limitations (Anonymous, 1987). Most critical is the complexity of the assay, which requires sophisticated technical expertise and expensive analytical equipment, and necessitates frequent recalibration and standardization. In addition, certain physicochemical properties of CsA itself complicate analysis: for example, maximum UV spectral absorption occurs at 195 nm while many HPLC methods use detection at 210–214 nm, and there are no easily derivatized groups to improve detection. For these reasons, HPLC is now normally employed as a reference procedure, or for specific analysis of drug metabolism.

The initial RIA method employed rabbit polyclonal antisera raised against protein-conjugated cyclosporine C (CsC) (Donatsch *et al.*, 1981), which cross-reacted by approximately 60% with the major metabolite M17. This was subsequently replaced by a polyclonal sheep antibody which exhibited a 32% cross-reactivity, and was widely employed for clinical measurement of CsA. With the development of monoclonal antibodies against the CsA molecule, however, the capability for specific and comprehensive monitoring by RIA has increased enormously. A library of monoclonal antibodies to parent CsA and metabolites were generated in mice using a lysyl-cyclosporine derivative coupled to guinea pig or chicken gammaglobulin. The two antibodies selected for clinical use recognize either the specific parent CsA molecule, or a framework determinant common to the parent and metabolite (Quesniaux *et al.*, 1986). Two principal RIA methods have evolved utilizing these monoclonal antibodies. The first, a ^{3}H-RIA (Sandoz Ltd) incorporates both specific and non-specific antibodies, and enables the measurement of both specific CsA concentration and total metabolite pool. The concentration of CsA measured by this technique correlated closely with that determined by HPLC even under the stringent conditions of cardiac and liver transplantation where marked expansion of the metabolite pool occurs (Ball *et al.*, 1988). A second ^{125}I-RIA (Cyclotrac-SP, INCStar Ltd) confers further technical advantages, eliminating the need for β scintillation counting and quench correction when using a whole blood matrix. However, because of iodination of the tracer, the specificity is somewhat less than with the ^{3}H-RIA and this assay has a consistent positive bias of approximately 10% compared with the ^{3}H-RIA and 10–20% compared with HPLC (Fig. 3.4) (Keown *et al.*, 1990). Nonetheless, it is sufficiently accurate for clinical use

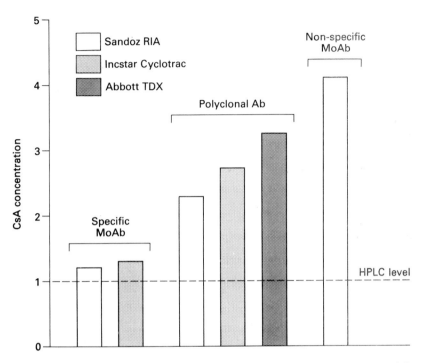

Fig. 3.4. Proportionate concentrations of CsA in human plasma as measured by HPLC, and polyclonal or monoclonal immunoassay ($n = 262$).

even in the early post-operative phase after heart or liver transplantation, and has quickly become the most widely used method for clinical CsA measurement.

Fluorescence polarization immunoassay (FPIA) is a recent technological development in which the antibody binding of a fluorescein-labelled CsA tracer in the immunoassay is reflected as a change in degree of polarization of incident light. This system offers advantages of simplicity, rapidity and technical accuracy with minimal technologist expertise, while the two major limitations have been cost and lack of specificity. Preliminary studies were performed utilizing a polyclonal anti-CsA antibody which cross-reacted extensively with both primary and secondary CsA metabolites, producing results which exceeded those of HPLC by over twofold in renal transplantation (Fig. 3.2). This discrepancy, and the inter-individual variability, were intensified by liver dysfunction, particularly common after heart or liver transplantation. The recent introduction of a CsA-specific monoclonal antibody has improved analytical accuracy, although a small degree (2–8%) of cross-reactivity persists, particularly against metabolites AM1 and AM4N (Wang et al., 1990). Other analytical methods are in a developmental phase, and clinical studies are currently under way. The automated analytical assay produced by DuPont Ltd is an affinity-column mediated immunometric assay which employs a β-galactosidase-coupled specific anti-CsA monoclonal antibody. The assay is rapid, simple and specific, with an analysis time of approximately 30 min. Preliminary results suggest that the sensitivity, accuracy and reproducibility are comparable to current assays and, like the FPIA, recalibration of the automated analytical equipment is required infrequently, further reducing operator time (Hansen et al., 1990). A non-isotopic semiautomated assay currently being developed by Syva Ltd employs an enzyme multiplied immunoassay technique (EMIT), which avoids the requirement for separation of bound and free components. CsA concentration is determined by spectrophotometric measurement of enzyme activity, with excellent accuracy and specificity. A more revolutionary approach has employed a cyclophilin binding assay to determine CsA receptor binding affinity. Preliminary studies using this approach appear promising, and it may offer an alternative and perhaps more relevant methodology for CsA measurement (Lorber et al., 1990).

Multi-centre quality assessment programmes have now been established world-wide to coordinate the therapeutic monitoring of CsA and to facilitate the definition of therapeutic operating ranges for different clinical indications. Principal among these are the UK Interlaboratory Quality Assessment Programme, the Swiss Interlaboratory CsA Testing Programme, the American Association for Clinical Chemistry service, the Pittsburgh Cyclosporine Survey and the Canadian Working Group on CsA Monitoring (Jonston et al., 1989; Wong et al., 1990). Each programme distributes unknown samples on a monthly basis to test the accuracy, reproducibility, sensitivity and specificity of all analytical methods.

Therapeutic monitoring has been extensively employed in the management of both solid organ transplantation and autoimmune disease following the initial retrospective studies which documented a clear relationship between adverse events and drug levels (Keown et al., 1981; Kahan et al., 1982). With increased sophistication in the use of CsA and the improved outcome in all forms of solid organ transplantation, documentation of a strict correlation has become more problematic. Aggressive reduction in CsA dosage, either alone or as a component of triple and quadruple immunosuppressive protocols, has progressively narrowed the therapeutic operating range of CsA in serum or whole blood, while the decrease in severity of organ toxicity, coupled with the imprecision in clinical discrimination from immunological graft injury, limits the specificity, sensitivity and predictive value of therapeutic monitoring (Stiller & Keown, 1990). Therapeutic monitoring is most useful for interpretation of acute events, and offers less assistance in the discrimination of chronic organ dysfunction where it is employed principally as a measure of compliance and drug interaction. Current studies with selective measurement of CsA concentration in whole blood confirm that acute graft rejection occurs predominantly with trough CsA concentrations below 200 μg/l, while organotoxicity is normally observed in conjunction with CsA levels above this threshold (Lindholm, 1990; Sridhar *et al.*, 1990; Taube *et al.*, 1990). Pharmacokinetic monitoring of AUC at steady state, though more complex, appears to provide a more accurate index of the biological effect of CsA, and limited sampling strategies have been developed to facilitate the broader application of this approach (Kahan *et al.*, 1988; Johnson *et al.*, 1990). Measurements *in vivo* in general confirm the limited biological relevance of CsA metabolites, with the possible exception of live transplantation where metabolite concentrations may be inordinately high and produce renal dysfunction (Wonigeit *et al.*, 1990). The factors of administered dose and individuality of response are equally important in regard to autoimmune disease, where three categories may be defined. CsA-induced nephrotoxicity is unusual with the doses currently employed in the treatment of psoriasis and similar immune disorders (< 5 mg/kg/day), and therapeutic monitoring is of limited value. In disorders such as diabetes mellitus and uveitis, however, the higher doses required for clinical efficacy entail an increased risk of adverse events. Both efficacy and toxicity appear to be concentration dependent, and therapeutic monitoring is considered essential (Feutren *et al.*, 1986; Canadian European Randomized Control Trial 1988; Feutren, 1990). Finally, rheumatoid arthritis and inflammatory bowel disease represent an intermediate category of risk/benefit, where measurement of CsA levels may provide supplementary information in cases of inadequate response, unexpected toxicity, or multiple drug therapy.

Acknowledgements

I am indebted to Dr M. Pacio for her invaluable editorial assistance in preparation of this manuscript.

References

Allen, R. D. M., Hunnisett, A. G. & Morris, P. J. (1985). Cyclosporin and rifampicin in renal transplantation. *Lancet* i, 980.

Anderson, J. E. & Blaschke, T. F. (1986). Ketoconazole inhibits cyclosporine metabolism *in vivo* in mice. *Journal of Pharmacology and Experimental Therapeutics* **236**, 671–674.

Anonymous. (1987). Critical issues in cyclosporine monitoring: report of the task force on cyclosporine monitoring. *Clinical Chemistry* **33**, 1269–1288.

Anonymous. (1990). Concensus document: Hawks Cay meeting on therapeutic drug monitoring of cyclosporine. *Transplantation Proceedings* **22**, 1357–1361.

Awni, W. M., Heim-Duthoy, K. & Kasiske. B. L. (1990). Impact of lipoproteins on cyclosporine pharmacokinetics and biological activity in transplant patients. *Transplantation Proceedings* **22**, 1193–1196.

Ball, P. E., Munzer, H., Keller, H. P., Abisch, E. & Rosenthaler, J. (1988). Specific ^{3}H radioimmunoassay with a monoclonal antibody for monitoring cyclosporine in blood. *Clinical Chemistry* **34**, 257–260.

Ballantyne, C., Podet, E., Patsch, W., Harati, Y., Appel, V., Gotto, A. & Young, J.

(1989). Effect of cyclosporine therapy on plasma lipoprotein levels. *Journal of American Medical Association* **262**, 53–58.

Behrens, O., Kohlhaw, K., Gunter, H., Wonigeit, H. & Niesert, S. (1989). Detection of cyclosporin in breast milk — is breast feeding contraindicated? *Geburtshilfe Und Fraunenheikunde* **49**, 207–209.

BenEzra, D & Maftzir, G. (1990). Ocular penetration of cyclosporine A in the rat eye. *Archives of Ophthalmology* **108**, 584–587.

BenEzra, D., Maftzir, G., de Courten, C. & Timonen, P. (1990). Ocular penetration of cyclosporine A. III: The human eye. *British Journal of Ophthalmology* **74**, 350–353.

Billaud, E. M., Guillemain, R., Fortineau, N., Kitzis, M. D., Dreyfus, G., Amrein, C., Kreft-Jalis, C., Husson, J. M. & Chretien, P. (1990). Interaction between roxithromycin and cyclosporin in heart transplant patients. *Clinical Pharmacokinetics* **19**, 499–502.

Birmele, B., Lebranchu, Y., Beliveau, F., Rateau, H. & Furet, Y. (1989). Absence of interaction between cyclosporine and spiramycin. *Transplantation* **47**, 927–928.

Brockmoller, J., Neumayer, H. H., Wagner, K., Weber, W., Heinemeyer, g., Kewitz, H. & Roots, I. (1990). Pharmacokinetic interaction between cyclosporine and diltiazem. *European Journal of Clinical Pharmacology* **38**, 237–242.

Brunner, L. J., Luke, D. R., Lautersztain, J., Williams, L. A. LeMaistre, C. F. & Yau, J. C. (1990). Single-dose cyclosporine pharmacokinetics in various biological fluids of patients receiving allogeneic marrow transplantation. *Therapeutic Drug Monitoring* **12**, 134–138.

Butman, S. M., Wild, J., Nolan, P., Fagan, T. & Mackle, M. (1989). Cyclosporine and concomitant ketoconazole after cardiac transplantation: intermediate term findings and potential savings. *Journal of American College of Cardiology* **13**, 6A.

Canadian-European Randomized Control Trial Group (1988). Cyclosporin-induced remission of IDDM after early intervention: association of 1 year of cyclosporin treatment with enhanced insulin secretion. *Diabetes* **37**, 1574–1582.

Canafax, D. M., Graves, N. M., Hilligoss, D. M., Carelton, B. C., Gardner, M. J. & Matas, A. J. (1991). Increased cyclosporine levels as a result of simultaneous fluconazole and cyclosporine therapy in renal transplant recipients: a double-blind, randomized pharmacokinetic and safety study. *Transplantation Proceedings* **23**, 1041–1042.

Cantarovich, M., Hisse, C., Lockiec, F., Charpentier, B. & Fries, D. (1987). Conformation of the interaction between cyclosporine and calcium channel blocker nicardipine in renal transplant patients. *Clinical Nephrology* **28**, 190–203.

Combalbert, J., Fabre, I., Fabre, G., Dalet, I., Derancourt, J., Cano, J. P. & Maurel, P. (1989). Metabolism of cyclosporin A. IV. Purification and identification of the rifampicin-inducible human liver cyctochrome P-450 (cyclosporin A oxidase) as a product of P450IIIA gene subfamily. *Drug Metabolism and Disposition* **17**, 197–207.

Copur, M. S., Tasdemir, I., Turgan, C., Yasavul, U. & Caglar, S. (1989). Effects of nitrendipine on blood pressure and blood cyclosporin A level in patients with post-transplant hypertension. *Nephron* **52**, 227–230.

Couet, W., Istin, B., Seniuta, P., Morel, D., Potaux, L. & Fourtillan, J. B. (1990). Effect of ponsinomysin on cyclosporin pharmacokinetics. *European Journal of Clinical Pharmacology* **39**, 165–167.

Coward, R. A., Raftery, A. T. & Brown, C. B. (1985). Cyclosporin and antituberculous therapy. *Lancet* i, 1342.

Diaz-Llopis, M. & Menezo, J. L. (1989). Penetration of 2% cyclosporine eye drops into aqueous humor. *British Journal of Ophthalmology* **73**, 600–603.

Donatsch, P., Abisch, E., Homberger, M., Traber, R., Trapp, M. & Voges, R. (1981). A radioimmunoassay to measure cyclosporin A in plasma and serum samples. *Journal of Immunoassay* **2**, 19–32.

Duncan, J. I., Payne, S., Winfield, A. J., Ormerod, A. D. & Thomson, A. W. (1990). Enhanced percutaneous absorption of a novel topical cyclosporin A formulation and assessment of its immunosuppressive activity. *British Journal of Dermatology* **123**, 631–640.

Ericzon, B. G., Todo, S., Lynch, S., Kam, I., Ptachcinski, R. J., Burchart, G. J., Van Thiel, D. H., Starzl, T. E. & Venkataramanan, R. (1987). Role of bile salts on cyclosporine absorption in dogs. *Transplantation Proceedings* **19**, 1248–1249.

Fabre, I., Fabre, G., Maurel, P., Bertault-Peres, P. & Cano, J. P. (1988). Metabolism of cyclosporin A. III. Interaction of macrolide antibiotic, erythromycin, using rabbit hepatocytes and microsomal fractions. *Drug Metabolism and Disposition* **16**, 296–301.

Fahr, A., Hiestand, P. & Ryffel, B. (1990). Studies on the biologic activities of Sandimmun metabolites in humans and in animal models: review and original experiments. *Transplantation Proceedings* **22**, 1116–1124.

Feutren, G. (1990). Summary on autoimmune diseases. *Transplantation Proceedings* **22**, 1355.

Feutren, G., Papoz, L., Assan, R., Vialettes, B., Karsenty, G., Vexiau, P., Du Rostu, H., Rodier, M., Sirmai, J. & Lallemand, A. (1986). Cyclosporin increases the rate and length of remissions in insulin-dependent diabetes of recent onset. *Lancet* **ii**, 119–124.

First, M. R., Weiskittel, P., Alexander, J. W., Schroeder, R. L. & Najarian, J. S. S. (1989). Concomitant administration of cyclosporin and ketoconazole in renal transplant recipients. *Lancet* **ii**, 1198–1201.

Flechner, S. M., Katz, A. R., Rogers, A. J., Van Buren, C. & Kahan, B. D. (1985). The presence of cyclosporine in body tissues and fluids during pregnancy. *American Journal of Kidney Diseases* **5**, 60–63.

Flechner, S. M., Kolbeinsson, M. C., Tam, J. & Lum, B. (1989). The effect of obesity on cyclosporine pharmacokinetics in uremic patients. *Transplantation Proceedings* **21**, 1446–1448.

Freeman, D. J. (1991). Pharmacology and pharmacokinetics of cyclosporine. *Clinical Biochemistry* **24**, 9–14.

Freeman, D. J., Laupacis, A., Keown, P. A., Carruthers, S. G. & Stiller, C. R. (1984). Evaluation of cyclosporine–phenytoin interaction with observations on cyclosporin metabolites. *British Journal of Clinical Pharmacology* **18**, 887–893.

Freeman, D. J., Martell, R., Carruthers, S. G., Heinrichs, D. & Keown, P. A. (1987). Cyclosporin–erythromycin interaction in normal subjects. *British Journal of Clinical Pharmacology* **23**, 776–778.

Gelb, A. W., Freeman, D., Robertson, K. M. & Zhang, C. (1991). Isoflurane alters the kinetics of oral cyclosporine. *Anesthesia and Analgesia* **72**, 801–804.

Gmur, D. J., Yee, G. C. & Kennedy, M. S. (1985). Modified column-switching high-performance liquid chromatographic methods for measurement of cyclosporine in serum. *Journal of Chromatography* **344**, 422–427.

Gupta, S. K., Bakran, A., Johnson, R. W. & Rowland, M. (1989). Cyclosporine–erythromycin interaction in renal transplant patients. *British Journal of Clinical Pharmacology* **27**, 475–481.

Gupta, S. K. & Benet, L. Z. (1990). High-fat meals increase the clearance of cyclosporine. *Pharmaceutical Research* **7**, 46–48.

Gupta, S. K., Manfro, R. C., Tomlanovich, S. J., Gambertoglio, J. G., Garovy, M. R. & Benet, L. Z. (1990). Effect of food on the pharmacokinetics of cyclosporine in healthy subjects following oral and intravenous administration. *Journal of Clinical Pharmacology* **30**, 643–653.

Hansen, J. B., Lau, H. P., Janes, C. J., Lehance, D. P. & Miller, W. K. (1990) A rapid and specific assay for du Pont aca discreet clinical analyzer, performed directly on whole blood. *Transplantation Proceedings* **22**, 1189–1192.

Henricsson, S. & Lindholm A. (1988). Inhibition of cyclosporine metabolism by other drugs *in vitro*. *Transplantation Proceedings* **20**, 569–571.

Hilbrands, L. B., Hoitsma, A. J., van den Berg, J. W. & Koene, R. A. (1991). Cyclosporine A blood levels during use of cyclosporine as oral solution or in capsules: comparison of pharmacokinetic parameters. *Transplant International* **4**, 125–127.

Hillebrand, G., Castro, L. A., van Scheidt, W., Beukelmann, D., Land, W. & Schmidt, D. (1987). Valproate for epilepsy in renal transplant recipients receiving cyclosporine. *Transplantation* **43**, 915–916.

Honcharik, N. (1991). The effect of food on cyclosporine absorption. *Clinical Biochemistry* **24**, 89–92.

Howard, P., Bixler, T. J. & Gill, B. (1985). Cyclosporine-rifampicin drug interaction. *Drug Intelligence and Clinical Pharmacy* **19**, 763–764.

Hoyer, P. F., Offner, G., Wonigeit, K., Brodehl, J. & Pichlmayer, R. (1984). Dosage of cyclosporin A in children with renal transplants. *Clinical Nephrology* **22**, 68–71.

Johnston, A., Marsdem, J. T. & Holt, D. W. (1989). The continuing need for quality assessment of cyclosporine measurement. *Clinical Chemistry* **35**, 1309–1312.

Johnston, A., Sketris, I., Marsden, J. T., Galustian, C. G., Fashola, T., Taube, D., Pepper, J. & Holt, D. W. (1990). A limited sampling strategy for the measurement of cyclosporine AUC. *Transplantation Proceedings* **22**, 1345–1346.

Jones, D. K., Hakim, M., Wallwork, J., Higenbottam, T. W. & White, D. J. G. (1986). Serious interaction between cyclosporin A and sulphadimide. *British Medical Journal* **292**, 728–729.

Kahan, B. D. (1989). Cyclosporine. *New England Journal of Medicine* **321**, 1725–1736.

Kahan, B. D. & Grevel, J. (1988). Optimization of cyclosporine therapy in renal transplantation by pharmacokinetic strategy. *Transplantation* **46**, 631–644.

Kahan, B. D., Kramer, W. G., Wideman, C., Flechner, S. M., Lorber, M. I. & Van Buren, C. T. (1986). Demographic factors affecting the pharmacokinetics of cyclosporine estimated by radioimmunoassay. *Transplantation* **41**, 459–464.

Kahan, B. D., Shaw, L. M., Holt, D., Grevel, J. & Johnston, A. (1990). Consensus document: Hawk's Cay Meeting on Therapeutic Drug Monitoring of Cyclosporine. *Clinical Chemistry* **36**, 1510–1516.

Kahan, B. D., Van Buren, C. T., Lin, S., Ono, Y., Agostino, G., Legrue, S., Boileau, M., Payne, W. & Kerman, R. (1982). Immunopharmacological monitoring of cyclosporin A treated recipients of cadaveric kidney allografts. *Transplantation* **34**, 36–45.

Karlsson, M. O. & Lindberg-Freijs, A. (1990). Comparison of methods to calculate cyclosporine A bioavailability from consecutive oral and intravenous doses. *Journal of Pharmacokinetics and Biopharmaceutics* **18**, 293–311.

Keown, P. A. (1990). Emerging indication for the use of cyclosporin in organ transplantation and autoimmunity. *Drugs* **40**, 315–325.

Keown, P. A., Glenn, J., Denegri, J., Maciejewska, U., Seccombe, D., Stawecki, M., Freeman, D., Stiller, C., Shackleton, C., Cameron, E. & Philips, D. (1990). Therapeutic monitoring of cyclosporine: impact of a change in standards on ^{125}I-monoclonal RIA performance in comparison with liquid chromatography. *Clinical Chemistry* **36**, 804–807.

Keown, P. A., Laupacis, A., Carruthers, S. G., Stawecki, M. & Koegler, J. (1984). Interaction between phenytoin and cyclosporine following organ transplantation. *Transplantation* **38**, 304–306.

Keown, P. A., Stiller, C. R., Ulan, R. A., Sinclair, N. R., Wall, W. J., Carruthers, G. & Howson, W. (1981). Immunological and pharmacological monitoring in the clinical use of cyclosporin A. *Lancet* **i**, 686–689.

Keown, P. A., Stiller, C. R., Laupacis, A. L., Howson, W., Coles R., Stawecki, M., Koegler, J., Carruthers, G., McKenzie, N. & Sinclair, N. R. (1982). The effects and side effects of cyclosporine: relationship to drug pharmacokinetics. *Transplantation Proceedings* **14**, 659–661.

Klintmalm, G. & Sawe, J. (1984). High dose methylprednisolone increases plasma cyclosporin levels in renal transplant recipients. *Lancet* **i**, 731.

Kolars, J. C., Merion, R. M., Awni, W. M. & Watkins, P. B. (1991). First-pass metabolism of cyclosporin by the gut. *Lancet* **338**, 1488–1490.

Kreft-Jais, C., Bilaud, E. M., Gaudry, C. & Bedrossian, J. (1987). Effect of josamycin on plasma cyclosporine levels. *European Journal of Clinical Pharmacology* **32**, 327–328.

Kronbach, T., Fisher, V. & Meyer, U. A. (1988). Cyclosporine metabolism in human liver: identification of a cytochrome P-450III gene family as the major cyclosporine-metabolizing enzyme explains interactions of cyclosporine with other drugs. *Clinical Pharmacology and Therapeutics* **43**, 630–635.

Landgraf, R., Landgraf-Leurs, N. M. C., Nusser, J., Hillebrand, G. & Illner, W. D. (1987). Effect of somatostatin analogue (SMS201-995) on cyclosporine levels. *Transplantation* **44**, 724–725.

Langhoff, E. & Madsen, S. (1983). Rapid metabolism of cyclosporin and prednisone in kidney transplant patient receiving tuberculostatic treatment. *Lancet* **ii**, 1303.

Lavrijsen, K., Van Houdt, J., Thijs, D. Meuldermans, W. & Heykants, J. (1987). Interaction of miconazole, ketoconazole and itraconazole with rat-liver microsomes. *Xenobiotica* **17**, 45–57.

Legg, B., Gupta, S. K., Rowland, M., Johnson, R. W. & Solomon, L. R. (1988). Cyclosporin: pharmacokinetics and detailed studies of plasma erythrocyte binding during intravenous and oral administration. *European Journal of Clinical Pharmacology* **31**, 451–460.

Lemaire, M., Fahr, A. & Maurer, G. (1990). Pharmacokinetics of cyclosporine: inter and intra-individual variations and metabolic pathways. *Transplantation Proceedings* **22**, 1110–1112.

Lemaire, M. & Tillement, J. P. (1982). Role of lipoproteins and erythrocytes in the in vitro binding and distribution of cyclosporin A in the blood. *Journal of Pharmacokinetics and Pharmacology* **34**, 715–718.

Lensmeyer, G., Wiebe, D. & Carlson, I. (1989). Distribution of cyclosporin A metabolites among plasma and cells in whole blood: effect of temperature, hematocrit, and metabolite concentration. *Clinical Chemistry* **35**, 56–63.

Lindholm, A. (1990). A prospective study of cyclosporine monitoring in renal transplantation. *Transplantation Proceedings* **22**, 1260–1263.

Lindholm, A. & Henricsson, S. (1989). Intra- and inter-individual variability in the free fraction of cyclosporine in plasma in recipients of renal transplants. *Therapeutic Drug Monitoring* **11**, 623–630.

Lindholm, A., Henricsson, S. & Dahlqvist, R. (1990). The effect of food and bile acid administration on the relative bioavailability of cyclosporine. *British Journal of Pharmacology* **29**, 541–548.

Lorber, M. I., Paul, K., Harding, M. W., Handschunmacher, R. E. & Marks, W. H. (1990). Cyclophilin binding: a receptor-mediated approach to monitoring cyclosporine immunosuppressive activity following organ transplantation. *Transplantation Proceedings* **22**, 1240–1244.

Martell, R., Heirichs, D., Stiller, C. R., Jenner, M. & Keown, P. A. (1986). The effect of erythromycin in patients treated with cyclosporine. *Annals of Internal Medicine* **104**, 660–661.

Maurer, G. & Lemaire, M. (1986). Biotransformation and distribution in blood of cyclosporine and its metabolites. *Transplantation Proceedings* **18**, 25.

Maurer, G., Looseli, H. R., Schreier, E. & Keller, B. (1984). Disposition of cyclosporine in several animal species and man. *Drug Metabolism Disposition* **12**, 120–126.

McCauley, J., Ptachcinski, R. J. & Shapiro, R. (1989). The cyclosporine-sparing effects of diltiazem in renal transplantation. *Transplantation Proceedings* **21**, 3955–3957.

McMillan, M. A. (1989). Clinical pharmacokinetics of cyclosporine. *Pharmacology and Therapeutics* **42**, 135–156.

Modry, D. L., Stinson, E. B., Oyer, P. E., Jamieson, S. W. & Baldwin, J. C. (1985). Acute rejection and massive cyclosporine requirements in heart transplant recipients treated with rifampicin. *Transplantation* **39**, 313–314.

Nandakumaran, M. & Eldeen, A. S. (1990). Transfer of cyclosporine in the perfused human placenta. *Developmental Pharmacology and Therapeutics* **15**, 101–105.

Naoumov, N. V., Tredger, J. M., Steward, C. M., O'Grady, J. G., Grevel, J., Niven, A., Whiting, B. & Williams, R. (1989). Cyclosporin A pharmacokinetics in liver transplant recipients in relation to biliary T-tube clamping and liver dysfunction. *Gut* **30**, 391–396.

Nashan, B., Bleck, J., Wonigeit, K., Vogt, P., Christians, U., Sewing, K-F., Beveridge, T., & Pichlmayer, R. (1988). Effect of the application form of cyclosporine on blood levels: comparison of oral solution and capsules. *Transplantation Proceedings* **20**, 637–639.

Niederberger, W., Schaub, P. & Beveridge, T. (1980). High performance liquid chromatographic determination of cyclosporin A in human plasma and urine. *Journal of Chromatography* **182**, 454–458.

Novakova, I., Donnelly, P., De White, T., De Pauw, B., Boezeman, J., & Veltman, G. (1987). Itraconazole and cyclosporin nephrotoxicity. *Lancet* **ii**, 920–921.

Offerman, G., Keller, F. & Molzahan, M. (1985). Low cyclosporin A blood levels and acute graft rejection in a renal transplant recipient during rifampicin treatment. *American Journal of Nephrology* **5**, 385–387.

Orme, M. L., Back, D. J. & Breckenridge, A. M. (1983). Clinical pharmacokinetics of oral contraceptive steroids. *Clinical Pharmacokinetics* **8**, 95–136.

Petric, R., Freeman, D., Wallace, C., McDonald, J., Stiller, C. & Keown, P. A. (1992). Amelioration of experimental cyclosporin nephrotoxicity by calcium channel inhibition. *Transplantation* (in press).

Ptachcinski, R. J., Venkataramanan, R., Burckart, G. J., Hakala, T. R., Rosenthal, J. R., Carpenter, B. J. & Taylor, R. J. (1987). Cyclosporine—high dose steroid interaction in renal transplant recipients: assessment by HPLC. *Transplantation Proceedings* **19**, 1728–1729.

Ptachcinski, R. J., Venkataramanan, R. & Burckart, G. J. (1986). Clinical pharmacokinetics of cyclosporin. *Clinical Pharmacokinetics* **11**, 107–132.

Quesniaux, V., Tees, R., Schreier, M. H., Wenger, R. M. & van Regenmortel, M. H. V. (1986). Monoclonal antibodies to ciclosporin. In Borel, J. F. (ed.) *Progress in Allergy* **38**, 108–122.

Renton, K. W. (1985). Inhibition of hepatic microsomal drug metabolism by the calcium channel blockers diltiazem and verapamil. *Biochemical Pharmacology* **34**, 2549–2553.

Ritschel, G. B., Adolph, S., Ritschel, G. B. & Schroeder, T. (1990). Improvement of peroral absorption of cyclosporine A microemulsions. *Methods and Findings in Experimental and Clinical Pharmacology* **12**, 127–134.

Rosano, T. G. (1985). Effect of hematocrit on cyclosporine (cyclosporin A) in whole blood and plasma of renal transplant patients. *Clinical Chemistry* **31**, 410–412.

Rosenberg, L., Dfoe, D. C., Schwartz, R., Campbell, D. A. & Turcotte, J. G. (1987). Administration of somatostatin analogue (SMS 201-995) in the treatment of a fistula occurring after pancreas transplantation. *Transplantation* **43**, 764–766.

Rowland, M. & Gupta, S. K. (1987). Cyclosporine–phenytoin interaction: re-evaluation using metabolite data. *British Journal of Clinical Pharmacology* **24**, 329–334.

Sabate, I., Grino, J. M., Castelao, A. M. & Ortola, J. (1988). Evaluation of cyclosporin-verapamil interaction, with observations on parent cyclosporin and metabolites. *Clinical Chemistry* **34**, 2151.

Sabate, I., Grino, J. M., Castelao, A. M., Huguet, J., Seron, D. & Blanco, A. (1989). Cyclosporin-diltiazem interaction: comparison of cyclosporin levels measured with monoclonal antibodies. *Transplantation Proceedings* **21**, 1460–1461.

Sandborn, W. J., Strong, R. M., Forland, S. C. & Chase, R. E. (1991). The pharmacokinetics and colonic tissue concentration of cyclosporine after i.v., oral and enema administration. *Journal of Clinical Pharmacology* **31**, 76–80.

Sangalli, L., Bortolotti, A., Jiritano, L. & Bonati, M. (1988). Cyclosporine pharmacokinetics in rats and interspecies comparison in dogs, rabbits, rats and humans. *Drug Metabolism and Disposition: the Biological Fate of Chemicals* **16**, 749–753.

Sangalli, L., Bortolotti, A., Passerini, F. & Bonati, M. M. (1990). Placental transfer, tissue distribution, and pharmacokinetics of cyclosporine in the pregnant rabbit. *Drug Metabolism and Disposition: the Biological Fate of Chemicals* **18**, 102–106.

Schmidt, H., Naumann, R., Jaschonek, K., Einsele, H., Dopfer, R. & Ehninger, G. (1989). Drug interaction between cyclosporin and phenytoin in allogeneic bone marrow transplantation. *Bone Marrow Transplantation* **4**, 212–213.

Schreiber, S. L. (1991). Chemistry and biology of the immunophilins and their immunosuppressive ligands. *Science* **251**, 283–288.

Shaw, L. M., Yatscoff, R. W., Bowers, L., Freeman, D. J., Jeffery, J. R., Keown, P. A., McGilverary, I. J., Rosanok T. G. & Wong, P. (1990). Canadian consensus meeting on cyclosporine monitoring: report of the consensus panel. *Clinical Chemistry* **36**, 1841–1846.

Shaw, M. A., Gumbleton, M. & Nicholis, P. J. (1987). Interaction of cyclosporin and itraconazole. *Lancet* **ii**, 637.

Sokol, R. J., Johnson, K. E., Karrer, F. M., Narkewics, M. R., Smith, D. & Kam, I. (1991). Improvement of cyclosporine absorption in children after liver transplantation by means of water-soluble vitamin E. *Lancet* **338**, 212–214.

Sridhar, N., Schroeder, T. J., Pesce, A. & First, M. R. (1990). Clinical correlations of cyclosporine HPLC and FPIA levels in renal recipients. *Transplantation Proceedings* **22**, 1257–1259.

Stiller, C. & Keown, P. A. (1990). Failure of ^{125}I-tracer selective monoclonal antibody levels on a whole blood matrix to predict rejection on nephrotoxic episodes in renal transplant patients under anti-lymphocyte globulin and prednisone therapy. *Transplantation Proceedings* **22**, 1253–1254.

Takaya, S., Zaghloul, I., Iwatsuki, S., Starzl, T. E., Toguchi, T. Ohmori, Y., Burchart, G. J., Ptachcinksi, R. J. & Venkataramanan, R. (1987). Effect of liver dysfunction on cyclosporine pharmacokinetics. *Transplantation Proceedings* **19**, 1246–1247.

Tarr, B. D. & Yalkowsky, S. H. (1989). Enhanced intestinal aborption of cyclosporine in rats through reduction of emulsion droplet size. *Pharmaceutical Research* **6**, 40–43.

Taube, D., Marsden, J., Palmer, A., Cairns, T., Johnston, A. & Holt, D. W. (1990). Value of cyclosporine measurements in renal transplant recipients immunosuppressed with triple therapy. *Transplantation Proceedings* **22**, 1251–1252.

Thompson, J. F., Chalmers, D. H., Hinnisett, A. G. W., Wood, R. F. M. & Morris, P. J. (1983). Nephrotoxicity of trimethoprim and cotrimoxazole in renal allograft recipients treated with cyclosporine. *Transplantation* **36**, 204–206.

Trenk, D., Brett, W., Jahnchen, A. & Birnbaum, D. (1987). Time course of cyclosporin itraconazole interaction. *Lancet* **ii**, 1335–1336.

Tufveson, G., Frodin, L. & Linberg, A. (1986). A longitudinal study of the pharmacokinetics of cyclosporine A and *in vitro* lymphocyte responses in renal transplant. *Transplantation Proceedings* **18**, 1264–1265.

Van Buren, D., Wideman, C. A., Ried, M., Gibbons, S. & Van Buren, C. T. (1984). The antagonistic effect of rifampicin upon cyclosporine bioavailability. *Transplantation Proceedings* **16**, 1642–1645.

Van den Berg, J. W. O., Verhoef, M. L., de Boer, A. J. H. & Schalm, S. W. (1985). Cyclosporin A assay: conditions for sampling and processing of blood. *Clinical Chimica Acta* **147**, 291–297.

Venkataram, S., Awni, W. M., Jordan, K. & Rahman, Y. E. (1990). Pharmacokinetics of two alternative dosage forms of cyclosporine: liposomes and intralipid. *Journal of Pharmaceutical Sciences* **79**, 216–219.

Vereestraeten, P., Thiry, P., Kinnaert, P. & Toussaint, C. (1987). Influence of erythromycin on cyclosporine pharmacokinetics. *Transplantation* **44**, 155–156.

Veremis, S. A., Maddux, M. S., Pollak, R. & Mozes, M. F. (1987). Sub-therapeutic cyclosporine concentrations during nafcillin therapy. *Transplantation* **43**, 913–915.

Wadhwa, N. K., Schroeder, T. J., O'Flaherty, E., Pesce, A. J., Myre, S. A. & First, M. R. (1987). The effect of oral metoclopramide on the absorption of cyclosporine. *Transplantation Proceedings* **19**, 1730–1733.

Wagner, K., Albrecht, S. & Neumayer, H-H. (1987). Prevention of post-transplant acute tubular necrosis by the calcium antagonist diltiazem: a prospective randomized study. *American Journal of Nephrology* **7**, 287–291.

Wagner, K., Philipp, T. H., Heinemeyer, G., Brockmuller, F., Roots, I. & Neumayer, H. H. (1989). Interaction of cyclosporine and calcium antagonists. *Transplantation Proceedings* **21**, 1453–1456.

Wang, P., Meucci, V., Simpson, E., Morrison, M., Lunette, S., Zajac, M. & Boeckx, R. (1990). A monoclonal antibody fluorescent polarization immunoassay for cyclosporine. *Transplantation Proceedings* **22**, 1203–1207.

Wassef, R., Cohen, Z. & Langer, B. (1985). Pharmacokinetic profiles of cyclosporine in rats. *Transplantation* **43**, 489–493.

Watkins, P. B., Wrighton, S. A., Scheutz, E. G., Molowa, D. T. & Guzelian, P. S. (1987). Identification of glucocorticoid-inducible cytochrome P-450 in the intestinal mucosa of rats and man. *Journal of Clinical Investigation* **80**, 1029–1036.

Wenger, R. M. (1990). Structures of cyclosporine and its metabolites. *Transplantation Proceedings* **22**, 1104–1109.

Wong, P. Y., Mee, A. V., Glenn, J. & Keown, P. A. (1990). Quality assessment of cyclosporine monitoring — Canadian validations. *Transplantation Proceedings* **22**, 1216–1217.

Wonigeit, K., Kohlhaw, K., Winkler, M., Schaefer, O. & Pinchmayr, R. (1990). Cyclosporine monitoring in liver allograft recipients: two distinct patterns of blood level derangement associated with nephrotoxicity. *Transplantation Proceedings* **22**, 1305–1311.

Yale, J. F., Ahmed, S. & Maharajh, G. (1991). Effects of SMS 201-995 on the pharmacokinetic profile and cellular immunity and toxic effects of cyclosporine in male Wister rats. *Transplantation* **52**, 336–340.

Yee, G. C. (1990). Pharmacokinetic interactions between cyclosporine and other drugs. *Transplantation Proceedings* **22**, 1203–1207.

Yee, G. C. & McGuire, T. R. (1990a). Pharmacokinetic drug interactions with cyclosporin (Part I). *Clinical Pharmacokinetics* **19**, 319–332.

Yee, G. C. & McGuire, T. R. (1990b). Pharmacokinetic interaction with cyclosporin (Part II). *Clinical Pharmacokinetics* **19**, 400–405.

Yee, G. C., McGuire, T. R., Gmur, D. J. Lennon, T. P. & Deeg, H. G. (1988). Blood cyclosporine pharmacokinetics in patients undergoing marrow transplantation: influence of age, obesity, and hematocrit. *Transplantation* **46**, 399–402.

Zara, G. P., Thompson, H. H., Pilot, M. A. & Ritchie, H. D. (1985). Effects of erythromycin on gastrointestinal motility. *Journal of Antimicrobial Chemotherapy* **16**, 175–179.

Chapter 4
The use of cyclosporin in organ transplantation

Anders Lindholm and Barry D. Kahan

Introduction

In 1973, cyclosporin A (CsA) was purified from fungal extracts of soil samples obtained at Hardanger Vidda in southern Norway. Five years later CsA was administered to a renal transplant recipient as an alternative to azathioprine for maintenance immunosuppressive therapy (Calne *et al.*, 1978). Even though it may be just one of several simultaneously administered drugs, CsA remains the cornerstone immunosuppressant in organ transplantation. The superior potency of CsA was documented in early multicentre studies in which CsA was administered as the sole drug, resulting in higher graft survival rates than in patients receiving azathioprine and prednisolone therapy (European Multicentre Trial Group, 1983; Shiel *et al.*, 1983). However, upon the suggestion of Starzl, CsA was combined with corticosteroids (Fig. 4.1) a dual combination that shows greater potency than treatment with azathioprine and corticosteroids (Starzl *et al.*, 1980), or azathioprine, steroids and antilymphocyte globulin (Najarian *et al.*, 1985).

In 1985 azathioprine was added to the immunosuppressive regimen in some centres (triple drug therapy; Fries *et al.*, 1985) in order to enable reduction in the CsA dose, thus minimize nephrotoxicity, and to possibly potentiate the immunosuppressive effects, especially in patients with

77

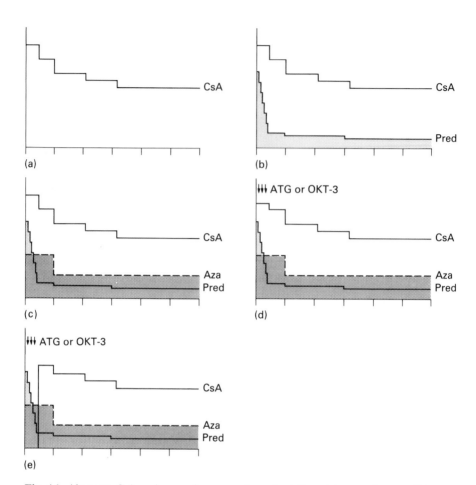

Fig. 4.1. Alternate CsA regimens after organ transplantation: (a) monotherapy; (b) double therapy; (c) triple therapy; (d) quadruple therapy; (e) sequential therapy.

severe rejection. However, in spite of the frequent use of triple drug immunosuppression in organ transplantation the prospective trials comparing double and triple drug therapy have failed to show a superiority for either treatment (Koote *et al.*, 1988; Ponticelli *et al.*, 1988b; Brinker *et al.*, 1990; Lindholm *et al.*, 1991), probably because CsA and azathioprine act only additively.

A fourth strategy to potentiate the immunosuppressive effect uses daily intravenous (i.v.) doses of antithymocyte globulin or monoclonal T-cell antibodies during the first post-transplantation week (quadruple immunosuppression; Fig. 4.1) or as a substitute for CsA as sequential therapy, thereby increasing immunosuppression in patients who are at high immunological risk or as a measure to avoid early CsA exposure and additive toxicity to the ischaemic injury following organ preservation (Bieber *et al.*, 1976; Cosimi *et al.*, 1981).

Several problems remain in the use of CsA in spite of impressive scientific research and clinical efforts. The drug has many side-effects. Most distressing is nephrotoxicity, which poses a particular problem in renal transplantation, where it is difficult to distinguish between graft rejection and CsA nephrotoxicity. Nephrotoxicity and hepatotoxicity may be life-threatening events in liver and heart transplantation. In all forms of solid organ transplantation, the dosing of CsA is a delicate balance between the pitfalls of rejection and toxicity. Knowledge of CsA pharmacokinetics and dosing guided by therapeutic drug monitoring may provide physicians with weapons for optimal patient treatment.

Pharmacokinetic features of CsA important in the clinical management of the transplanted patient

The clinical pharmacological properties of CsA have been described in detail in the previous chapter. This chapter will describe specific problems pertaining to the use of CsA after organ transplantation as outlined in Fig. 4.2.

Absorption

In transplant recipients the absorption of CsA after oral administration is slow, incomplete and highly variable. Peak blood or plasma levels are

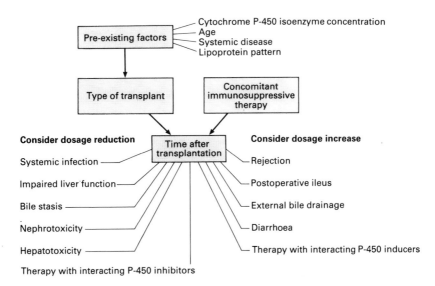

Fig. 4.2. Some points of consideration when selecting the dose of CsA.

usually reached between 1 and 8 h after oral administration, but may occur even later. A marked interindividual variation in the bioavailability has been observed with a range of 2–89% and a mean of 30% reported in recipients of various transplants (Kahan et al., 1983; Bertault-Pérès et al., 1985; Ptachcinski et al., 1985a; Burckart et al., 1986a; Frey et al., 1988).

In early post-transplantation there is impaired absorption of CsA (Kahan et al., 1983; Tufveson et al., 1986) related to post-operative ileus, which may continue for the first post-transplantation week(s). In renal allograft recipients the bioavailability increased from 24.2% at transplantation ($n = 170$) to 51.4% 2–4 weeks after transplantation ($n = 63$; Kahan et al., 1986a). Insufficient CsA levels may be prevented by giving pre-operative loading doses (routinely performed in living related kidney transplantation), by i.v. administration of CsA during the first post-transplantation days and/or by giving adjunctive immunosuppressants such as high corticosteroid doses and/or monoclonal T-cell antibodies.

CsA and its oil vehicle are absorbed as micelles formed with bile. The importance of bile flow for CsA absorption has been documented in liver transplant patients upon external drainage of bile. Thus absorption of CsA can be increased up to fivefold by clamping the T-tube (Venkataramanan et al., 1985b; Ptachcinski et al., 1986b; Andrews et al., 1987; Mehta et al., 1988). Furthermore, in liver transplant recipients hepatic function may be poor immediately after transplantation, and bile production and flow may be reduced to one-third of normal production (Venkataramanan et al., 1985c; Burckart et al., 1986b; Busuttil et al., 1986). However, impaired hepatic function may reduce CsA clearance and thus counteract the effect of reduced absorption (see below). A peroral test dose during continuous intravenous therapy may determine if the absorption is sufficient (Kahan Grevel, 1988). Such a test can assure sufficient drug absorption to avert early, frequently irreversible, rejection episodes.

The absorption of CsA is impaired in patients with diarrhoea (Burckart et al., 1985; Andrews et al., 1987). Atkinson et al. (1983) found the area through a dosing interval (AUC) of CsA in bone marrow transplant recipients with diarrhoea ($> 500 \, \text{ml}/72 \, \text{h}$) to be 38% of that in patients without diarrhoea. Bouts of gastroenteritis can trigger late acute rejection episodes resulting in graft loss.

Although several studies on the role of food on CsA absorption suggest different conclusion, it seems likely that a small breakfast has no influence on CsA absorption, while a high fat content meal may increase the absorption (Ptachcinski et al., 1985b; Keogh et al., 1988; Penouil et al., 1988; Gupta et al., 1990; Lindholm et al., 1990b). Other studies have shown that there is no influence on the absorption by the diluent (water, juice or chocolate milk; Ota, 1983; Johnston et al., 1986) or dosage form (mixture or capsules; Grevel et al., 1985; Bleck et al., 1990). Ingestion of alcohol may impair CsA absorption (Ota, 1983).

Distribution

Since CsA is highly lipophilic, it is highly distributed throughout the body. In renal transplant recipients the mean volume of distribution was 2.9 to 4.7 litre/kg (Ptachcinski *et al.*, 1985a; Morse *et al.*, 1988) and in bone marrow transplant recipients 4.4 (adults) to 8.1 (children; Yee *et al.*, 1988a).

Pharmacological theory predicts that the unbound fraction in plasma is the portion responsible for the therapeutic effect. CsA is highly lipophilic and the free fraction of CsA (f_u) in plasma is only 1–2% (Lemaire & Tillement, 1982; Lindholm & Henricsson, 1989). The free fraction of CsA co-varies with serum albumin, bilirubin, high density lipoprotein (HDL)-cholesterol and apolipoprotein A1. In transplant recipients, the free fraction was highest immediately after transplantation, in connection with episodes of infection and higher in diabetics than in non-diabetics. The free fraction decreased significantly at the time of an acute rejection episode, as compared to 1 week before. However, monitoring of free drug in plasma did not improve the correlation with clinical events as compared to total concentrations (Lindholm, 1991).

Since CsA binds to lipoproteins, mainly HDL, changes in these moieties may alter the kinetics of CsA. Thus, in patients with lipoprotein disorders, for example in patients with type V hyperlipoproteinaemia the CsA levels should be maintained at a higher level (Nemunaitis *et al.*, 1986). After renal transplantation, hypercholesterolaemia develops, with or without hypertriglyceridaemia (Chan *et al.*, 1981; Hodel *et al.*, 1986). The fact that low density lipoprotein (LDL)-cholesterol is high and HDL-cholesterol is low indicates an increased risk of atherosclerosis (Hodel *et al.*, 1986). In fact, cardiovascular disease is the major cause of death after the first post-transplantation year in transplanted patients aged over 55 years (Lindholm *et al.*, 1991).

CsA *per se* may give increased levels of serum cholesterol LDL-cholesterol and apolipoprotein B as demonstrated in a non-transplant population (Ballantyne *et al.*, 1989). In renal transplant patients Vathsala *et al.*, (1989) found corticosteroids made the greatest primary contribution to the elevated cholesterol level with CsA contributing more significantly to the increased triglycerides. However, assessment of lipid profiles in renal transplant recipients is complicated by the impaired renal function as well as concomitant medication.

Metabolism

CsA is extensively metabolized in the liver by isoenzymes of the cytochrome P-450IIIA subfamily (Kronbach *et al.*, 1988; Aoyama *et al.*, 1989; Combalbert *et al.*, 1989) and is mainly excreted as metabolites via the bile

(Beveridge *et al.*, 1981; Maurer, 1985). CsA is a low-to-intermediate clearance drug (Ptachcinski *et al.*, 1986b). In renal transplant patients, the clearance is reported to range almost 40-fold, from 0.63 ml/min/kg to 23.9 ml/min/kg in adult patients (Ptachcinski *et al.*, 1985a) with a mean of 5.7 ml/min/kg and a mean half-life of 10.7 h. In adult bone marrow transplant recipients the mean clearance is 10.3 ml/min/kg (Yee *et al.*, 1988a).

The large interindividual variability in the capacity to metabolize CsA depends to a large extent on the inherited variability in the concentration of the responsible cytochrome P-450 isoenzymes. For example, Kronbach *et al.* (1988) found a 25-fold variation in the metabolizing capacity in 15 different human livers. This inborn variability in clearance is one of the main reasons for the interindividual variability in the kinetics of CsA. One approach to individualize the dose of CsA is the performance of pre-transplant intravenous pharmacokinetic evaluations, which may accurately predict the individual CsA clearance rate and thus the dose needed post-transplantation (Kahan & Grevel, 1988).

The clearance of CsA is higher in paediatric than in adult patients and the dose required to achieve the same steady state concentration or AUC may be several times higher in paediatric than adult organ transplant recipients (Ptachcinski *et al.*, 1985a, 1986a; Burckart *et al.*, 1986a; Yee *et al.*, 1986). Thus, infants may require CsA administration three times daily in doses as high as 30 mg/kg/day (Ptachcinski *et al.*, 1985a, 1986a; Yee *et al.*, 1986).

Since CsA is metabolized in the liver, patients with impaired liver function should be expected to clear the drug more slowly. The clearance of CsA is decreased by 25–33% in transplant patients with signs of hepatic impairment (Yee *et al.*, 1984; Kahan *et al.*, 1988a). Frequent monitoring and extended dosage intervals are often necessary in these cases.

Some known cytochrome P-450 inducers may increase the clearance of CsA (Yee & McGuire, 1990) including the common convulsants phenytoin, phenobarbitol, carbamazepine and the antibiotics rifampicin and isoniazide. These interactions may produce subtherapeutic drug levels, leading to subsequent graft loss and even death. If for example, phenytoin is to be introduced, the CsA dose may have to be increased by two- to fourfold and/or dosing intervals reduced during the first 2 weeks. Close monitoring of CsA levels is mandatory. Another alternative in this case is to use valproic acid, an antiepileptic drug that does not induce CsA metabolism (Pichard *et al.*, 1990).

Several drugs inhibit CsA metabolism resulting in increased trough CsA levels (Yee & McGuire, 1990), including ketoconazole, erythromycin, josamycin, nafcillin, pristinamycin and the calcium channel blockers diltiazem, nicardipine and verapamil (but not nifedipine!). In this instance the dose of CsA may have to be reduced or the dosing interval extended, manoeuvres that are usually done when accumulation has been demonstrated by increased trough levels. First *et al.* (1989) suggest the routine use of ketoconazole as a strategy to reduce the necessary CsA dose and therefore the cost of therapy; however, the variable extent of the effect as well as possible adverse effects of accumulated metabolites require intensive monitoring of the effects of this strategy on CsA levels.

Side-effects of CsA of special importance in the transplanted patient

Nephrotoxicity

Nephrotoxicity remains the most common complication of CsA treatment. All patients treated with CsA (Myers *et al.*, 1984; Berg *et al.*, 1986) display a reduced glomerular filtration rate, as indicated by a reduction in creatinine clearance of between 20 and 30%, a level that is referred to as drug-induced renal dysfunction. The incidence of CsA nephrotoxicity, that is a greater impairment of function, occurs in 30–74% of the patients depending on the immunosuppressive protocol (Gordon *et al.*, 1985; Klintmalm *et al.*, 1985; Sutherland *et al.*, 1985).

The exact mechanism leading to nephrotoxicity is not known. Renal blood flow is reduced by a direct vasoconstrictive effect of CsA on afferent glomerular arterioles (English *et al.*, 1987; Lamb & Webb 1987; Dieperink, 1989). This vasoconstrictor effect may be due to the capacity of CsA to enhance vascular endothelial uptake of and sensitivity to calcium (Meyer-Lehnert & Schrier, 1989), to potentiate endothelin generation and/or to inhibit transcription of cytokine relaxation factors. One hypothesis proposes that this glomerular hypoperfusion is compensated by autoregulation involving glomerular prostaglandin production and renin-angiotensin activation (Baxter 1982; Coffman *et al.*, 1987). Proximal fractional reabsorption increases and tubular flow rate decreases. The tubular hypoperfusion leads to cell injury. Although the vasoconstriction may be at least partially reversible, the interstitial fibrosis resultant from chronic ischaemia is persistent (Dieperink *et al.*, 1988, 1989).

Clinically, nephrotoxicity presents as a reduced glomerular filtration rate with an elevated serum creatinine and a disproportionate increase in blood urea nitrogen in spite of preserved urine volume and increased sodium reabsorption. Hyperkalaemia, hyperuricaemia and hypertension frequently develop with the not infrequent picture of hyperkalaemic hyperchloraemic renal tubular acidosis (Kahan, 1986).

In renal transplantation, the diagnosis of acute nephrotoxicity is mainly based on the absence of signs of acute rejection along with the presence of toxic pathological changes in renal biopsies. Chronic nephrotoxicity may present with a biopsy picture of irreversible fibrosis, particularly in a striped pattern, and atrophy (Klintmalm et al., 1984). However, interstitial fibrosis is also seen in azathioprine-treated renal transplants (Wilczek et al., 1988), and, indeed, some studies showed no histological findings specific for CsA nephrotoxicity (Farnsworth et al., 1984; d'Ardenne et al., 1986). In contrast, Mihatsch et al. (1986) suggests that the mucoid deposits in endothelial cells accompanied by arteriolar smooth muscle necrosis are pathognomonic for the CsA injury.

Several drugs may potentiate nephrotoxicity independent of changes in CsA drug concentrations, including aminoglucosides, melphalan, amphotericin B, sulindac, diclofenac and non-steroidal anti-inflammatory drugs (Harris et al., 1988). The most common offenders are cotrimoxazole and trimethoprim. However, the mechanism of the trimethoprim effect is probably not reduced glomerular filtration rate, but rather inhibited renal tubular secretion of creatinine (Myre et al., 1987).

Management of nephrotoxicity

Acute or subacute nephrotoxicity usually occurs in the first 3–6 months after transplantation, presenting with a rapid increase in serum creatinine (within a few days), in renal transplantation indistinguishable from acute rejection (Kahan, 1986). In contradistinction a chronic form shows a persistent increase in serum creatinine and irreversible morphological changes (Klintmalm et al., 1984). In the acute, but not in the chronic form, the severity is related to the dose and concentration of CsA (Kahan et al., 1982; Klintmalm et al., 1985). Thus, CsA dose reduction is the first (and often the only necessary) measure to be taken in cases of acute nephrotoxicity.

Interestingly, several groups report a protective effect of calcium channel blockers on CsA nephrotoxicity, which may be related to a disruption of the vasoconstrictive effect of CsA on the autoregulatory mechanisms involving glomerular prostaglandin production and renin-angiotensin activation (Dieperink et al., 1986; Wagner et al., 1986; Sumpio et al., 1987). The protective effect is observed in patients receiving calcium channel blockers from the day of transplantation, in spite of the higher CsA blood levels (due to the inhibition of CsA metabolism) compared to control patients.

In addition to these deleterious effects on functioning grafts, CsA has been associated with a higher percentage of non-functioning kidneys than azathioprine, especially when the cold ischaemia time is longer than 24 h (Lundgren et al., 1986), possibly due to an additive effect of ischaemia and toxicity (Devineni et al., 1983). However, because primary non-function occurs more commonly in sensitized patients, early rejection is probably a more common cause for primary non-function (Karuppan et al., 1991).

With the lower doses of CsA presently used in immunosuppressive therapy nephrotoxicity has become a less important problem (Kasiske *et al.*, 1988; Lindholm *et al.*, 1990c). Most of the studies addressing the question of whether chronic nephrotoxicity is progressive have found impaired but stable renal function in CsA-treated recipients of renal transplants followed for more than 5 years after transplantation (Lewis *et al.*, 1988; Ponticelli *et al.*, 1988a; Linder *et al.*, 1991).

Other acute side-effects

Potentially life-threatening side-effects that may occur early after transplantation include hepatotoxicity, neurological symptoms and infections. All three are more common after liver and bone marrow transplantation than after renal transplantation. These three side-effects often coincide; examples of this are simultaneous cytomegaloviral hepatitis and CsA hepatotoxicity or disseminated fungal infection with hepatic involvement necessitating the simultaneous use of hepatotoxic antifungal drugs and CsA.

Dose-related hepatic impairment, including hyperbilirubinaemia and an increase in alkaline phosphatase and transaminases, occurs mainly during the first month after transplantation (Lorber *et al.*, 1987). The mechanism of CsA-induced cholestasis remains unknown. In present day renal transplant practice, hepatotoxicity is infrequent due to the lower CsA doses used. However, in hepatic transplantation CsA-induced hepatotoxicity may compound the liver impairment necessitating temporary discontinuation of CsA with substitution of monoclonal antibodies and/or high steroid doses.

The neurological toxicity of CsA may present in mild, moderate or severe forms with paresthesias, tremor, irritability, seizures, confusion, hallucinations, amnesia and cortical blindness (Wilczek *et al.*, 1984; Rubin, 1989). Neurological toxicity is more common after hepatic transplantation (Tollemar *et al.*, 1988), possibly related to changes in lipoprotein concentrations with low serum cholesterol levels (de Groen *et al.*, 1987) and/or toxicity from the polyoxyethylated castor oil (Cremophor EL) in i.v. administered CsA (Hoefnagels *et al.*, 1988). CsA-induced hypomagnesaemia may lower the seizure threshold (Thompson *et al.*, 1984). Thus, careful monitoring of magnesium levels with prompt replacement in cases of hypomagnesaemia is recommended.

In contrast with the experience in autoimmune disease, opportunistic infection is the primary cause of death during the first year after organ transplantation (Frödin *et al.*, 1987). The overall incidence of infections is equal between CsA and corticosteroid compared with azathioprine and corticosteroid treatment (Kahan *et al.*, 1985; Canafax *et al.*, 1986). Trimethoprim-cotrimoxazole prophylaxis renders *Pneumocystis carinii* infection no longer a problem (Fox *et al.*, 1990). Mortality and morbidity from cytomegaloviral infection has been reduced with the use of gancyclovir or immune-globulin preparations (Mai *et al.*, 1989; Davis, 1990; Freeman *et al.*, 1990).

Chronic and late side-effects

Hypertension requiring antihypertensive drug treatment is more frequent than nephrotoxicity, probably due to increased vascular resistance and local activation of the renin–angiotensin system (Schachter, 1988). Hypertension in transplant recipients is often treated with calcium channel blockers in spite of a pharmacokinetic drug interaction that may occur, in order to reduce calcium influx into anoxic or damaged endothelial cells.

In a clinical study 70% of the patients had gingival hyperplasia and of these 17% had a severe form (Daley *et al.*, 1986). It is of note that nifedipine produces an additive effect on this side-effect (Slavin & Taylor, 1987) as does phenytoin. The mechanism regulating gingival hyperplasia is not known. The treatment consists of regular dental care and in severe cases gingivectomy.

CsA does not appear to be mutagenic in animal toxicological studies *in vitro* and *in vivo* (Matter *et al.*, 1982; Ryffel *et al.*, 1983), but has mutagenic potential for human lymphocytes (Yuzawa *et al.*, 1986). The incidence of malignancies usually increases following organ transplantation, but the overall incidence is not altered by CsA and prednisolone treatment as compared to azathioprine and prednisolone treatment (Cockburn, 1987). On the one hand, skin cancers comprised 40% of the tumours in patients treated with azathioprine as compared to 16% in patients treated with CsA (Penn, 1987). On the other hand, non-Hodgkin's lymphoma may occur during CsA treatment, an effect thought to be induced by Epstein-Barr viral infection (Crawford *et al.*, 1980). The incidence of lymphoma increases with CsA therapy and was estimated to be 0.7% in 5500 CsA-treated organ transplant recipients (Beveridge *et al.*, 1984). Kaposi's sarcoma is also over-represented in patients treated with CsA. After organ transplantation, the patients must be made aware of the potential danger of excessive sunbathing. Furthermore, regular dermatological examinations may be added to the ordinary post-transplantation surveillance. Fortunately, CsA does not seem to alter the malformation rate of CsA and many transplanted mothers have given birth to healthy children (Cockburn *et al.*, 1989). However, as a safety precaution, it is usually recommended that pregnancy should be avoided during the first post-transplantation year.

CsA has several other side-effects, of which hypertrichosis, gynaecomastia and hyperglycaemia should be mentioned (Gunnarsson *et al.*, 1984; Lindholm *et al.*, 1988; Kahan, 1989). CsA induces platelet aggregation and release of thromboxane A_2 (Coffman et al., 1987, Grace et al., 1987). Some studies suggest that CsA increases the incidence of thromboembolic complications (Vanrenterghem et al., 1985a), whereas others find no support for this suggestion (Brunkwall et al., 1987).

Therapeutic drug monitoring of CsA

Therapeutic monitoring of CsA is often considered mandatory in organ transplantation ever since the first reports of an association between CsA concentrations in blood and clinical events of renal graft rejection and nephrotoxicity (Keown et al., 1981; Kahan et al., 1982).

Analysis of CsA by a specific method in whole blood has been recommended as the routine measurement method (Shaw et al., 1987). The main reasons for this are firstly that the levels in plasma may be under the limit of detection in spite of therapeutic immunosuppression (Klintmalm et al., 1985; Lindholm et al., 1990c). Secondly, plasma separation is technically difficult since the equilibrium of CsA between plasma and blood cells is highly temperature dependent (Niederberger et al., 1983; Humbert et al., 1990). Thirdly, it has been demonstrated that the immunosuppressive effect of CsA is mainly exerted by the parent compound and most known metabolites are inactive. The most potent metabolite, AM1, is estimated to possess only 5–10% of the immunosuppressive activity of CsA (Copeland et al., 1990; Rosano et al., 1990).

The clinician must not rely on the result of CsA analysis, and should never trust a single determination. Mistakes in sample collection may give completely false results, such as collection from an indwelling line through which CsA has been administered, a state of contamination persists at least 2 weeks after the drug has been administered in such a line (Blifeld & Ettenger, 1987). Furthermore, topical skin contamination by CsA may give falsely high CsA levels in capillary samples (Lindholm et al., 1990a).

Since interleukin production and release in vitro are almost totally blocked at 100 ng/ml (Bunjes et al., 1981), it is tempting to accept this as the threshold CsA concentration throughout the dosing interval, thus avoiding triggering of the rejection process. However, it is not known whether the trough, mean or peak concentration or the AUC is the most important factor for optimal CsA treatment evaluation. Traditionally trough concentrations are monitored, i.e. 12 or 24 h after dosage and just before the next dose.

Studies performed with specific analysis of CsA suggest that occurrence of an acute rejection episode is more likely if the 12-hour trough concentration of CsA is below 125–200 ng/ml during the first month after renal transplantation (Moyer et al., 1988; Holt et al., 1989; Lindholm et al., 1990c). On the other hand empirical experience has shown that lower trough concentrations of CsA are compatible with stable graft function later after transplantation. For example, in a cohort of 162 Swedish renal transplant patients with functioning grafts at 5 years after transplantation the median CsA dose and whole blood concentration were 2.92 mg/kg and 75 ng/ml, respectively (5 to 95 percentiles 1.56–5.19 mg/kg and 33–162 ng/ml, respectively).

In the first reports using therapeutic monitoring of CsA an association was found not only with rejection but also between high trough concentrations of CsA and nephrotoxicity (Kahan et al., 1982; Irschik et al., 1984). However, considerable overlap is observed and acute nephrotoxicity may occur at any concentration of CsA (Kahan et al., 1984; Klintmalm et al., 1985; Holt et al., 1989).

In some centres CsA concentrations are obtained at additional time-points, such as 6 h after dosage (Cantarovich et al., 1988), or as complete 24-hour AUC studies (Kahan & Grevel, 1988). Thus, Cantarovich et al. (1988) suggest that measurements of CsA at 6 h after dosage are more useful than trough concentrations as correlates of clinical events, particularly to nephrotoxicity.

Two studies described an association between the occurrence of acute rejection and the average steady-state concentrations, but not trough levels, of CsA (Kasiske et al., 1988; Grevel et al., 1991). However, this approach has its limitations because, for practical reasons, only a limited number of AUCs may be collected.

Recently, Johnston et al. (1990) suggested that measurement of CsA at three time points during a 12-hour dosing interval may accurately predict the true AUC. This approach may prove useful in a clinical setting, especially regarding the possible relationship between the concentration of CsA/CsA metabolites and nephrotoxicity. In a report from a single centre Sewing et al. (1990) recently claimed a correlation between nephrotoxicity and the concentration of the double hydroxylated metabolites of CsA and cyclized metabolite 26 but not with CsA itself. This potential association between nephrotoxicity and specific metabolites requires further investigation.

CsA dosing strategies in organ transplantation

Renal transplantation

In renal transplantation CsA is usually introduced at a fixed mg/kg body weight dose, and successively tapered according to preset acceptable blood concentration windows. Experience has shown that high doses of immunosuppressants are required immediately after transplantation, whereas smaller maintenance doses are adequate after the first 3–6 post-transplantation months. However, since cadaveric organs with ischaemic damage may be susceptible to the additive effect of the CsA toxicity, otherwise therapeutic initial concentrations may be excessive in some individuals. Furthermore, the large interindividual variability in the kinetics of the drug favours an individual approach in the dosing strategy although Bayesian forecasting has not been successful to predict initial i.v. CsA doses post-transplantation (Kahan et al., 1986b).

As performed at the transplantation unit in Houston, a 3 mg/kg body weight i.v. and a 14 mg/kg oral dose are administered on two occasions pre-transplantation. Blood is sampled for 24 h after each dose, in order to calculate the individual patient average concentration during a dosing interval, clearance rate, terminal half-life and bioavailability. Based upon the target value the post-transplantation doses are calculated. Due to post-operative ileus, absorption may be poor during the first post-transplant week. Therefore, oral test doses are administered to determine when absorption is sufficient so that the i.v. CsA may be discontinued (Kahan & Grevel, 1988). With this test dose method the post-transplantation i.v. dose was correctly predicted in 73% of the patients, whereas the peroral dose only correctly predicted the post-transplant absorption in 41% of the patients. Further studies and/or better drug formulations may be required to improve the prediction rate for the oral dosage of CsA.

Heart (heart–lung) transplantation

Traditionally, and as a consequence of the vital function of the transplanted organ and the absence of myocardiotoxicity of CsA, the CsA dose is higher and target blood levels are higher in cardiac than in renal transplantation. In heart transplantation intraoperative ischaemia often causes reversible renal impairment, and during the initial experience, haemodialysis was not infrequent during the first post-transplant week. Furthermore, some heart transplant recipients experienced end-stage renal disease from irreversible nephrotoxicity of CsA (Myers et al., 1984). However, with the reduced doses of CsA used today, post-transplantation uraemia and end-stage renal disease rarely occur. At present triple drug immunosuppression is the most common immunosuppressive therapy in cardiac transplantation (McCarthy et al., 1989).

Some studies have demonstrated an association between CsA blood levels and the risk of acute cardiac graft rejection. In a small paediatric series, eight of 12 episodes of rejection occurred in the presence of CsA concentrations of below half the recommended 200 ng/ml concentration. Half of these rejection episodes occurred in adolescents who stopped immunosuppressive medication (Braunlin et al., 1990). Indeed, mild cases of rejection diagnosed by endomyocardial biopsy may be treated by increasing the oral CsA dose and/or intravenous course of CsA (Radovancevic & Frazier, 1986).

Liver transplantation

In liver transplantation it may be difficult to introduce oral CsA therapy post-transplantation. As already mentioned, this is especially the case if the patient has a T-tube externally draining the bile. A second problem is that the transplanted organ metabolizes the CsA and thus the dosage required is dependent on the function of the new organ. Pre-transplantation evaluations are non-informative. Generally the doses administered are higher than those in renal transplantation and the target concentrations are set higher than for renal transplants.

Few studies have documented a relationship between CsA blood levels and the outcome of liver transplantation. In a cohort of 50 patients those with significantly lower CsA concentrations displayed signs of moderate to severe acute rejection on day 7 compared to patients with no or mild rejection, the median concentrations being 126 ng/ml and 150 ng/ml, respectively ($P < 0.01$; Gunson et al., 1990). In another study the CsA concentrations were lower 7 days prior to rejection than during the rest of follow-up (Haven et al., 1989).

Bone marrow transplantation

In bone marrow transplantation CsA is given to reduce graft-versus-host disease (GVHD). Combined with methotrexate acute GVHD may be almost totally prevented in allogeneic haploidentical transplantations (Storb et al., 1989). The price, however, is an increased risk of recurrence of the leukaemia. CsA is usually given for the first 6-12 months after transplantation and/or for therapy of chronic GVHD.

Most studies on the possible correlation between CsA concentrations and efficacy in bone marrow transplant recipients have failed to find any relationship between CsA concentrations and the occurrence of GVHD (Barrett et al., 1982; Gratwohl et al., 1983; Biggs et al., 1985; Lindholm et al., 1987). However, in the most recent study in 179 bone marrow recipients Yee et al. (1988b) found that low mean trough CsA concentrations during a given week were associated with an increased risk of the occurrence of acute GVHD during the following week, a finding that was significant only when the data for all weeks were pooled ($P = 0.03$).

Nephrotoxicity is easily recognized in bone marrow transplant recipients (Gratwohl et al., 1983; Lindholm et al., 1987) and may be observed at any dosage of CsA even though it is more common in the measure of high blood concentrations (Kennedy et al., 1985).

Conclusion

There is no doubt that clinical transplantation has made great progress as a direct effect of the discovery and clinical introduction of CsA. However, now that 10 years have passed since these events we still do not know how to use the drug with maximum efficiency and a minimum of side-effects.

This chapter has emphasized some of the problems that may be encountered when CsA is used after organ transplantation. Unfortunately there are no absolute rules to guide drug administration. Each situation and patient is unique and individualized dosages of CsA are required. Thus, several dosage schedules and combinations of immunosuppressants been used concurrently and may be of equal efficacy. Future improvements in the CsA dosing strategy will probably rely on further individualization based on the pharmacokinetics and pharmacodynamics of CsA.

An alternative approach seeks to develop synergistic immunosuppressive drug combinations. Whereas azathioprine only exerts an additive effect with CsA, and FK 506 has an antagonistic effect, rapamycin shows synergistic immunosuppressive properties with CsA (Kahan et al., 1991). While CsA and FK 506 prevent T-cell progression from the G_0 to the G_1 phase of the cell cycle, rapamycin acts at the late G_1 stage, blocking T cells from entering the S phase of the cell cycle (Dumont et al., 1990; Metcalf & Richards, 1990). Such a drug combination of CsA with rapamycin would enable dose reduction of CsA with intact immunosuppressive potency but less toxicity.

Acknowledgements

This work was supported by NIDDK (DK38016), the Swedish Medical Research Council (B92-17R-9812) and the Swedish Society of Medicine (91-554).

References

Andrews, W., Iwatsuki, S., Shaw, B. W. & Starzl, T. E. (1985). Letter. *Transplantation* **39**, 338.

Andrews, W., Fyock, B., Gray, S., Coln, D., Hendricse, W., Siegel, I., Belknap, B., Hogge, A., Benser, M. & Lennard, B. (1987). Pediatric liver transplantation: The Dallas experience. *Transplantation Proceedings* **19**, 3267–3276.

Aoyama, T., Yamano, S., Waxman, D. J., Lapenson, D. P., Meyer, U. A., Fischer, V., Tyndale, R., Inaba, T., Kalow, W., Gelboin, H. V. & Gonzales, F. J. (1989). Cytochrome P-450 hPCN3, a novel cytochrome P-450 IIIA gene product that is differentially expressed in adult human liver. *Journal of Biology and Chemistry* **264**, 10388–10395.

Atkinson, K., Britton, K., Paull, P., Farrell, C., Concannon, A., Dodds, A. & Biggs, J. (1983). Detrimental effect of intestinal disease on absorption of orally administered cyclosporine. *Transplantation Proceedings* **15** (supp 1), 2446–2449.

Ballantyne, C. M., Podet, E. J., Patsch, W. P., Harati, Y., Appel, V., Gotto, A. M. Jr. & Young, J. B. (1989). Effects of cyclosporine therapy on plasma lipoprotein levels. *Journal of the American Medical Association* **262**, 53–56.

Barrett, A. J., Kendra, J. R., Lucas, C. F., Joss, D. V., Joshi, R., Pendharkar, P. & Hugh-Jones, K. (1982). Cyclosporin A as prophylaxis against graft-versus-host disease in 36 patients. *British Medical Journal* **285**, 162–166.

Baxter, C. R., Duggin, G. G., Willis, N. S., Hall, B. M., Horvath, J. S. & Tiller, D. J. (1982). Cyclosporin A-induced increases in renin storage and release. *Research Communications in Chemistry, Pathology and Pharmacology* **37**, 305–312.

Berg, K. J., Förre, Ö., Bjerkhoel, F., Amundsen, E., Djöseland, O., Rugstad, H. E. & Westre, B. (1986). Side effects of cyclosporin A treatment in patients with rheumatoid arthritis. *Kidney International* **29**, 1180–1187.

Bertault-Pérès, P., Maraninchi, D., Carcassonne, Y., Cano, J. P. & Barbet, J. (1985). Clinical pharmacokinetics of ciclosporin A in bone marrow transplantation patients. *Cancer Chemotherapy and Pharmacology* **15**, 76–81.

Beveridge, T., Gratwohl, A., Michot, F., Niederberger, W., Nüesch, E., Nussbaumer, K., Schaub, P. & Speck, B. (1981). Cyclosporin A: pharmacokinetics after a single dose in man and serum levels after multiple dosing in recipients of allogeneic bone-marrow grafts. *Current Therapeutic Research* **30**, 5–18.

Beveridge, T., Krupp, P. & McKibbin, C. (1984). Lymphomas and lymphoproliferative lesions developing under cyclosporin therapy. *Lancet* **i**, 788.

Bieber, C. P., Griepp, R. B., Oyer, P. E., Wong, J. & Stinson, E. B. (1976). Use of rabbit antithymocyte globulin in cardiac transplantation: relationship of serum clearance rates to clinical outcome. *Transplantation* **22**, 478–488.

Biggs, J. C., Atkinson, K., Britton, K. & Downs, K. (1985). The use of cyclosporine in human marrow transplantation: absence of a therapeutic window. *Transplantation Proceedings* **17**, 1239–1241.

Bleck, J. S., Nashan, B., Christians, U., Schottmann, R., Wonigeit, K. & Sewing, K. F. (1990). Single dose pharmacokinetics of cyclosporin and its main metabolites after oral cyclosporin as oily solution or capsule. *Drug Research* **40**, 62–64.

Blifield, C. & Ettenger, R. B. (1987). Measurement of cyclosporine levels in samples obtained from peripheral sites and indwelling lines. *New England Journal of Medicine* **317**, 509.

Braunlin, E. A., Canter, Olivari, M. T., Ring, W. S., Spray, T. L. & Bolman, R. M. (1990). Rejection and infection after pediatric cardiac transplantation. *Annals of Thoracic Surgery* **49**, 385–390.

Brinker, K. R., Dickerman, R. M., Gonwa, T. A., Hull, A. R., Langley, J. W., Long, D. L., Nesser, D. A., Trevino, G. & Velez, R. L. (1990). A randomized trial comparing double-drug and triple-drug therapy in primary cadaveric renal transplantation. *Transplantation* **50**, 43–49.

Brunkwall, J., Bergqvist, D., Bergentz, S. E., Bornmyr, S. & Husberg, B. (1987). Postoperative deep venous thrombosis after renal transplantation. *Transplantation* **43**, 647–649.

Bunjes, D., Hardt, C., Röllinghoff, M. & Wagner, H. (1981). Cyclosporin A mediates immunosuppression of primary cytotoxic T cell responses by impairing the release of interleukin 1 and interleukin 2. *European Journal of Immunology* **11**, 657–661.

Burckart, G., Starzl. T. E., Williams, L., Sangvi, A., Gartner, C., Venkataramanan, R., Zitelli, B., Malatack, I., Urbach, A., Diven, W., Ptachcinski, R., Shaw, B. & Iwatsuki, S. (1985). Cyclosporine monitoring and pharmacokinetics in pediatric liver transplant patients. *Transplantation Proceedings* **17**, 1172–1175.

Burckart, G. J., Venkataramanan, R., Ptachcinski, R. J., Starzl, T. E., Gartner, J. C. Jr, Zitelli, B. J., Malatack, J. J., Shaw, B. W., Iwatsuki, S & van Thiel, D. H. (1986a). Cyclosporine absorption following orthotopic liver transplantation. *Journal of Clinical Pharmacology* **26**, 647–651.

Burckart, G. J., Venkataramanan, R., Ptachcinski, R. J., Starzl, T. E., Griffith, B. P., Hakala, T. R., Rosenthal, J. T., Hardesty, R. L., Iwatsuki, S & Brady, J. (1986b).

Cyclosporine pharmacokinetic profiles in liver, heart and kidney transplant patients as determined by high-performance liquid chromatography. *Transplantation Proceedings* **18** (suppl 5), 129–136.

Busuttil, R. W., Goldstein, L. I., Danovitch, M., Ament, M. E. & Memsic, L. D. F. (1986). Liver transplantation today. *Annals of Internal Medicine* **104**, 377–389.

Calne, R. Y., White, D. J. G., Thiru, S., Evans, D. B., McMaster, P., Dunn, D. C., Craddock, G. N., Pentlow, B. D. & Rolles, K. (1978). Cyclosporin A in patients receiving renal allografts from cadaver donors. *Lancet* **ii**, 1323–1327.

Canafax, D. M., Simmons, R. L., Sutherland, D. E. R., Fryd, D. S., Strand, M. H., Ascher, N. L., Payne, W. D. & Najarian, J. S. (1986). Early and late effects of two inmmunosuppressive drug protocols on recipients of renal allografts: results of the Minnesota randomized trial comparing cyclosporine versus antilymphocyte globulin azathioprine. *Transplantation Proceedings* **18** (suppl 2), 192–196.

Cantarovich, F., Bizollon, Ch., Cantarovich, D., Lefrancois, N., Dubenard, J. M. & Traeger, J. (1988). Cyclosporine plasma levels six hours after oral administration: a useful tool for monitoring therapy. *Transplantation* **45**, 389–394.

Chan, M. K., Varghese, Z. & Moorhead, J. F. (1981). Lipid abnormalities in uremia, dialysis, and transplantation. *Kidney International* **19**, 625–637.

Cockburn, I. (1987). Assessment of the risks of malignancy and lymphomas developing using Sandimmun. *Transplantation Proceedings* **19**, 1804–1807.

Cockburn, I., Krupp, P. & Monka, C. (1989). Present experience of Sandimmun in pregnancy. *Transplantation Proceedings* **21**, 3730–3732.

Coffman, T. M., Carr, D. R., Yarger, W. E. & Klotman, P. E. (1987). Evidence that renal prostaglandin and thromboxane production is stimulated in chronic cyclosporine nephropathy. *Transplantation* **43**, 282–285.

Combalbert, J., Fabre, I., Dalet, I., Derancourt, J., Cano, J. P. & Maurel, P. (1989). Metabolism of cyclosporin A. IV. Purification and identification of the rifampicin-inducible human liver cytochrome P-450 (cyclosporin A oxidase) as a product of P450IIIA gene subfamily. *Drug Metabolism and Disposition* **17**, 197–220.

Copeland, K. R., Yatscoff, R. & McKenna, R. (1990). Immunosuppressive activity of cyclosporine metabolites compared and characterized by mass spectroscopy and nuclear magnetic resonance. *Clinical Chemistry* **36**, 225–229.

Cosimi, A. B., Colvin, R. B., Burton, R. C., Rubin, R. H., Goldstein, G., Kung, P., Hansen, W. P., Delmonico, F. L. & Russell, P. S. (1981). Use of monoclonal antibodies to T-cell subsets for immunologic monitoring and treatment in recipients of renal allografts. *New England Journal of Medicine* **305**, 308–314.

Crawford, D. H., Thomas, J. A., Janossy, G., Sweny, P., Fernando, O. N., Moorhead, J. F. & Thompson, J. H. (1980). Epstein Barr virus nuclear antigen positive lymphoma after cyclosporin A treatment in patient with renal allograft. *Lancet* **i**, 1355–1356.

d'Ardenne, A. J., Dunhill, M. S., Thompson, J. F., McWhinnie, D., Wood, R. F. M. & Morris, P. J. (1986). Cyclosporin and renal graft histology. *Journal of Clinical Pathology* **39**, 145–151.

Daley, T. D., Wysocki, G. P. & Day, C. (1986). Clinical and pharmacologic correlations in cyclosporine-induced gingival hyperplasia. *Oral Surgery, Oral Medicine, and Oral Pathology* **62**, 417–421.

Davis, C. L. (1990). The prevention of cytomegalovirus disease in renal transplantation. *American Journal of Kidney Disease* **16**, 175–188.

Devineni, R., McKenzie, N., Duplan, J., Keown, P., Stiller, C. & Wallace, A. C. (1982). Renal effects of cyclosporine: clinical and experimental observations. *Transplantation Proceedings* **15**, 2695–2698.

Dieperink, H. (1989). Cyclosporine A nephrotoxicity. *Danish Medical Bulletin* **36**, 235–248.

Dieperink, H., Leyssac, P., Starklint, H., Jörgensen, K. A. & Kemp, E. (1986).

Antagonist capacities of nifedipine, captopril, phenoxybenzamine, prostacyclin and indomethacin on cyclosporin A induced impairment of rat renal function. *European Journal of Clinical Investigation* **16**, 540–548.

Dieperink, H., Leyssac, P., Starklint, H. & Kemp, E. (1988). Long-term cyclosporin A nephrotoxicity in the rat. Effects on renal function and morphology. *Nephrology, Dialysis and Transplantation* **3**, 317–326.

Dumont, F. J., Staruch, M., Koprak, S. L., Melino, M. R. & Sigal, N. H. (1990). Distinct mechanisms of suppression of murine T cell activation by the related macrolides FK506 and rapamycin. *Journal of Immunology* **144**, 251–258.

English, J., Evan, A., Houghton, D. C. & Bennett, W. M. (1987). Cyclosporine-induced acute renal dysfunction in the rat. *Transplantation* **44**, 135–141.

European Multicenter Trial Group (1983). Cyclosporin in cadaver renal transplantation: one-year follow-up of a multicentre trial. *Lancet* **ii**, 986–989.

Farnsworth, A., Hall, B. M., Ng, A. B. P., Duggin, G. G., Horvath, J. S., Shell, A. G. R. & Tiller, D. J. (1984). Renal biopsy morphology in renal transplantation. *American Journal of Surgery and Pathology* **8**, 243–252.

First, M. R., Schroeder, T. J., Weiskittel, P., Myre, S. A. Alexander, J. W. & Pesce, A. J. (1989). Concomitant administration of cyclosporin and ketoconazole in renal transplant recipients. *Lancet* **ii**, 1198–1201.

Fox, B. C., Sollinger, H. W., Belzer, F. O. & Maki, D. G. (1990). A prospective, randomized, double-blind study of trimethoprim-sulfamethoxazole for prophylaxis of infection in renal transplantation. Clinical efficacy, absorption of trimethoprim-sulfamethoxazole, effects on the microflora, and the cost-benefit of prophylaxis. *American Journal of Medicine* **89**, 255–274.

Freeman, R., Gould, F. K. & McMaster, A. (1990). Management of cytomegalovirus antibody negative patients undergoing heart transplantation. *Journal of Clinical Pathology* **43**, 373–376.

Frey, F. J., Horber, F. F. & Frey, B. M. (1988). Trough levels and concentration time curves of cyclosporine in patients undergoing renal transplantation. *Clinical Pharmacology and Therapeutics* **43**, 55–62.

Fries, D., Kechrid, C., Charpentier, B., Hammouche, M. & Moulin, B. (1985). A prospective study of a triple association: Cyclosporine, corticosteroids, and azathioprine in immunologically high-risk renal transplantation. *Transplantation Proceedings* **17**, 1231–1234.

Frödin, L., Backman, U., Brekkan, E., Claesson, K., Flatmark, A., Gäbel, H., Larsson, A., Lundgren, G., Persson, H., Sjöberg, O., Tufveson, G. & Wahlberg, J. A. (1987). Causes of graft loss and mortality in cyclosporine-treated cadaveric kidney graft recipients. *Transplantation Proceedings* **19**, 1831–1832.

Gordon, R. D., Iwatsuki, S., Shaw, B. W. & Starzl, T. E. (1985). Cyclosporine-steroid combination therapy in 84 cadaveric renal transplants. *American Journal of Kidney Disease* **5**, 307–312.

Grace, A. A., Barradas, M. A., Mikhailidis, D. P., Jeremy, J. Y., Moorhead, J. F., Sweny, P. & Dandona, P. (1987). Cyclosporine A enhances platelet aggregation. *Kidney International* **32**, 889–895.

Gratwohl, A., Speck, B., Wenk, M., Forster, I., Müller, M., Osterwalder, B., Nissen, C. & Follath, F. (1983). Cyclosporine in human bone marrow transplantation: serum concentration, graft-versus-host disease, and nephrotoxicity. *Transplantation* **36**, 40–44.

Grevel, J., Kutz, K., Abisch, E. & Nüesch, E. (1985). A study on the relative bioavailability of Sandimmun in normal volunteers (soft gelatine capsules versus an oral solution). *Sandoz internal document.*

Grevel, J., Napoli, K. L., Welsh, M. S., Atkinson, N. E. & Kahan, B. D. (1991).

Prediction of acute graft rejection in renal transplantation: the utility of cyclosporine blood concentrations. *Pharmaceutical Research* **8**, 278–281.

Groen, P. C., de, Aksamit, A. J., Rakela, J., Forbes, G. S. & Krom, R. A. F. (1987). Central nervous system toxicity after liver transplantation: the role of cyclosporine and cholesterol. *New England Journal of Medicine* **317**, 861–866.

Gunnarsson, R., Klintmalm, G., Lundgren, G., Tydén, G., Wilczek, H., Östman, J. & Groth, C. G. (1984). Deterioration in glucose metabolism in pancreatic transplant recipients after conversion from azathioprine to cyclosporine. *Transplantation Proceedings* **16**, 709–712.

Gunson, B., K., Jones, S. R., Buckles, J. A. C., Jain, A. B. & McMaster, P. (1990). Liver transplantation in Birmingham — use of cyclosporine — clinical correlations with drug measurements. *Transplantation Proceedings* **22**, 1312–1318.

Gupta, S. K., Manfro, R. C., Tomlanovich, S. J., Gambertoglio, J. G., Garovoy, M. R. & Benet, L. Z. (1990). Effect of food on the pharmacokinetics of cyclosporine in healthy subjects following oral and intravenous administration. *Journal of Clinical Pharmacology* **30**, 643–653.

Harris, K. P. G., Jenkins, D. & Walls, J. (1988). Nonsteroidal anti-inflammatory drugs and cyclosporine: a potentially serious adverse interaction. *Transplantation* **46**, 598–599.

Haven, M. C., Sobeski, L. M., Earl, R. A. & Markin, R. S. (1989). Comparison of cyclosporine immunoassay methods: examination of rejection and nephrotoxic episodes in liver transplantation (abstract). *Clinical Chemistry* **35**, 1183.

Hodel, K., Mordasini, R. C., Brunnre, F. P. & Thiel, G. (1986). Cyclosporin A und Hyperlipidämie nach Nierentransplantation. *Schweiz Medicinal Wochenschrift* **116**, 885–888.

Hoefnagels, W. A. J., Gerritsen, E. J. A., Brouwer, O. F. & Souverijn, J. H. M. (1988). Cyclosporin encephalopathy associated with fat embolism induced by the drug's solvent. *Lancet* **ii**, 901.

Holt, D. W., Marsden, J. T., Johnston, A. & Taube, D. H. (1989). Cyclosporine monitoring with polyclonal and specific monoclonal antibodies during episodes of renal allograft dysfunction. *Transplantation Proceedings* **21**, 1482–1484.

Humbert, H., Vernillet, L., Cabiac, M. D., Barradas, J. & Billaud, E. (1990). Influence of different parameters for the monitoring of cyclosporine. *Transplantation Proceedings* **22**, 1210–1215.

Irschik, E., Tilg, H., Niederwieser, D., Gastl, G., Huber, Ch. & Margreiter, R. (1984). Cyclosporin blood levels do correlate with clinical complications. *Lancet* **ii**, 692–693.

Johnston, A., Marsden, J. T., Hla, K., Henry, J. A. & Holt, D. W. (1986). The effect of vehicle on the oral absorption of cyclosporine. *British Journal of Clinical Pharmacology* **21**, 331–333.

Johnston, A., Sketris, I., Marsden, J. T., Galustian, C. G., Fashola, T., Taube, D., Pepper, J. & Holt, D. W. (1990). A limited sampling strategy for the measurement of cyclosporin AUC. *Transplantation Proceedings* **22**, 1345–1346.

Kahan, B. D. (1986). Cyclosporine nephrotoxicity: pathogenesis, prophylaxis, therapy, and prognosis. *American Journal of Kidney Disease* **8**, 323–331.

Kahan, B. D. (1989). Cyclosporine. *New England Journal of Medicine* **321**, 1725–1738.

Kahan, B. D., Gibbons, S., Tejpal, N., Stepkowski, S. M. & Chou, T. C. (1991). Synergistic interactions of cyclosporine and rapamycin to inhibit immune performances of normal human peripheral blood lymphocytes *in vitro*. *Transplantation* **51**, 232–239.

Kahan, B. D. & Grevel, J. (1988). Optimization of cyclosporine therapy in renal transplantation by a pharmacokinetic strategy. *Transplantation* **46**, 631–644.

Kahan, B. D., Kramer, W. G., Wideman, C., Flechner, S. M., Lorber, M. I. & van Buren,

C. T. (1986a). Demographic factors affecting the pharmacokinetics of cyclosporine estimated by radioimmunoassay. *Transplantation* **41**, 459–464.

Kahan, B. D., Kramer, W. G., Williams, C. & Wideman, C. A. (1986b). Application of Bayesian forecasting to predict appropriate cyclosporine dosing regimens for renal allograft recipients. *Transplantation Proceedings* **18** (Suppl. 5), 200–203.

Kahan, B. D., Ried, M. & Newburger, J. (1983). Pharmacokinetics of cyclosporine in human renal transplantation. *Transplantation Proceedings* **15**, 446–453.

Kahan, B. D., van Buren, C. T., Flechner, S. M., Jarowenko, M., Yasumura, T., Rogers, A. J., Yoshimura, N., LeGrue, S., Drath, D. & Kerman, R. H. (1985). Clinical and experimental studies with cyclosporine in renal transplantation. *Surgery* **97**, 125–140.

Kahan, B. D., van Buren, C. T., Lin, S. N., Ono, Y., Agostino, G., LeGrue, S. J., Boileua, M., Payne, W. D. & Kerman, R. H. (1982). Immunopharmacologic monitoring of cyclosporin A treated recipients of cadaveric kidney allografts. *Transplantation* **34**, 36–45.

Kahan, B. D., Wideman, C. A., Reid, M., Gibbons, S., Jarowenko, M., Flechner, S. & van Buren, C. T. (1984). The value of serial serum trough cyclosporine levels in human renal transplantation. *Transplantation Proceedings* **16**, 1195–1199.

Karuppan, S., Lindholm, A. & Möller, E. (1991). Improved graft survival with flow cytometric crossmatching in renal transplantation. *Transplantation* (in press).

Kasiske, B. L., Heim-Duthoy, K., Rao, K. V. & Awni, W. M. (1988). The relationship between cyclosporine pharmacokinetic parameters and subsequent acute rejection in renal transplant recipients. *Transplantation* **46**, 716–722.

Kennedy, M. S., Yee, G. C., McGuire, T. R., Leonard, T. M., Crowley, J. J. & Deeg, H. J. (1985). Correlation of serum cyclosporine concentration with renal dysfunction in marrow transplant recipients. *Transplantation* **40**, 249–253.

Keogh, A., Day, R., Critchley, L., Duggin, G. & Baron, D. (1988). The effect of food and cholestyramin on the absorption of cyclosporine in cardiac transplant recipients. *Transplantation Proceedings* **20**, 27–30.

Keown, P. A., Ulan, R. A., Wall, W. J., Stiller, C. R., Sinclair, N. R., Carruthers, G. & Howson, W. (1981). Immunological and pharmacological monitoring in the clinical use of cyclosporin A. *Lancet* **i**, 686–689.

Klintmalm, G., Bohman, S. O., Sundelin, B. & Wilczek, H. (1984). Interstitial fibrosis in renal allografts after 12 to 40 months of cyclosporin treatment. *Lancet* **ii**, 950–954.

Klintmalm, G., Säwe, J., Ringdén, O., von Bahr, C. & Magnusson, A. (1985). Cyclosporine plasma levels in renal transplant patients: association with renal toxicity and allograft rejection. *Transplantation* **39**, 132–137.

Kootte, A. M. M., Lensen, L. M., van Bockel, J. H., van Es, L. A. & Paul, L. C. (1988). High- and low-dose regimens of cyclosporin in renal transplantation: immunosuppressive efficacy and side-effects. *Nephrology, Dialysis and Transplantation* **3**, 666–670.

Kronbach, T., Fischer, V. & Meyer, U. A. (1988). Cyclosporine metabolism in human liver: Identification of a cytochrome P-450III gene family as the major cyclosporine-metabolizing enzyme explains interactions of cyclosporine with other drugs. *Clinical Pharmacology and Therapeutics* **43**, 630–635.

Lamb, F. S. & Webb, R. C. (1987). Cyclosporine augments reactivity of isolated blood vessels. *Life Sciences* **40**, 2572–2578.

Lemaire, M. & Tillement, J. P. (1982). Role of lipoproteins and erythrocytes in the *in vitro* binding and distribution of cyclosporin A in the blood. *Journal of Pharmacy and Pharmacology* **34**, 715–718.

Lewis, R. M., Janney, R. P., Van Buren, C. T., Kerman, R. H., Herson, J., Kerr, N. A., Golden, D. A. & Kahan, B. D. (1988). A retrospective analysis of long-term renal allograft function associated with cyclosporine-prednisone immunosuppressive therapy. *Transplantation Proceedings* **20** (suppl 3), 534–539.

Linder, R., Lindholm, A., Restifo, A., Duraj, F. & Groth, C. G. (1991). Long-term renal allograft function under maintenance immunosuppression with cyclosporin A or azathioprine — A single center, five-year follow-up study. *Transplant International* (in press).

Lindholm, A. (1991). Monitoring of the free concentration of cyclosporine in plasma in man. *European Journal of Clinical Pharmacology* **40**, 571–576.

Lindholm, A., Albrechtesen, D., Tufveson, G., Karlberg, I., Persson, N. H. & Groth, C. G. (1991). A randomized trial of cyclosporine and prednisolone versus cyclosporine, azathioprine and prednisolone in primary cadaveric renal transplantation. *Transplantation*, submitted.

Lindholm, A., Elinder, C. G. & Ekqvist, B. (1990a). Falsely high cyclosporine concentrations in capillary samples due to topical contamination. *Therapeutic Drug Monitoring* **12**, 211–213.

Lindholm, A., Henricsson, S. & Dahlqvist, R. (1990b). The effect of food and bile acid administration on the relative bioavailability of cyclosporin. *British Journal of Clinical Pharmacology* **29**, 541–548.

Lindholm, A. & Henricsson, S. (1989). Intra- and interindividual variability in the free fraction of cyclosporine in plasma in recipients of renal transplants. *Therapeutic Drug Monitoring* **11**, 623–630.

Lindholm, A., Henricsson, S., Groth, C. G. & Sjöqvist, F. (1990c). A prospective study of cyclosporin concentration in relation to its therapeutic effect and toxicity after renal transplantation. *British Journal of Clinical Pharmacology* **30**, 443–452.

Lindholm, A., Poussete, Å., Carlström, K. & Klintmalm, G. (1988). Ciclosporin-associated hypertrichosis is not related to sex hormone levels following renal transplantation. *Nephron* **50**, 199–204.

Lindholm, A., Ringdén, O. & Lönnqvist, B. (1987). The role of cyclosporine doses and plasma levels in efficacy and toxicity in bone marrow transplant recipients. *Transplantation* **43**, 680–684.

Lorber, M. I., van Buren, C. T., Flechner, S. M., Willaims, C. & Kahan, B. D. (1987). Hepatobiliary complications of cyclosporine therapy following renal transplantation. *Transplantation Proceedings* **19**, 1808–1810.

Lundgren, G., Groth, C. G., Albrechtsen, D., Brynger, H., Flatmark, A., Frödin, L., Gäbel, H., Husberg, B., Klintmalm, G., Maurer, W., Persson, H. & Thorsby, E. (1986). HLA-matching and pretransplant blood transfusions in cadaveric renal transplantation — a changing picture with cyclosporin. *Lancet* **ii**, 66–69.

Mai, M., Nery, J., Sutker, W., Husberg, B., Klintmalam, G. & Gonwa, T. (1989). DHPG (Gancyclovir) improves survival in CMV pneumonia. *Transplantation Proceedings* **21**, 2263–2265.

Matter, B. E., Donatsch, P. P., Racube, R. R., Schmid, B. & Schmid, W. (1982). Genotoxicity evaluation of cyclosporin A, a new immunosuppressive agent. *Mutation Research* **105**, 257.

Maurer, G. (1985). Metabolism of cyclosporine. *Transplantation Proceedings* **17** (suppl. 1), 19–26.

McCarthy, P. M., Starnes, V. A. & Shumway, N. E. (1989). Heart and heart-lung transplantation: the Stanford experience. In Terasaki, P. I. (ed.) *Clinical Transplants 1989*, pp. 63–71. UCLA Tissue Typing Laboratory, Los Angeles.

Mehta, M. U., Ventakaramanan, R., Burckart, G. J., Ptachcinski, R. J., Delamos, B., Stachak, S., van Thiel, D. H., Iwatsuki, S. & Starzl, T. E. (1988). Effects of bile on cyclosporin absorption in liver transplant patients. *British Journal of Clinical Pharmacology* **25**, 579–584.

Metcalfe, S. M. & Richards, F. M. (1990). Cyclosporine, FK506, and rapamycin: some effects on early activation events in serum-free, mitogen-stimulated mouse spleen cells. *Transplantation* **49**, 798–802.

Meyer-Lehnert, L. H. & Schrier, R. W. (1989). Potential mechanism of cyclosporine A-induced vascular smooth muscle contraction. *Hypertension* **13**, 352–360.

Mihatsch, M. J., Thiel, G. & Ryffel, B. (1986). Morphology of ciclosporin nephropathy. *Progress in Allergeology* **38**, 447–465.

Morse, G. D., Holdsworth, M. T., Venuto, R. C., Gerbasi, J. &. Walshe, J. J. (1988). Pharmacokinetics and clinical tolerance of intravenous and oral cyclosporine in the immediate postoperative period. *Clinical Pharmacology and Therapeutics* **44**, 654–664.

Moyer, T. P., Post, G. R., Strerioff, S. & Anderson, C. F. (1988). Cyclosporine nephrotoxicity is minimized by adjusting dosage on the basis of drug concentration in blood. *Mayo Clinical Proceedings* **63**, 241–247.

Myers, B. D., Ross, J., Newton, L., Luetscher, J. & Perlroth, M. (1984). Cyclosporine-associated chronic nephropathy. *New England Journal of Medicine* **311**, 699–705.

Myre, S. A., McCann, J., First, M. R. & Cluxton, R. J. Jr (1987). Effect of trimethoprim on serum creatinine in healthy and chronic renal failure volunteers. *Therapeutic Drug Monitoring* **9**, 161–165.

Najarian, J. S., Fryd, D. S., Strand, M., Canafax, D. M., Ascher, N. L., Payne, W. D., Simmons, R. L. & Sutherland, D. E. R. (1985). A single institution, randomized, prospective trial of cyclosporin versus azathioprine-antilymphocyte globulin for immunosuppression in renal allograft recipients. *Annals of Surgery* **201**, 142–157.

Nemunaitis, J., Deeg, H. J. & Yee, G. C. (1986). High cyclosporin levels after bone marrow transplantation associated with hypertriglyceridaemia. *Lancet* **ii**, 744–745.

Niederberger, W., Lemaire, M., Maurer, G., Nussbaumer, K. & Wagner, O. (1983). Distribution and binding of cyclosporine in blood and tissues. *Transplantation Proceedings* **15**, 203–205.

Ota, B. (1983). Administration of cyclosporine. *Transplantation Proceedings* **15** (suppl. 1), 3111–3123.

Penn, I. (1987). Cancers following cyclosporine therapy. *Transplantation Proceedings* **19**, 2211–2213.

Penouil, F., Morel, D., Saux, M. C., Brachet-Liermain. A., Potaux, L. & Aparicio, M. (1988). Résorption de la ciclosporine administrée par voie orale à des transplantés rènaus. *Therapie* **43**, 15–19.

Pichard, L., Fabre, I., Fabre, G., Domergue, J., Saint-Aubert, B., Mourad, B., Mourad, G. & Maurel, P. (1990). Cyclosporin A drug interactions. Screening for inducers and inhibitors of cytochrome P-450 (cyclosporin A oxidase) in primary cultures of human hepatocytes and in liver microsomes. *Drug Metabolism and Disposition* **18**, 595–606.

Ponticelli, C., Minetti, L., DiPalo, F. Q., Vegeto, A., Belli, L., Corbetta, G., Tarantino, A. & Civati, G. (1988a). The Milan clinical trial with cyclosporine in cadaveric renal transplantation. *Transplantation* **45**, 908–913.

Ponticelli, C., Tarantino, A., Montagnino, G., Aroldi, A. K., Banfi, G. DeVecchi, A., Zubani, R., Berardinelli, L. & Vegeto, A. (1988b). A randomized trial comparing triple-drug and double-drug therapy in renal transplantation. *Transplantation* **45**, 913–918.

Ptachcinski, R. J., Burckart, G. J., Rosenthal, J. T., Venkataramanan, R., Howrie, D. L., Taylor, R. J., Avner, E. D., Ellis, D. & Hakala, T. R. (1986a). Cyclosporine pharmacokinetics in children following cadaveric renal transplantation. *Transplantation Proceedings* **18**, 766–767.

Ptachcinski, R. J., Venkataramanan, R. & Burckart, G. J. (1986b). Clinical pharmacokinetics of cyclosporin. *Clinical Pharmacokinetics* **11**, 107–132.

Ptachcinski, R. J., Venkataramanan, R., Rosenthal, J. T., Burckart, G. J., Taylor, R. J. & Hakala, T. R. (1985a). Cyclosporine kinetics in renal transplantation. *Clinical Pharmacology and Therapeutics* **38**, 296–300.

Ptachcinski, R. J., Venkataramanan, R., Rosenthal, J. T., Burckart, G. J., Taylor, R. J. &

Hakala, T. R. (1985b). The effect of food of cyclosporine absorption. *Transplantation* **40**, 174–176.

Radovancevic, B. & Frazier, O. H. (1986). Treatment of moderate heart allograft rejection with cyclosporine. *Journal of Heart Transplantation* **5**, 307–311.

Rosano, T. G., Brooks, C. A., Dybas, M. T., Cramer, S. M., Stevens, C. & Freed, B. M. (1990). Selection of an optimal assay method for monitoring of cyclosporine therapy. *Transplantation Proceedings* **22**, 1125–1128.

Rubin, A. M. (1989). Transient cortical blindness and occipital seizures with cyclosporine toxicity. *Transplantation* **47**, 572–573.

Ryffel, B., Donatsch, P., Madorin, M., Matter, B. E., Ruttimann, G., Schon, H., Stoll, R. & Wilson, J. (1983). Toxicological evaluation of cyclosporin A. *Archives of Toxicology* **53**, 107–141.

Schachter, M. (1988). Cyclosporine A and hypertension. *Journal of Hypertension* **6**, 511–516.

Sewing, K. F., Christians, U., Kohlhaw, K., Radeke, H., Strohmeyer, S., Kownatzki, R., Budniak, J., Schottman, R., Bleck, J. S., Almeida, V. M. F., Deters, M., Wonigeit, K. & Pichlmayre, R. (1990). Biologic activity of cyclosporine metabolites. *Transplantation Proceedings* **22**, 1129–1134.

Shaw, L. M., Bowers, L., Demers, L., Freeman, D., Moyer, T., Sanghvi, A., Seltman, H. & Venkataramanan, R. (1987). Critical issues in cyclosporine monitoring: report of the task force on cyclosporine monitoring. *Clinical Chemistry* **33**, 1269–1288.

Sheil, A. G. R., Hall, B. M., Tiller, D. J., Stephen, M. S., Harris, J. P., Duggin, G. G., Horvath, J. S., Johnson, J. R., Rogers, J. R. & Boulas, J. (1983). Australian trial of cyclosporine in cadaveric donor renal transplantation. *Transplantation Proceedings* **15** (suppl 1), 2485–2489.

Slavin, J. & Taylor, J. (1987). Cyclosporin, nifedipine, and gingival hyperplasia. *Lancet* **ii**, 739.

Starzl, T. E., Weil, R., Iwatsuki, S., Klintmalm, G., Schröter, G. P. J., Koep, L. J., Iwaki, Y., Terasaki, P. I. & Porter, K. A. (1980). The use of cyclosporin A and prednisone in cadaver kidney transplantation. *Surgery, Gynecology and Obstetrics* **151**, 17–26.

Storb, R., Deeg, H. J., Pepe, M., Appelbaum, F., Anasetti, C., Beatty, P., Bensinger, W., Berenson, R., Buckner, C. D., Clift, R., Doney, K., Longton, G., Hansen, J., Hill, R., Loughran, T., Martin, P., Singer, J., Sanders, J., Stewart, P., Sullivan, K., Witherspoon, R. & Thomas, D. (1989). Methotrexate and cyclosporine versus cyclosporine alone for prophylaxis of graft-versus-host disease in patients given HLA-identical marrow grafts for leukemia: long-term follow-up of a controlled trial. *Blood* **73**, 1729–1734.

Sumpio, B. E., Baue, A. E. & Chaudry, I. H. (1987). Alleviation of cyclosporine nephrotoxicity with verapamil and ATP–MgC12. *Annals of Surgery* **206**, 655–660.

Sutherland, D. E. R., Fryd, D., Strand, M. H., Canafax, D. M., Ascher, N. L., Payne, W. D., Simmons, R. L. & Najarian, J. S. (1985). Results of the Minnesota randomized prospective trial of cyclosporine versus azathioprine-antilymphocyte globulin for immunosuppression in renal allograft recipients. *American Journal of Kidney Disease* **5**, 318–327.

Thompson, C. B., Sullivan, K. M., June, C. H. & Thomas, E. D. (1984). Association between cyclosporin neurotoxicity and hypomagnesemia. *Lancet* **ii**, 1116–1120.

Tollermar, J., Ringdén, O., Ericzon, B. G. & Tydén, G. (1988). Cyclosporine-associated central nervous system toxicity. *New England Journal of Medicine* **318**, 788–789.

Tufveson, G., Odlind, B., Sjöberg, O., Lindberg, A., Gabrielsson, J., Lindström, B., Lithell, H., Selinus, I., Tötterman, T. & Dahlberg, J. (1986). A longitudinal study of the pharmacokinetics of cyclosporine A and *in vitro* lymphocyte responses in renal transplant patients. *Transplantation Proceedings* **18** (suppl 5), 16–24.

Vanrenterghem, Y., Roels, L. Lerut, T., Gruwez, J., Michielsen, P., Gresele, P.,

Deckmyn, H., Colucci, M., Arnout, J. & Vermylen, J. (1985a). Thromboembolic complications and haemostatic changes in cyclosporin-treated cadaveric kidney allograft recipients. *Lancet* **i**, 999–1002.

Vathsala, A., Weinberg, R. B., Schoenberg, L., Grevel, J., Goldstein, R. A., van Buren, C. T., Lewis, R. M. & Kahan, B. D. (1989). Lipid abnormalities in cyclosporine-prednisone-treated renal transplant recipients. *Transplantation* **48**, 37–43.

Venkataramanan, R., Burckart, G. J. & Ptachcinski, R. J. (1985a). Pharmacokinetics and monitoring of cyclosporine following orthotopic liver transplantation. *Seminars in Liver Disease* **5**, 357–368.

Venkataramanan, R., Starzl, T. E., Yang, S., Burckart, G. J., Ptachcinski, R. J., Shaw, B. W., Iwatsuki, S., van Thiel, D. H., Sanghivi, A. & Seltman, H. (1985b). Biliary excretion of cyclosporine in liver transplant patients. *Transplantation Proceedings* **17**, 286–289.

Wagner, K., Albrecht, S. & Neumayer, H. H. (1986). Prevention of delayed graft function by a calcium antagonist — a randomized trial in renal graft recipients on cyclosporine A. *Transplantation Proceedings* **18**, 1269–1271.

Wilczek, H., Bohman, S. O., Klintmalm, G. & Groth, C. G. (1988). Five-year serial renal graft biopsy study in cyclosporine-treated patients. *Transplantation Proceedings* **20** (suppl 3), 812–815.

Wilczek, H., Ringdén, O. & Tydén, G. (1984). Cyclosporin-associated central nervous system toxicity after renal transplantation. *Transplantation* **39**, 110.

Yee, C. G. & McGuire, T. R. (1990). Pharmacokinetic drug interactions with cyclosporin. *Clinical Pharmacokinetics* **19**, 319–332, 400–415.

Yee, G. C., Kennedy, M. S., Storb, R. & Thomas, E. D. (1984). Pharmacokinetics of intravenous cyclosporine in bone marrow transplant patients. *Transplantation* **38**, 511–513.

Yee, G. C., Lennon, T. P., Gmur, D. J., Kennedy, M. S. & Deeg, H. J. (1986). Age-dependent cyclosporine pharmacokinetics in marrow transplant recipients. *Clinical Pharmacology and Therapeutics* **40**, 438–443.

Yee, G. C., McGuire, T. R., Gmur, D. J., Lennon, T. P. & Deeg, H. J. (1988a). Blood cyclosporine pharmacokinetics in patients undergoing marrow transplantation. *Transplantation* **46**, 399–402.

Yee, G. C., Self, S. G., McGuire, T. R., Carlin, J., Sanders, J. E. & Deeg, H. J. (1988b). Serum cyclosporine concentrations and risk of acute graft-versus-host disease after allogeneic marrow transplantation. *New England Journal of Medicine* **319**, 65–70.

Yuzawa, K., Kondo, I., Fukao, K., Iwasaki, Y. & Hamaguchi, H. (1986). Mutagenicity of cyclosporine: Induction of sister chromatid exchange in human cells. *Transplantation* **42**, 61–63.

Chapter 5
The use of cyclosporin in autoimmune diseases

Gilles Feutren

Introduction

After the superiority of cyclosporin A (CsA) (Sandimmun[®], Sandoz) had been demonstrated over conventional therapy in organ transplantation, it appeared logical to investigate its effect in autoimmune diseases.

However, in human autoimmune diseases where the abnormal immune reaction is always fully ongoing at the time of immunointervention by CsA, the mechanism of drug action is not as easy to understand as when CsA is given at the time of antigenic challenge such as in transplantation. Cytotoxic T lymphocytes that are already differentiated are not modified by CsA (Fig. 5.1) (Di Padova, 1989). The same holds true with B lymphocytes and antibody production. In addition, it is known that CsA has little, if any, direct effect on neutrophil and macrophage functions. Hence, it could be speculated that the effect of CsA on autoimmunity should mainly involve the inhibition of inflammatory and cytotoxic lymphokines at the level of T helper cells (Fig. 5.1). Additionally, through inhibition of gamma-interferon production, the expression of major histocompatibility antigens may also be diminished, thereby inhibiting both inducer and effector mechanisms (Autenried & Halloran, 1985). CsA could also prevent the expansion of new autoreactive clones in diseases which have a fluctuating course.

Finally, it cannot be ruled out that CsA may also act through mechanisms not related to B- or T-cell immunity, e.g. the inhibition of

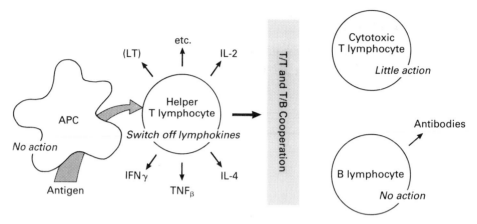

Fig. 5.1. Mode of action of CsA (actions given in italic). IL, interleukin; IFNγ, gamma interferon; TNF$_\beta$, tumour necrosis factor-beta; LT, lymphotoxin; APC, antigen-presenting cell.

basophile degranulation (Hultsch *et al.*, 1990), or the inhibition of some non-lymphoid cells such as keratinocytes (Nickoloff *et al.*, 1988).

Animal models of autoimmune diseases

The results of CsA treatment in animal models of autoimmunity correlate with our knowledge of the mechanisms of action of the drug (reviewed in Borel & Gunn, 1986) because it is more effective on T-cell mediated than on B-cell mediated diseases.

Preventive treatment

Experimental autoimmune diseases induced by the injection of purified autoantigen were in most cases completely prevented by the administration of CsA given at the time of antigen injection. This is the case for T-cell-mediated diseases such as rat arthritis induced by Freund's ajuvant (Borel *et al.*, 1976) or type-II collagen sensitization, rat uveitis following the injection of retinal S antigen (Nussenblatt *et al.*, 1981), or experimental allergic encephalomyelitis following immunization against the encephalitogenic basic protein (Bolton *et al.*, 1982). CsA also prevented the appearance of autoantibodies and the related disease in experimental myasthenia gravis (Drachman *et al.*, 1985), Heyman's nephritis, acute serum sickness of the rabbit, and autoimmune haemolytic anaemia of the mouse. In some cases short-term CsA treatment resulted in the long-term prevention of the disease, and in the rat uveitis model it was possible to demonstrate the existence of antigen-specific suppressor T cells.

Similar features were found in spontaneous models of autoimmune diseases. The continuous administration of CsA before the age of onset of the disease resulted in the prevention of insulin-dependent diabetes mellitus in the BB rat (Laupacis *et al.*, 1983) or NOD mouse (Mori *et al.*, 1986), and of systemic lupus in (NZB × W) F1 (Israel-Biet *et al.*, 1983) or MLR lpr/lpr mice (Mountz *et al.*, 1987). On the other hand, no effect was detected in spontaneous thyroiditis of the obese chicken (Wick *et al.*, 1982), which is a purely B-lymphocyte-mediated disease since it is prevented by bursectomy and not by thymectomy.

Curative treatment

The effect of CsA given as a curative treatment in cases of established autoimmune diseases is less clear-cut. Even when it is effective, as in the cases of T-lymphocyte-mediated disease, the effect is sometimes difficult to demonstrate if the active immunological aggression results in irreversible lesions which do not have any chance to improve, even when the immunological process is stopped by CsA. This was obviously the case for insulin-dependent diabetes mellitus in the BB rat or NOD mouse.

In most instances, once a disease directly mediated by autoantibodies is established, no effect of CsA is observed either on autoantibody levels or on the symptoms or the lesions, as shown in experimental myasthenia gravis. The case is more complicated in MLR lpr/lpr lupus mice (Mountz *et al.*, 1987). CsA administration resulted in a histologically proven improvement of joints, kidneys and lymph nodes, although humoral abnormalities (anti-DNA antibodies, immune complexes, rheumatoid factor, immunoglobulin levels) remained unchanged. This suggests that in some diseases known to be antibody-mediated, CsA-sensitive cellular immune effectors may be involved and lead to clinical improvement.

Clinical trials in autoimmune diseases

Clinical indications were selected on the basis of the experimental results in animal models of autoimmunity and on medical need, as therapy is still unsatisfactory in some indications. It is important to differentiate between clinical trials intended to study the 'efficacy' of CsA and those which aimed at evaluating 'benefit'. For instance, the fact that CsA decreases serum alkaline phosphatase levels in patients with primary biliary cirrhosis may indicate efficacy. However, assessing the beneficial aspect of this effect would consist of showing an altered natural course of the disease (progression of histological alteration, reduction of mortality).

At the present time, the efficacy and the clinical benefit of CsA therapy have been demonstrated for severely affected patients in four diseases: rheumatoid arthritis, autoimmune uveitis, idiopathic nephrotic syndrome and psoriasis.

Rheumatoid arthritis

The first attempt to treat arthritic patients with CsA was in 1978 (Herrman & Müller, 1979), when appreciable improvement was obtained in five out of six patients treated with CsA for up to 10 months.

In controlled studies with a CsA dose of 5–10 mg/kg/day, dose-dependent improvements were reported in pain and morning stiffness by 43–87% of patients, joint tenderness (Ritchie or ARA joint index) by 38–67%, and grip strength by 15–98%, with an average 'responder rate' of 70%. The reduction of concomitant steroid dosage reported in some studies suggested the possible use of the drug in a 'steroid sparing' capacity. Cessation of treatment in responsive patients was followed by recurrence of symptoms within 2–10 weeks in most of them.

This positive effect of CsA was confirmed in three double-blind studies (van Rijthoven et al., 1986; Dougados et al., 1988; Tugwell et al., 1990). On 5 mg/kg/day CsA, the overall responder rate was 54% on CsA and 7% on placebo. Interestingly, this clinical effect was observed despite the absence of change in erythrocyte sedimentation rate (ESR), rheumatoid factor or immunoglobulin concentration. In the Canadian study of 6 months duration (Tugwell et al., 1990), CsA was started at a low dose (2.5 mg/kg/day) and then progressively increased to 5 mg/kg/day in cases of insufficient clinical response. The optimal effect was observed at an average dose of 3.8 mg/kg/day CsA, resulting in a very good response rate of 31% compared to 8% on placebo (reduction of the number of inflammatory joints by 50% of more). The improvement on CsA was slower than in other diseases. The difference in the efficacy of CsA compared to placebo was apparent after 4 months, and the optimal effect was sometimes obtained after 6 months of treatment.

However, even if CsA is efficacious in the treatment of active rheumatoid arthritis (RA), its place in the hierarchy of drug treatment in RA still remains to be determined.

Autoimmune uveitis

The main subgroups of endogenous uveitis where the effect of CsA have been investigated are Behçet's disease involving the posterior segment of the eye, 'idiopathic' uveitis, pars planitis, retinal vasculitis, Vogt-Koyanagi-Harada uveitis, birdshot chorio-retinopathy and sarcoid uveitis. Patients included in trials with CsA were suffering from severe sight-threatening uveitis (Nussenblatt et al., 1983; Ben Ezra et al., 1988; Le Hoang et al., 1988). CsA was given at an initial loading dose of 5–10 mg/kg/day followed by a dose reduction according to ocular inflammatory activity and tolerability. Improvement of intraocular inflammation and visual acuity was observed in over 60% of patients within the first 2–4 weeks. However, in many cases relapses of the inflammatory processes were observed when rapid discontinuation of CsA was attempted.

In Behçet's disease with ocular involvement, CsA has a remarkable therapeutic effect on the intraocular inflammatory progress, prolonging the periods of remission and thereby arresting the inevitable gradual loss of vision (Ben Ezra, 1986). This effect was confirmed by a double-masked trial of 4 months duration were 48% of the patients responded well on CsA versus 13% in the control group who received colchicine (Masuda et al., 1989). The beneficial effects on the systemic manifestations of the disease, however, are less obvious and may require combining CsA with low dose steroids.

Idiopathic nephrotic syndrome

Clinical studies with CsA in idiopathic nephrotic syndrome (NS) (reviewed by Meyrier, 1989) have been performed in either steroid-resistant (mostly focal segmental glomerulosclerosis (FSGS)) or steroid-dependent patients (mostly minimal change nephropathy (MCN)), in adults (Clasen et al., 1988; Meyrier et al., 1991) and in children (Brodehl et al., 1988; Tejani et al., 1988; Niaudet et al., 1991). Many of these patients were also resistant to alkylating agents.

In steroid-dependent idiopathic NS, the starting dose of CsA averaged 6 mg/kg/day (or 150 mg/m^2/day) in children, and 5 mg/kg/day in adults. Treatment duration ranged from 3 to 24 months. A drop in proteinuria was detected within 1 or 2 weeks after starting CsA, and complete remission was reported in over 80% of patients after a median duration of treatment of 2 months. In the majority of these patients, steroid-induced remissions could be maintained by CsA despite the withdrawal of steroids. In steroid-resistant idiopathic NS, complete remissions were achieved on CsA monotherapy in 14%, and partial remissions in an additional 12%. However, with the combination of CsA and steroids, the rates of complete and partial remission were 24% and 24%, respectively, a result which is considered relevant in these patients previously unresponsive to steroids. After CsA was discontinued, most of the patients relapsed in a few weeks. The lowest, still effective dose seems to be in the range of 2–5 mg/kg/day and shows inter-patient variability.

The side-effect profile of CsA in NS is similar to that in other autoimmune diseases (Collaborative Study Group of Sandimmun in Nephrotic Syndrome, 1991). However, several patients with FSGS, especially if renal function was abnormal at the start of CsA therapy, showed marked deterioration of renal function, which in some cases did not improve on discontinuation of CsA. It is difficult to assess whether this was due to CsA or to the natural course of the disease.

Renal biopsies have been performed in 42 patients after 2–18 months of continuous CsA therapy. In one series (Niaudet *et al.*, 1991), slight to moderate changes suggestive of CsA nephrotoxicity were reported in five of 22 biopsies in children, whereas no relevant changes were reported in other series. However, in some biopsies, progression of FSGS was recorded despite CsA therapy.

Many questions relating to the optimal use of CsA in NS remain open. Despite this, it now appears that CsA can provide benefit for steroid-sensitive patients with steroid toxicity and that therapeutic testing of CsA can be considered in steroid-resistant NS.

At the moment results are too scarce to support the use of CsA in glomerulonephritides other than MCN and FSGS.

Psoriasis and other dermatological disorders

It is unclear whether the hyperproliferative epidermis, which is the hallmark of psoriasis, represents a primary defect in keratinocyte growth regulation or is of immunological origin.

The clinical effect of CsA in psoriasis was detected by pure chance (Müller & Herrman, 1979) in patients treated with CsA in a trial in psoriatic arthropathy. Following this original observation, studies have been conducted in patients with severe, generalized plaque-form psoriasis. Most of them had longstanding disease and had been treated previously with either Psoralen-UV-A therapy, methotrexate or/and retinoids. In placebo-controlled studies, remission ($\geqslant 75\%$ improvement) was observed in 55% of patients after only 4 weeks CsA treatment at a dose of 5 mg/kg/day compared with 3% of patients on placebo (van Joost *et al.*, 1988). In dose-finding studies, a clear dose–response remission rate was observed. After 8 weeks of treatment, patients who were rated as being clear or almost clear of lesions represented 0% on placebo, 36% on 3 mg/kg/day CsA, 65% on 5 mg/kg/day CsA and 80% on 7.5 mg/kg/day CsA (Ellis *et al.*, 1991). In another study, the rate of very good response (75% improvement of psoriasis or more) was 50% after 3 months on 2.5 mg/kg/day and 92% on 5 mg/kg/day CsA (Timonen *et al.*, 1990).

Unfortunately, most patients brought into remission relapsed within 2–10 weeks after therapy was withdrawn (Higgins *et al.*, 1989). This indicates the need for continued maintenance treatment of psoriasis by low doses of CsA.

In addition to psoriasis, CsA has been administered in many dermatological diseases (reviewed in Ho *et al.*, 1990). In dermatomyositis, a marked steroid-sparing effect, as well as an improvement in muscle strength has been reported (Heckmatt *et al.*, 1989). In severe atopic dermatitis, a cross-over study in 33 patients showed significant improvement after 2 weeks on 5 mg/kg/day in comparison to placebo (Sowden *et al.*, 1991). After 8 weeks treatment, the average improvement of the disease score was 50% on CsA, but was unchanged on placebo. As observed in psoriasis, a relapse occurred shortly after stopping CsA. No change in IgE concentration in serum was detected.

Other autoimmune diseases

Insulin-dependent diabetes mellitus

The hypothesis that autoimmune mechanisms are involved in the destruction of pancreatic beta-cells in insulin-dependent diabetes mellitus (IDDM) (Eisenbarth, 1986; Bach, 1987) and the observation that immune intervention with CsA is capable of modifying the natural course of the disease in animal models have led to an exciting new era in clinical research on IDDM. The problem of immune intervention in overt IDDM is that extensive beta-cell destruction has already occurred when the clinical diagnosis is made. The aim is to prevent the autoimmune destruction of the few remaining beta-cells.

Two double-blind placebo-controlled studies (Feutren et al., 1986; Canadian-European Multicentre Trial, 1988) have confirmed the initial pilot study data in adults (Stiller et al., 1984; Assan et al., 1985) and children (Bougnères et al., 1988): with CsA doses of 7.5–10 mg/kg/day significantly more patients attained complete remission (defined as good metabolic control without exogenous insulin) at 12 months than patients treated with placebo — 17–32% on CsA versus 0–10% on placebo. Clinical remission in CsA-treated patients was associated with a sustained increase in the endogenous secretion of insulin as assessed by C-peptide measurements.

The major problem in all patient series was that clinical remissions were progressively lost even on continuous CsA therapy sometimes despite sustained C-peptide levels (Assan et al., 1990), suggesting the concomitant development of purely metabolic abnormalities such as insulin-resistance. For this reason, CsA therapy of recent onset IDDM must still be regarded as an experimental procedure only justified within a limited number of controlled clinical trials (Rubenstein & Pyke, 1987).

Gastroenterology, hepatology

Results of several pilot studies in Crohn's disease suggested that oral doses of CsA ranging from 5 to 15 mg/kg/day were effective in most, but not all, patients with chronic active disease, but a rapid relapse was seen after stopping therapy. The efficacy of CsA in chronic active Crohn's disease was confirmed by a placebo-controlled study in which 6–8 mg/kg/day CsA orally was associated with a success rate of 59% compared with 32% on placebo after 3 months of treatment (Brynskov et al., 1989a).

Only uncontrolled experience has been reported with the use of CsA in ulcerative colitis. In 15 patients with severe, active disease, intravenous CsA (4 mg/kg/day for 10 days) resulted in a 73% improvement rate (Lichtiger & Present, 1990). The improvement was maintained on oral CsA (6–8 mg/kg/day) over 6 months in 60%. Of interest has been the use of a CsA enema in patients with chronic proctitis (Brynskov et al., 1989b).

Several studies with CsA were conducted in primary biliary cirrhosis. As early as 1980, improved liver function had been reported in six patients receiving 5–10 mg/kg/day CsA, but substantial toxicity occurred (Routhier et al., 1980). A placebo-controlled study in 29 patients has confirmed the improvement of clinical symptoms and decreased laboratory liver abnormalities after 1 year of treatment (Wiesner et al., 1990). A large placebo-controlled, long-term study (more than 300 patients followed for 2–5 years) is ongoing with the aim of evaluating whether disease progression can be influenced.

Neurology

Three double-blind, randomized studies enrolling a total of more than 700 patients have been completed in multiple sclerosis. Two trials compared CsA to placebo (Rudge et al., 1989, Multiple Sclerosis Group, 1990) and the third CsA to azathioprine (Kappos et al., 1988). Treatment duration was 2 years. No significant difference between CsA and the control group was detected in the incidence of relapses or in the rate of progression of the disease in either study. One of the reasons for such poor efficacy may be the low penetration of CsA through the blood/brain barrier resulting in a low concentration in the brain tissue and in the cerebral spinal fluid.

A placebo-controlled study in patients with progressively worsening generalized myasthenia gravis (MG) who had not yet been treated with thymectomy, steroids or other immunosuppressants, showed that patients on CsA (6 mg/kg/day) had significantly greater improvement in strength after 6 months of therapy than patients on placebo (Tindall et al., 1987). More studies are needed to define more clearly the potential of CsA in MG, and to define its place in relation to corticosteroids and azathioprine. It is of interest that in most responders the titres of antiacetylcholine receptor antibodies did not fall.

Asthma

The effect of CsA in steroid-dependent chronic severe asthma has recently been reported in a 12-week cross-over study in which 33 patients received 5 mg/kg/day CsA or placebo (Alexander et al., 1992). A significant improvement by 12-18% was observed on CsA over the placebo response using various measures of respiratory function such as forced expiratory volume (1 s), or peak expiratory flow, or frequency of disease exacerbations. Overall 64% of the patients reported an improvement on CsA compared to 24% on placebo. These results may suggest a role for activated T lymphocytes in the pathogenesis of asthma. However, these result may also be explained by a CsA-induced inhibition of mediator release from mast cells and basophils (Civillo *et al.*, 1990). These findings are encouraging but the place of CsA in the armamentarium of antiasthmatic drugs still needs to be defined.

Haematology

In several very limited series of patients with severe aplastic anaemia treated with CsA the response rate on CsA seemed to be similar to that reported with antilymphocyte globulins (ALG). It is interesting that some non-responders to ALG went into remission on CsA. Full efficacy was mostly obtained within the first 3 months. Relapses frequently occurred within 3 months of stopping CsA. A further randomized study of 84 patients compared the combination of ALG plus steroids to CsA plus ALG plus steroids (Frickhofen *et al.*, 1991). After 3 months, 65% responded in the CsA group compared to 39% in the control group.

The limited numbers of patients treated with CsA in other haematological autoimmune diseases precludes a definitive conclusion concerning efficacy.

Varia

Improvement or steroid sparing effect was reported in several open studies with CsA in systemic lupus erythematosus (SLE). In two studies, which included a total of 54 patients, the CsA dose was 5 mg/kg/day (Feutren *et al.*, 1987; Miescher *et al.*, 1988). No relevant changes were found in anti-DNA titres. Hypertension and reversible renal dysfunction were the most serious side-effects. The available experience with CsA in SLE is still quite limited. However, it seems that steroid sparing could be a substantial benefit of CsA therapy in this disease.

In Sjögren's disease 5 mg/kg/day CsA did not exert relevant clinical effects in a placebo-controlled study (Drosos *et al.*, 1986). The use of CsA has also been reported in many other diseases. But the results are too uncertain or the experience is too limited to draw any conclusion. This is the case for Grave's ophthalmopathy, Wegener's granulomatosis, pulmonary sarcoidosis, male autoimmune infertility, relapsing polychondritis, giant cell arteritis and myocarditis.

Adverse reactions

The safety documentation on the use of CsA in autoimmune diseases is based on more than 3700 patients included in the various studies conducted by Sandoz in this field where detailed documentation is available. The main adverse reactions and the incidence of treatment discontinuation resulting from adverse reactions are summarized in Table 5.1. Adverse reactions affecting the kidney limit the therapeutic potential of CsA the most.

Renal dysfunction

The impairment of renal dysfunction induced by CsA is characterized by a reduction in the renal plasma flow and subsequently in the glomerular filtration rate resulting in increased serum creatinine and urea. Increased potassium and uric acid, as well as decreased serum magnesium, may also occur in relation to an impairment of tubular function, but are seldom relevant clinically.

Renal dysfunction has been analysed in large numbers of autoimmune patients (Dieterle *et al.*, 1988; Feutren *et al.*, 1990). A dose-dependent fall in renal function starts within the first 2 weeks of CsA therapy and reaches a plateau at month 2. When the dose of CsA does not exceed 5 mg/kg/day, renal dysfunction is mild and serum creatinine remains within normal limits in most patients. No further decline of renal dysfunction is observed,

Table 5.1. Adverse drug reactions of CsA (dose $\leq$ 6 mg/kg/day) in autoimmune diseases

	Psoriasis ($n = 631$)	Nephrotic syndrome ($n = 661$)	Rheumatoid arthritis ($n = 378$)
Discontinuation because of:			
Renal dysfunction	1.9%	3.7%	6.1%
Hypertension	1.0%	0.6%	2.9%
Other	4.5%	3.1%	20.6%
Hypertension[1]	12.0%	14.0%	15.0%
CsA-nephropathy	Risk < 5.0%	Risk < 5.0%	Risk < 5.0%
Malignancies			
Lymphoma	Risk $\leq$ 0.1%	Risk $\leq$ 0.1%	Risk $\leq$ 0.1%
Squamous cell carcinoma	1.0%	0%	0%
Kaposi's sarcoma	0%	0%	0%

[1]WHO/ISH definition of mild hypertension.

indicating that the functional disturbance is not progressive for up to 2 years of continuous therapy. Renal dysfunction is worsened by concomitant medication with nephrotoxic compounds, including non-steroidal anti-inflammatory drugs (Ludwin et al., 1988).

After stopping CsA, renal dysfunction is fully reversible when the dose of CsA did not exceed 5 mg/kg/day and when the dose had been adjusted to avoid large rises of serum creatinine.

Morphological kidney alterations

More relevant than functional and reversible renal dysfunction are the histological lesions that have been found in renal biopsies of CsA-treated autoimmune patients (so-called CsA nephropathy). CsA nephropathy has been described as a combination of arteriolopathy, acellular interstitial fibrosis (striped form) and tubular atrophy within areas of fibrosis (Mihatsch, 1985).

Results of over 300 renal biopsies are available in IDDM, SLE, RA, uveitis, NS, psoriasis and various other diseases. More than 'minimal' or 'slight' lesions (which cannot be attributed with certainty to CsA) were found in 22% of the patients, with reported frequencies ranging from 0 to 100% (Palestine et al., 1986; Miescher et al., 1987; Feutren, 1988). This large variation is most likely due to the different treatment dosages used. When analysing the entire data, it appears that the risk of developing CsA-nephropathy is low (less than 5%) when CsA dose does not exceed 5 mg/kg/day and when the dose is decreased in order to avoid rises in serum creatinine of more than 30% above the patient's own baseline level. In these series where the biopsy had been performed after a mean period of 15 months on CsA therapy, morphological changes were neither related to the treatment duration nor to the cumulative dose of CsA (Feutren & Mihatsch, 1992).

Malignancies

Malignancies associated with immunosuppression have been observed in CsA in autoimmune diseases (Arellano & Krupp, 1991). Lymphoproliferative disorders have a low incidence ($\leqslant 0.1\%$) but may occur even in patients treated with a dose of CsA as low as 2.5 mg/kg/day. As observed in transplantation (Starzl et al., 1984), the lymphoproliferation may be reversible when it is diagnosed early and when immunosuppression is then interrupted. Squamous cell skin carcinomas have mainly been observed in psoriasis patients where the incidence is around 1%. This special sensitivity is perhaps related to previous antipsoriasis therapy, especially radiation therapy with UV-A.

Infections

Infections have been surprisingly infrequent and follow an uncomplicated course. In long-term controlled studies in diabetes and multiple sclerosis, the frequency of urinary, skin and respiratory tract infections was not significantly higher in CsA-treated patients than in those on placebo (Feutren *et al.*, 1986; Canadian-European Control Trial Group, 1988).

Other adverse events

Mild to moderate hypertension developed in 10–15% of patients, usually within 1 or 2 months after starting CsA. Hypertension is reversible after stopping CsA. If therapy was required, conventional treatment of various kinds was successful. In the light of experimental data, calcium channel inhibitors not interfering with CsA pharmacokinetics such as isradipidine or nifedipine should be tried first.

Among other adverse events, unspecific gastrointestinal disturbances (nausea, discomfort, diarrhoea) accounted for the majority of the cases of treatment discontinuation, especially in rheumatoid arthritis (Table 5.1). Because a lower dose of CsA is used in autoimmune diseases than in transplantation, hypertrichosis, gingival hyperplasia, paresthesia and tremor, rises in bilirubin or falls in haemoglobin have a low incidence and are usually mild.

Optimal use of CsA in autoimmune diseases

Patients

Only patients who have a chance of responding to CsA should be selected. This implies excluding diseases where no convincing effect by CsA is observed, as well as potentially responsive diseases where organ failure is likely to be irreversible, e.g. blindness in patients with uveitis. The use of CsA should be limited to patients with severe disease, especially when conventional therapy is ineffective, inappropriate or not well tolerated.

Dose of CsA

The effective dose of CsA depends on the disease. On the one hand, good results are obtained with 2.5 or 3 mg/kg/day CsA in psoriasis, whereas doses of 5–7 mg/kg/day are necessary in endogenous uveitis (Table 5.2). In all instances, the dosage must be adjusted later on the basis of individual response and tolerability. The lowest effective maintenance dose should be used. The dose of CsA should be decreased when serum creatinine is increased at two consecutive control visits by more than 30% over the patient's own pre-CsA level.

Table 5.2. Efficacy of CsA monotherapy in autoimmune diseases

Disease	Initial dose of CsA (mg/kg/day)	% Very good efficacy[1]	Onset of effect	Time to maximal effect
Psoriasis	2.5	50	2 weeks	2–4 months
	5.0	90	2 weeks	2–3 months
Nephrotic syndrome	5.0		2 weeks	3–4 months
Steroid-resistant		20		
Steroid-dependent		80		
Rheumatoid arthritis	3.0	30	2 months	6 months
Crohn's disease	5.0–7.0	30	1 month	3–4 months
Uveitis	5.0–7.0	60	2 weeks	3 months

[1]Definition of very good efficacy: psoriasis, $\geq 75\%$ improvement; nephrotic syndrome, proteinuria < 0.5 g/day; rheumatoid arthritis, $\geq 50\%$ reduction in joint count; Crohn's disease, grading score sum ≥ 4; uveitis, improved or stabilized vision.

When the optimal improvement is not achieved by 5 mg/kg/day CsA, it is recommended to combine CsA with low dose steroids instead of further increasing the dose of CsA; this is especially relevant for endogenous uveitis and steroid-resistant nephrotic syndrome.

Treatment duration

CsA should be stopped as soon as possible in patients who do not show a relevant clinical effect at a maximum dose of 5 mg/kg/day, or at their highest individual tolerable dose. The minimal duration of treatment for deciding whether therapy is efficient or not differs from one disease to another (Table 5.2). In most indications the onset of the effect is very quick and consequently CsA should not be administered for more than about 3 months in the absence of a relevant clinical response. RA is an exception to this rule because the rate of improvement is low and patients are still improving 4–6 months after starting treatment. Other exceptions are diseases such as primary biliary cirrhosis where CsA prevents the natural course towards spontaneous worsening and organ failure, and where it may not be possible to assess the clinical response to CsA before 1 or 2 years of therapy.

In patients who respond well to CsA, the disease usually recurs in the weeks following treatment interruption but responds again when CsA is reintroduced. Consequently, long-term therapy is necessary in most instances.

Monitoring

Permanent monitoring is mandatory as long as CsA therapy is continued, at a frequency of twice a month during the first 3 months and thereafter once every 1-2 months during the maintenance period. The monitoring is based on clinical examinations, including blood pressure, and simple laboratory tests, especially serum creatinine. In contrast to transplantation, the routine measurement of CsA blood levels is not necessary in autoimmune diseases (Ludwin, 1991), but is still mandatory in cases of drug interactions (Cockburn *et al.*, 1989) or liver dysfunction since CsA is metabolized by the liver and excreted in the bile.

Provided that these recommendations are observed, CsA may be safely used even in the long-term treatment of selected autoimmune diseases.

References

Alexander, A. G., Barnes, N. C. & Kay, A. B. (1992). Trial of cyclosporin in corticosteroid-dependent chronic severe asthma. *Lancet* **339**, 324-328.

Arellano, F. & Krupp, P. The risk of malignancies in patients treated with Sandimmun®. *Journal of Autoimmunity* (in press).

Assan, R., Feutren, G., Debray-Sachs, M., Quiniou-Debrie, M. C., Laborie, C., Thomas, G., Chatenond, L. & Bach, J.-F. (1985). Metabolic and immunological effects of cyclosporin in recently diagnosed type 1 diabetes mellitus. *Lancet* **i**, 67-71.

Assan, R., Feutren, G., Sirmai, J., Laborie, C., Boitard, C., Vexiau, P., du Rostu, H., Rodier, M., Figoni, M., Vague, P., Hors, J. & Bach, J.-F. (1990). Plasma C-peptide levels and clinical remissions in recent-onset type I diabetic patients treated with cyclosporin A and insulin. *Diabetes* **39**, 768-774.

Autenried, P. & Halloran, P. F. (1985). Cyclosporine blocks the induction of class I and class II MHC products in mouse kidney by graft-versus-host disease. *Journal of Immunology* **135**, 3922-3928.

Bach, J. F. (1988). Mechanisms of autoimmunity in insulin-dependent diabetes mellitus. *Clinical Experimental Immunology* **72**, 1-8.

Ben Ezra, D. (1986). Cyclosporin A in Behçet's disease — an overview. In Lehner, T. & Barnes, C. G. (eds) *Recent Advances in Behçet's Disease*, pp. 319-325. Royal Society of Medicine Services, London.

Ben Ezra, D., Cohen, E., Rakotomalala, M., de Courten, C., Harris, W., Chajek, T., Friedman, G. & Matamoros, N. (1988). Treatment of endogenous uveitis with cyclosporin A. *Transplantation Proceedings* **20** (suppl. 4), 122-127.

Bolton, C., Borel, J. F., Cuzner, M. L., Davison, A. N. & Turner, A. M. (1982). Immunosuppression by cyclosporin A of experimental allergic encephalomyelitis. *Journal of Neurological Sciences* **56**, 147-153.

Borel, J. F., Feurer, C., Gubler, H. U. & Stähelin, H. (1976). Biological effects of cyclosporin A: a new antilymphocyte agent. *Agents and Actions* **6**, 468-475.

Borel, J. F. & Gunn, H. (1986). Cyclosporine as a new approach to therapy. *Annals of the New York Academy of Sciences* **475**, 307-319.

Bougnères, P. F., Carel, J. C., Castano, L., Boitard, C., Gardin, J. P., Landais, P., Hors, P., Mihatsch, M. J., Paillard, M., Chaussain, J. L. & Bach, J.-F. (1988). Factors associated with early remission of type I diabetes in children treated with cyclosporin. *New England Journal of Medicine* **381**, 663-670.

Brodehl, J., Hoyer, P. F., Oemar, B. S., Helmchen, U. & Wonigeit, K. (1988). Cyclosporin treatment of nephrotic syndrome in children. *Transplantation Proceedings* **20** (suppl. 4), 269–274.

Brynskov, J., Freund, L., Rasmussen, S. N., Lauritsen, R., Schaffalitzky de Muckadell, O., Williams, N., MacDonald, A. S., Tanton, R., Molina, F., Campanini, M. C., Bianchi, P., Ranzi, T., Quarto di Palo, F., Malchow-Moller, A., Ostergaard Thomsen, O., Tage-Jensen, U., Binder, V. & Riis, P. (1989a). A placebo-controlled, double-blind, randomized trial of cyclosporine therapy in active chronic Crohn's disease. *New England Journal of Medicine* **321**, 845–850.

Brynskov, J., Freund, L., Thomsen, O., Andersen, C. B., Norby Rasmussen, S. & Binder, V. (1989b). Treatment of refractory ulcerative colitis with cyclosporin enemas. *Lancet* **i**, 721–722.

Canadian-European Randomized Control Trial Group. (1988). Induction of remission of type 1 diabetes mellitus by cyclosporin is dependent on early intervention and associated with maintained enhancement of insulin secretion through one year of treatment. *Diabetes* **37**, 1574–1582.

Clasen, W., Kindler, J., Mihatsch, M. J. & Sieberth H. G. (1988). Long-term treatment of minimal-change nephrotic syndrome with cyclosporin: as control biopsy study. *Nephrology, Dialysis, Transplantation* **3**, 733–737.

Cockburn, I. T. R. & Krupp, P. (1989). An appraisal of drug interactions with Sandimmun®. *Transplant Proceedings* **21**, 3845–3850.

Collaborative Study Group of Sandimmun® in Nephrotic Syndrome (1991). Safety and tolerability of cyclosporin A (Sandimmun®) in idiopathic nephrotic syndrome. *Clinical Nephrology* **35** (suppl.), S48–S60.

Civillo, R., Triggiani, M., Siri, L. *et al.* (1990). Cyclosporin A rapidly inhibits mediator release from human basophils presumably by interacting with cyclophilin. *Journal of Immunology* **144**, 3891–3897.

Dieterle, A., Abeywickrama, K. & von Graffenried, B. (1988). Nephrotoxicity and hypertension in patients with autoimmune diseases treated with cyclosporine. *Transplantation Proceedings* **20** (suppl. 4), 349–355.

Di Padova, F. (1989). Pharmacology of cyclosporine (Sandimmun®)—Pharmacological effect on immune function: *in vitro* studies. *Pharmacological Reviews* **41**, 373–405.

Dougados, M., Awada, H. & Amor, B. (1988). Cyclosporin in rheumatoid arthritis: a double-blind controlled study in 52 patients. *Annals of Rheumatic Disease* **47**, 127–133.

Drachman, D. B., Adams, R. N., McIntosh, K. & Pestronk, A. (1985). Treatment of experimental myasthenia gravis with cyclosporin A. *Clinical Immunology and Immunopathology* **34**, 174–188.

Drosos, A. A., Skopouli, F. N., Costopoulos, J. S., Papadimitrious, C. S. & Moutsopoulos, M. H. (1986). Cyclosporin A in primary Sjögren's syndrome: a double-blind study. *Annals of Rheumatic Disease* **45**, 731–735.

Ellis, C. N., Fradin, M. S., Messana, J. M., Brown, M. D., Siegal, M. T., Hartley, A. H., Rocher, L. L., Wheeler, S., Hamilton, T. A., Parish, T. G., Ellis-Madu, M., Duell, E., Annesley, T. M., Cooper, K. D. & Voorhees, J. J. (1991). Cyclosporine for plaque-type psoriasis. Results of a multidose, double-blind trial. *New England Journal of Medicine* **324**, 277–284.

Eisenbarth, G. S. (1986). Type 1 diabetes mellitus. A chronic autoimmune disease. *New England Journal of Medicine* **314**, 1360–1368.

Feutren, G. (1988). Functional consequences and risk factors of chronic cyclosporin nephrotoxicity in type 1 diabetes trials. *Transplantation Proceedings* **20** (suppl. 4), 356–366.

Feutren, G. & Mihatsch, M. J. (1992). Risk factors of cyclosporine-induced nephropathy in patients with autoimmune diseases. *New England Journal of Medicine* **326**, 1654–1660.

Feutren, G., Papoz, L., Assan, R., Vialettes, B., Karsenty, G., Vexiau, P., du Rostu, H., Rodier, M., Sirmai, J., Lallemand, A. & Bach, J. F. (1986). Cyclosporin increases the rate and length of remissions in insulin-dependent diabetes of recent onset. *Lancet* **ii**, 119–124.

Feutren, G., Querin, S., Noel, L. H., Chatenoud, L., Beaurain, G., Tron, F., Lesavre, P. & Bach, J.-F. (1987). Effects of cyclosporin in severe systemic lupus erythematosus. *Journal of Pediatrics* **111**, 1063–1068.

Feutren, G., Abeywickrama, K., Friend, D. & von Graffenried, B. (1990). Renal function and blood pressure in psoriatic patients treated with cyclosporin A. *British Journal of Dermatology* **122** (suppl. 36), 57–69.

Frickhofen, N., Kaltwasser, J. P., Schrezenmeier, H., Raghavar, A., Vogt, H. G., Hermann, F., Freund, M., Meusers, P., Salama, A., Heimpal, H. & the German Aplastic Anemia Group. (1991). Treatment of aplastic anemia with antilymphocyte globulin and methylprednisolone with or without cyclosporine. *New England Journal of Medicine* **324**, 1297–1304.

Heckmatt, J., Hasson, N., Saunders, C., Thompson, N., Peters, A. M., Cambridge, G., Rose, M., Hyde, S. A. & Dubowitz, V. (1989). Cyclosporin in juvenile dermatomyositis. *Lancet* **i**, 1063–1066.

Herrmann, B. & Müller, W. (1979). Die Therapie der chronischen Polyarthritis mit Cyclosporin A, einem neuen Immunosuppressivum. *Aktuelle Rheumatologie* **4**, 173–186.

Higgins, E., Munroe, C., Marks, J., Friedmann, P. S. & Shuster, S. (1989). Relapse rates in moderately severe chronic psoriasis treated with cyclosporin A. *British Journal of Dermatology* **121**, 71–74.

Ho, V., C., Lui, H. & McLean, D. L. (1990). Cyclosporine in non-psoriatic dermatoses. *Journal of the American Academy of Dermatology* **23** (suppl.), 1248–1259.

Hultsch, T., Rodriguez, J. L., Kaliner, M. A. & Hohman, R. (1990). Cyclosporin A inhibits degranulation of rat basophilic leukemia cells and human basophils. *Journal of Immunology* **144**, 2659–2664.

Israel-Biet, D., Noel, L. H., Bach, M. A., Dardenne, M. & Bach, J. F. (1983). Marked reduction of DNA antibody production and glomerulopathy in thymulin (FTS-Zn) or cyclosporin A treated NZB × NZW F1 mice. *Clinical and Experimental Immunology* **54**, 359–363.

Kappos, L., Patzold, U., Dommasch, D., Poser, S., Haas, J., Krauseneck, P., Malin, J. P., Fierz, W., von Graffenried, B. & Gugerli, U. S. (1988). Cyclosporin vs. azathioprine in the long term treatment of multiple sclerosis — results of the German multicenter study. *Annals of Neurology* **23**, 56–63.

Laupacis, A., Stiller, C. R., Gardell, C., Keown, P., Dupré,. J., Wallace, A. C. & Thibert, P. (1983). Cyclosporin prevents diabetes in BB Wistar rats. *Lancet* **i**, 10–12.

Le Hoang, P., Girard, B., Deray, G., Le Minh, H., de Kozak, Y. Thillaye, B., Faure, J. P. & Rousselie, F. (1988). Cyclosporine in the treatment of birdshot retinochoroidopathy. *Transplantation Proceedings* **20** (suppl. 4), 128–130.

Lichtiger, S. & Present, D. H. (1990). Preliminary report: cyclosporin in treatment of severe active ulcerative colitis. *Lancet* **336**, 16–19.

Ludwin, D., Bennett, K. J., Grau, E. M., Buchanan, W. W., Bensen, W., Bombardier, C. & Tugwell, P. X. (1988). Nephrotoxicity in patients with rheumatoid arthritis treated with cyclosporine. *Transplantation Proceedings* **20** (suppl. 4), 367–370.

Ludwin, D. (1991). Cyclosporine monitoring in autoimmune and other diseases. *Clinical Biochemistry* **34**, 97–99.

Masuda, K., Nakajima, A., Urayama, A., Nakae, K., Kagure, M. & Inaba, G. (1989).

Double-masked trial of cyclosporin versus colchicine and long-term open study of cyclosporin in Behçet's disease. *Lancet* **i**, 1093–1096.

Meyrier, A. (1989). Treatment of glomerular disease with cyclosporin A. *Nephrology, Dialysis, Transplantation* **4**, 923–931.

Meyrier, A., Condamin, M. C., Broneer, D., The Collaborative Group of the French Society of Nephrology (1991). Treatment of adult idiopathic nephrotic syndrome with cyclosporin A: minimal-change disease and focal-segmental glomerulosclerosis. *Clinical Nephrology* **35** (suppl.), S37–S42.

Miescher, P. A., Favre, H., Mihatsch, M. J., Chatelenat, F., Huang, Y. P. & Zubler, R. (1988). The place of cyclosporin A in the treatment of connective tissue diseases. *Transplantation Proceedings* **20** (suppl. 4), 224–237.

Mihatsch, M. J. (1985). International workshop in cyclosporine nephropathy. *Clinical Nephrology* **24**, 107–119.

Mori, Y., Suko, M., Okudaira, H., Matsuba, I., Tsuruoka, A., Saski, A., Yokoyama, H., Tanase, T., Shida, A., Nishimura, M., Terada, E. & Ikeda, Y. (1986). Preventive effect of cyclosporin in diabetes in NOD mice. *Diabetologia* **29**, 244–247.

Mountz, J. D., Smith, H. R., Wilder, R. L., Reeves, J. P. & Steinberg, A. D. (1987). CS-A therapy in MRL-lpr/lpr mice: amelioration of immunopathology despite autoantibody production. *Journal of Immunology* **138**, 157–163.

Müller, W. & Herrmann, B. (1979). Cyclosporin A for psoriasis. *New England Journal of Medicine* **301**, 555.

Multiple Sclerosis Study Group. (1990). Efficacy and toxicity of cyclosporine in chronic progressive multiple sclerosis: a randomized, double-blinded, placebo-controlled clinical trial. *Annals of Neurology* **27**, 591–605.

Niaudet, P., Broyer, M. & Habib, R. (1991). Treatment of idiopathic nephrotic syndrome with cyclosporin A in children. *Clinical Nephrology* **35** (suppl.), S31–S36.

Nickoloff, B. J., Fischer, G. J., Mitra, R. S. & Voorhees, J. J. (1988). Additive and synergistic antiproliferative effects of cyclosporin A and gamma interferon on cultured human keratinocytes. *American Journal of Pathology* **131**, 12–18.

Nussenblatt, R. B., Rodgrigues, M. M. & Wacker, W. B. (1981). Cyclosporin A-inhibition of experimental auto-immune uveitis in Lewis rats. *Journal of Clinical Investigation* **67**, 1228–1231.

Nussenblatt, R. B., Rook, A. H., Wacker, W. B., Palestine, A. G., Scher, I. & Gery, I. (1983). Treatment of intraocular inflammatory disease with cyclosporin A. *Lancet* **ii**, 235–238.

Palestine, A. G., Austin, H. A., Balow, J. E., Antonovych, T. T., Sabnis, S. G., Preuss, H. G. & Nussenblatt, R. B. (1986). Renal histopathologic alterations in patients treated with cyclosporin for uveitis. *New England Journal of Medicine* **314**, 1293–1298.

Routhier, G., Epstein, O., Janoss, G., Thomas, A. C. & Sherlock, S. (1980). Effects of cyclosporin A on suppressor and inducer T-lymphocytes in primary biliary cirrhosis. *Lancet* **ii**, 1223–1225.

Rubenstein, A. H. & Pyke, D. (1987). Immunosuppression in the treatment of insulin-dependent (type 1) diabetes. *Lancet* **i**, 436–437.

Rudge, P., Koetsier, J. C., Mertin, J., Mispelblom Beyer, J., van Walbeek, H. K., Jones, C. R., Harrison, J., Robinson, K., Mellein, B., Poole, T., Stokuis, J. C. J. M. & Timonen, P. (1989). Randomized double-blind controlled trial of cyclosporin in multiple sclerosis. *Journal of Neurology Neurosurgery and Psychiatry* **52**, 559–565.

Sowden, J. M., Berth-Jones, J., Ross, J. S., Motley, R. J., Marks, R., Finlay, A. Y., Salek, M. S., Graham-Brown, R. A. C., Allen, B. R. & Camp, R. D. R. (1991). Double-blind, controlled, crossover study of cyclosporin in adults with severe refractory atopic dermatitis. *Lancet* **338**, 137–140.

Starzl, T. E., Nalesnik, M. A., Porter, K. A., Ho, M., Iwatsuki, S., Griffith, B. P.,

Rosenthal, J. T., Hakala, T. R., Shaw, B. W., Hardesty, R. L., Atchison, R. W., Jaffe, R. & Bahnson, H. T. (1984). Reversibility of lymphomas and lymphoproliferative lesions developing under cyclosporin-steroid therapy. *Lancet* **ii**, 583–587.

Stiller, R., Dupré, J., Gent, M., Jenner, M. R., Keown, P. A., Laupacis, A., Martell, R., Rodger, R., von Graffenried, B. & Wolfe, B. M. J. (1984). Effects of cyclosporin immunosuppression in insulin-dependent diabetes mellitus of recent onset. *Science* **223**, 1362–1367.

Tejani, A., Butt, K. & Trachtman, H. (1988). Cyclosporin A induced remission of relapsing nephrotic syndrome in children. *Kidney International* **33**, 729–734.

Timonen, P., Friend, D., Abeywickrama, K., Laburte, C., von Graffenried, B. & Feutren, G. (1990). Efficacy of low-dose cyclosporin A in psoriasis: results of dose-finding studies. *British Journal of Dermatology* **122** (suppl. 36), 33–39.

Tindall, R. S. A., Rollins, J. A., Phillips, J. T., Greenlee, R. G., Wells, L. & Belendiuk, G. (1987). Preliminary results of a double-blind, randomized, placebo-controlled trial of cyclosporin in myasthenia gravis. *New England Journal of Medicine* **316**, 719–724.

Tugwell, P., Bombardier, C., Gent, M., Bennett, K. J., Bensen, W. G., Carette, S., Chalmers, A., Esdaile, J. M., Klinkhoff, A. V., Kraag, G. R., Ludwin, D. & Roberto, R. S. (1990). Low-dose cyclosporin versus placebo in patients with rheumatoid arthritis. *Lancet* **35**, 1051–1055.

Van Joost, T. H., Bos, J. D., Heule, F. & Meinardi, M. M. H. M. (1988). Low-dose cyclosporin A in severe psoriasis. A double-blind study. *British Journal of Dermatology* **118**, 183–190.

Van Rijthoven, A. W. A. M., Dijkamns, B. A. C., Goeithe, H. S., Hermans, J., Montnor-Beckers, Y. L. M. B., Jacobs, P. C. G. & Cats, A. (1986). Cyclosporin treatment for rheumatoid arthritis: a placebo controlled, double blind, multicentre study. *Annals of Rheumatic Disease* **45**, 726–731.

Wiesner, H., Ludwig, J., Lindor, D., Jorgensen, A., Baldus, P., Homburger, A. & Dickson, E. (1990). A controlled trial of cyclosporine in the treatment of primary biliary cirrhosis. *New England Journal of Medicine* **322**, 1419–1424.

Wick, H. G., Müller, P. U. & Schwary, S. (1982). Effect of cyclosporin A on spontaneous auto-immune thyroiditis of obese strain (os) chickens. *European Journal of Immunology* **12**, 877–881.

Part 2
FK 506

Chapter 6
FK 506: pharmacology and molecular action

Angus W. Thomson, Jacky Woo, John Fung and
Thomas E. Starzl

Historical perspective

During routine screening of the fermentation broths of soil fungi (*Strepto-myces* spp.) for specific inhibitory effects on mouse mixed lymphocyte reactions (MLR), investigators of the Fujisawa Pharmaceutical Co., Ltd., Osaka, Japan, 1982–1983, identified a product of *Streptomyces tsukubaen-sis*, which exhibited powerful antilymphocytic and immunosuppressive activity (Goto *et al.*, 1987). The isolated product, designated FK 506, although classified as a macrolide antibiotic, exhibited no growth inhibitory effect on bacteria or yeast and showed only limited antifungal activity against *Aspergillus fumigatus* and *Fursarium oxysporum* (Kino *et al.*, 1987a). Early investigations revealed that FK 506 was very effective in suppressing immune responses both *in vivo* and *in vitro* and that the effective concentration was usually 10 to 100 times lower than that of cyclosporin A (CsA) (Goto *et al.*, 1987; Kino *et al.*, 1987a,b). An initial report on the capacity of FK 506 to prevent organ (heart) allograft rejection in rats was presented by T. Ochiai at the 11th International Congress of the Transplantation Society held in Helsinki in August, 1986 (Ochiai *et al.*, 1987). Since then, there has been rapid progress in elucidating the mode of action of FK 506 and in characterizing its immunosuppressive properties, including its effects on allograft survival in various animal models (reviewed by Thomson, 1989, 1990). This has led to the clinical evaluation of FK 506 in human organ (liver, kidney, heart, small bowel) transplantation in the University of Pittsburgh (Starzl *et al.*, 1989a,b, 1990; Todo *et al.*, 1990a,b; Armitage *et al.*, 1991; Shapiro *et al.*, 1991) and more recently, in 20 other centres in the United States, Europe and Japan. These centres are presently conducting prospective, random-ized controlled trials of FK 506 in primary liver transplantation.

FK 506 shares many of the properties of CsA, a structurally unrelated fungal metabolite, but the former drug is considerably more potent. The two drugs share a very similar mode of action (Sawada *et al.*, 1987; Zeevi *et al.*, 1987; Tocci *et al.*, 1989) which inhibits the activation of CD4$^+$T (helper) lymphocytes and the secretion of cytokines crucial to the induction and expression of immune reactivity. What follows is an overview of the pharmacology and molecular action of FK 506. The molecular action of FK 506 was recently reviewed by Schreiber (1991) and Schreiber and Crabtree (1992).

Physicochemical properties of FK 506

FK 506 is a white crystalline powder at room temperature and dissolves readily in non-polar solvents, such as methanol, ethanol and chloroform (Tanaka *et al.*, 1987) but it is insoluble in polar solvents. The molecular formula of FK 506, deduced by elemental analysis and mass spectrometry, is $C_{44}H_{69}NO_{12}H_2O$ (molecular weight 822) (Tanaka *et al.*, 1987). Infrared spectral analysis has revealed the presence of hydroxy groups (3530/cm), carbonyl groups (1750, 1730, 1710/cm) and an amide group (1650/cm). Further detailed structural analysis by nuclear magnetic resonance has identified two ketones, one lactone, one hemiketal, three *O*-methyls and five *C*-methyls with the remainder being 12 methylenes and 13 methines. The structure of FK 506 is shown in Fig. 6.1. FK 506, a lactone with sugar substituents differs totally in structure from CsA, a cyclic peptide comprising 11 amino acids.

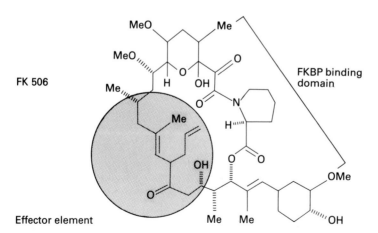

Fig. 6.1. The structure of FK 506 showing the immunophilin (FKBP) binding domain and the effector element. CsA is structurally dissimilar to FK 506.

FK 506 is relatively stable under normal laboratory conditions and has a melting point of 127–129°C. Maximal activity of FK 506 is retained after storage for 6 months at 40°C, 3 months at 82% relative humidity, 3 months under 500 Lux fluorescent light exposure and 24 months at room temperature (Tanaka *et al.*, 1987). Reports of its synthesis first appeared in 1989 (Harding *et al.*, 1989; Siekierka *et al.*, 1989).

Pharmacokinetics of FK 506 in animals and man

FK 506 is quantified in body fluids, following extraction of drug, by an enzyme-linked immunosorbant assay (ELISA), in which either a monoclonal or polyclonal antibody is employed. In blood, most of the FK 506 is bound to erythrocytes (mean trough blood:plasma ratio 10:1). The sensitivity limit is 20 pg/ml in plasma (Tamura *et al.*, 1987). A modified ELISA, using a solid phase extraction method and a mouse monoclonal anti-FK 506 antibody for quantitation of FK 506 in human plasma, has been described more recently (Cadoff *et al.*, 1990). The extent to which the antibody cross-reacts with FK 506 metabolites is unknown.

Monitoring of plasma FK 506 concentrations in the dog (Tamura *et al.*, 1987) has shown that, at immunosuppressive doses (1.0 mg/kg per os) the trough level lies between 0.08 and 0.4 ng/ml, while at non-immunosuppressive doses, a lower trough concentration is observed. This indicates that the effective, prophylactic plasma trough level is between 0.1 and 0.4 ng/ml (Todo *et al.*, 1988; Ochiai *et al.*, 1989). Coadministration of FK 506 with CsA can reduce the threshold effective FK 506 trough level (Ochiai *et al.*, 1989) and this may explain the synergy exhibited between these two drugs in experimental animals (Murase *et al.*, 1987; Todo *et al.*, 1987; Ochiai *et al.*, 1989) and reported earlier in *in vitro* models (Sawada *et al.*, 1987). In canine kidney recipients undergoing rejection, reduction in serum creatinine level and attenuation or disappearance of the cellular infiltrate during rejection was observed in FK 506-treated animals and was shown to correlate with an increase in FK 506 trough level (Ochiai *et al.*, 1989).

FK 506 is absorbed slowly after oral administration and distributed in various organs, including lung, spleen, heart and kidney (Venkataramanan *et al.*, 1990). Whilst absorption of CsA appears to be dependent on availability of bile in the gut, bile is unnecessary for FK 506 absorption (Jain *et al.*, 1990). The majority of FK 506 appears to be metabolized by *N*-demethylation and hydroxylation in the liver and is then excreted in bile, urine and faeces within 48 h of administration (Venkataramanan *et al.*, 1990, 1991). Activity of cytochrome P-450, the mixed function oxidase system of isoenzymes that metabolizes CsA, is downregulated by FK 506 both *in vivo* (Venkataramanan *et al.*, 1990) and *in vitro* (Burke *et al.*,

1990). This implies a possible mechanism whereby FK 506 affects the pharmacokinetics of CsA, which also depends on this degradation system.

Studies aimed at determining the optimal route of administration and dosage of FK 506 for clinical study were hampered by the severe toxic effects of the drug in dogs. Fortunately, the choice of method of drug delivery in the first clinical trial, i.e. 0.15 mg/kg intravenous (i.v.) over an hour soon after liver revascularization, followed by 0.075 mg/kg/12 h until the patient could eat, then oral doses of 0.15 mg/kg/12 h, was reasonably well tolerated (Todo et al., 1990a). With i.v. therapy, continuous instead of 4-h infusions reduce the associated risks of transient renal and neurological dysfunctions, especially in high-risk patients (Abu-Elmagd et al., 1991a,b). The i.v. doses used in man have required downward revision (Starzl et al., 1991a; Abu-Elmagd et al., 1991a,b). Peak plasma concentration is observed at the end of the infusion and then levels decline slowly over the next 24 h (Venkataramanan et al., 1990, 1991). Plasma trough levels tend to be about 1 ng/ml, the effective immunosuppressive concentration in vitro. The half-life ranges from 3.5 to 40.5 h, with a mean of 8.7 h (Venkataramanan et al., 1990). Drug absorption following oral administration is highly variable. The mean bioavailability is about 25% (range 6–57%). A peak plasma level of 0.4–3.7 ng/ml is reached after 1–4 h of an oral dose at 0.15 mg/kg (Venkataramanan et al., 1990). The half-life of CsA is prolonged in patients receiving FK 506, from a normal 6–15 h to 26–74 h. This indicates that FK 506 may affect CsA metabolism, a phenomenon demonstrated recently in vitro (Burke et al., 1990).

Experience gained from studies in CsA-treated liver transplant patients indicates that alterations in the absorption and metabolism of CsA occur with changing liver function (Grevel & Kahan, 1989). Since FK 506 and CsA share similar physical properties, the same issues might be expected to arise for FK 506. In five jaundiced patients with liver dysfunction, peak and trough FK 506 levels were higher than in patients with good hepatic function. Moreover, the half-life of FK 506 was increased and its clearance was reduced in patients with hepatic dysfunction (Jain et al., 1990). As a result, the overall bioavailability of FK 506 was expected to increase because of the greatly reduced intrinsic clearance (Venkataramanan et al., 1990, 1991).

The full impact of hepatic dysfunction on FK 506 pharmacokinetics was not appreciated until clinical trials were well established (Abu-Elmagd et al., 1991a; Starzl et al., 1991a). In liver transplant recipients, whose grafts do not function well initially and/or fail to recover quickly, the daily i.v. dose of 0.15 mg/kg quickly leads to enormously high trough plasma levels (> 100 ng/ml has been recorded), complete renal failure and neurotoxicity, which can progress to mutism, convulsions and coma. Prompt dose reduction is required and guidance for this is provided by rapid turn around time in the plasma assays. Dose control of the i.v. FK 506 is easier if the drug is given by constant infusion instead of the 2-h bolus, which was originally used.

Even with well-functioning liver grafts, or in kidney and heart recipients whose hepatic function is normal, the University of Pittsburgh patients are now given a smaller i.v. dose of 0.075 or 0.10 mg/kg/day, instead of the 0.15 mg/kg originally employed. The larger doses cause unacceptable increases in plasma levels and can cause acute renal failure or neurotoxicity (Abu-Elmagd et al., 1991a; Starzl et al., 1991a). Failure to make these revisions constitutes an unnecessary risk. Plasma levels of 3–5 ng/ml can be accepted during the peri-operative period of constant drug infusion, if there is no evidence of toxicity, but otherwise the doses should be reduced to < 3 ng/ml.

A number of interactions of FK 506 with other drugs have been observed. Trough plasma concentrations of FK 506 are increased by co-administration of erythromycin, fluconazole and clotrimazole, whilst the effects of phenytoin, phenobarbital and acyclovir on FK 506 pharmaco-kinetics are currently being investigated.

Antilymphocytic activity of FK 506

The effects of FK 506 on T-cell responses, *in vitro* and *in vivo*, and the influence of the drug on gene expression and cytokine production are summarized in Table 6.1. Studies that are aimed at elucidating the immunosuppressive action of FK 506 have shown that the drug is very effective in suppressing both alloantigen- and T-cell mitogen-induced lymphocyte proliferation. The 50% inhibitory concentrations (IC_{50}) of FK 506 and CsA for human MLR are 0.21 nM and 20 nM respectively and for phytohaemagglutinin (PHA)-induced responses 8.6 nM and 750 nM respectively (Thomson, 1989; Yoshimura et al., 1989a). Thus, compared with PHA-induced T-cell responses, those evoked by alloantigens are more FK 506-sensitive (Yoshimura et al., 1989a; Woo et al., 1990b; Zeevi et al., 1990). In contrast, anti-CD28-induced responses are FK 506 insensitive (Kay & Benzie, 1990; Bierer et al., 1991). Taken together, these observations reflect inherent differences between CD3- and CD28-activation pathways and their differential sensitivities to FK 506. Like CsA, FK 506 inhibits T-cell activation mediated not only by the T-cell receptor–CD3 complex, but also via another cell surface molecule, CD2 (Bierer et al., 1991).

Delay in the addition of FK 506 to mitogen-stimulated cultures results in reduction of its antilymphocytic activity (Kay et al., 1989), indicating a selective influence of FK 506 on early events in T-cell activation. The latter appear to include Ca^{2+} mobilization, protein kinase C (PKC) activation, cytokine gene transcription, cytokine secretion and cytokine-receptor expression, all of which occur within the first 2 h of T-

Table 6.1. Effects of FK 506 on T cells

Phenomenon	Effect	Reference
Lymphocyte responses in vitro		
MLR (human, mouse)	↓	Kino *et al.*, 1987b; Sawada *et al.*, 1987; Yoshimura *et al.*, 1989a
Con A, PHA-induced lymphocyte proliferation	↓	Sawada *et al.*, 1987; Yoshimura *et al.*, 1989a; Woo *et al.*, 1990b
Tc induction	↓	Sawada *et al.*, 1987; Yoshimura *et al.*, 1989a
Tc function	↓	Sawada *et al.*, 1987; Yoshimura *et al.*, 1989a
Ts induction	↓	Yoshimura *et al.*, 1989a
Cell-mediated immunity		
DTH (MBSA)	↓	Kino *et al.*, 1987a
Graft-versus-host disease	↓	Kino *et al.*, 1987a
Host-versus-graft popliteal lymph node assay	↓	Morris *et al.*, 1989
T-dependent humoral response:		
Alloantibody	↓	Propper *et al.*, 1990
Anti-SRBC Ab	↓	Woo *et al.*, 1990a
Ex vivo Con A-induced spleen cell proliferation	↓	Woo *et al.*, 1990c
Lymphokine production		
IL-1	?	
IL-2	↓	Kino *et al.*, 1987b; Sawada *et al.*, 1987
IL-3	↓	Kino *et al.*, 1987b
IL-4	?	
IL-5	?	
IL-6	NC	Yoshimura *et al.*, 1989b
INFγ	↓	Kino *et al.*, 1987b
GM-CSF	↓	Kino *et al.*, 1987b
Lymphokine receptor expression		
IL-2R	↓	Kino *et al.*, 1987b; Yoshimura *et al.*, 1989a,b; Woo *et al.*, 1990b

Table 6.1. *Continued*

Phenomenon	Effect	Reference
MHC antigen expression		
HLA-DR on activated T cells	↓	Woo *et al.*, 1990b
HLA-DR on monocytes	NC	Woo *et al.*, 1990b
Gene expression		
IL-1α, β	NC	Tocci *et al.*, 1989
IL-2	↓	Tocci *et al.*, 1989
IL-3	↓	Tocci *et al.*, 1989
IL-4	↓	Tocci *et al.*, 1989
IL-10	NC	Wang *et al.*, 1991
GM-CSF	↓	Tocci *et al.*, 1989
TNFα	↓	Tocci *et al.*, 1989
IFNγ	↓	Tocci *et al.*, 1989
c-*myc*	↓	Tocci *et al.*, 1989
c-*fos*	NC	Tocci *et al.*, 1989
TfR	NC	Tocci *et al.*, 1989
IL-2R α-chain	NC	Tocci *et al.*, 1989
TNFβ	NC	Tocci *et al.*, 1989
MHC class I HLA B-7	NC	Tocci *et al.*, 1989
FKBP	?	
TCRβ-chain	↑	Kay *et al.*, 1989

Abbreviations: ↓, decrease; ↑, increase; NC, no change; ?, unclear; DTH, delayed-type hypersensitivity; TfR, transferrin receptor; FKBP, FK 506-binding protein; MLR, mixed lymphocyte reaction; SRBC, sheep red blood cells.

cell activation.

The generation of cytotoxic T lymphocytes (CTL) and suppressor T cells during human MLR is inhibited by FK 506 (Yoshimura *et al.*, 1989a), but the cytolytic activity of CTL against target cells during the effector phase is FK 506 resistant (Sawada *et al.*, 1987; Yoshimura *et al.*, 1989a). This indicates that FK 506 affects only the early induction phase of CTL development and has no effect on antigen recognition by CTL or on the cytolytic mechanism which results in target-cell destruction. Moreover, Zeevi *et al.* (1990) have reported that FK 506 does not affect human CTL differentiation or maturation from pre-effector to effector CTL. The recent finding that FK 506 has little or no effect on natural killer (NK) cell numbers or function or on antibody-dependent cytotoxicity (Markus *et al.*, 1991; Wasik *et al.*, 1991), suggests beneficial sparing of natural immunity against infectious agents.

Information concerning effects of FK 506 on processing and presentation of antigen by antigen-presenting cells (APC), is presently very limited.

Nevertheless, FK 506 concentrations which strongly inhibit antigen purified protein derivative (PPD)-induced human T-cell proliferation, have little effect on antigen processing and presentation by human blood monocytes (Woo et al., 1990a). There is evidence, however, that FK 506 may impair alloantigen processing/presentation in human MLR (Thomas et al., 1990). Cooper et al. (1991) observed that any effect of FK 506 on the presentation of microbial (Listeria) antigens by murine macrophages could be ascribed to drug carryover to the readout system (T-cell proliferation).

Experimental data concerning the inhibitory effect of FK 506 on mitogen- and alloantigen-induced T-cell responses in culture, indicate that FK 506, like CsA, exerts its primary influence on CD4$^+$ (helper) T cells, with consequent effects on other cell types. Several studies have demonstrated that FK 506 inhibits the expression of the activation molecules interleukin (IL)-2R, MHC class II antigens and transferrin receptor (TfR), in a dose-dependent manner (Yoshimura et al., 1989a; Woo et al., 1990b). These effects, however, may be secondary to the potent inhibitory action of FK 506 on IL-2 production and to the reduction of its consequent, autocrine effect on the expression of IL-2R. Considered in conjunction with the reported failure of FK 506 to inhibit IL-2R mRNA expression (Tocci et al., 1989), these observations suggest post-transcriptional inhibition of IL-2R expression by the drug.

Effects of FK 506 on early T-cell activation genes

FK 506 strongly inhibits expression of mRNA for early T-cell-activation genes, including those encoding IL-2, IL-3, IL-4, IFNγ, granulocyte-monocyte-colony-stimulating factor (GM-CSF) and c-myc (Tocci et al., 1989; Dumont et al., 1990b; Metcalfe & Richards, 1990). It is likely that the generation or transmission of a common activation signal for these genes is inhibited by FK 506, as prevention of gene expression by the drug is unaffected by the nature of the inducers used. On the other hand, recent studies have shown that FK 506 does not inhibit production of human IL-6 (Yoshimura et al., 1989b) and may spare IL-10 (cytokine synthesis inhibitory factor) gene transcription by cloned murine helper T cells (T$_{H2}$) in vitro, whilst suppressing concomitant IL-4 mRNA production by these cells (Wang et al., 1991). Thus, differential interference with cytokine gene expression may be an important mechanism whereby FK 506 and CsA inhibit immune-cell activation. Inhibition of gene expression by FK 506 is specific to early genes. No inhibition of constitutively expressed T-cell receptor (TCR)-β, MHC class I human leukocyte antigen (HLA)-B7, GPDH or late-phase genes, like IL-2R, TfR and tumour necrosis factor (TNF)-β (Kay et al., 1989; Tocci et al., 1989) is observed. Inhibition and superinduction, respectively, of krox 20 and krox 24 mRNA by FK 506 in murine lymphocytes (Metcalfe & Richards, 1990) may be of particular significance, since these genes encode proteins which are likely to regulate gene expression. In contrast to its influence on lymphokine gene expression and protein secretion, no inhibitory action of FK 506 on monokine gene expression (including IL-1α or IL-1β mRNA synthesis) or monokine production (TNFα and IL-6) after lipopolysaccharide (LPS) stimulation or human monocytes has been observed (Tocci *et al.*, 1989).

Experiments designed to ascertain the influence of FK 506 prior to gene transcription have shown that FK 506 does not affect Ca^{2+} mobilization (Bierer *et al.*, 1990), phosphatidylinositol turnover (Fujii *et al.*, 1989) or PKC activities (Gschwendt *et al.*, 1989) following binding of the antigen receptor. The target of FK 506 is thus probably a later event elicited by the T-cell antigen receptor (TCR) pathway and/or a separate activation pathway distinct from phosphoinositol breakdown.

Influence of FK 506 on gene transcription

The precise molecular events which occur in the cytosol during T-cell activation and lead eventually to gene activation within the nucleus are still unclear. Following cytoplasmic biochemical changes, one or more signals pass into the nucleus to influence the IL-2 gene, expression of which is regulated by a transcription initiation site (Durand *et al.*, 1987; Williams *et al.*, 1988). The nucleic acid sequence of the IL-2 enhancer (regulatory) region has been identified and several *cis*-acting transcriptional segments of this region that bind different nuclear factors have been investigated (Williams *et al.*, 1988; Muegge & Durum, 1990). Two sequences of this enhancer, − 285 to − 255 and − 93 to − 63 activate a linked promoter in response to signals generated from the antigen receptor (Durand *et al.*, 1987) (Fig. 6.2.). These two regions are bound by two distinct nuclear factors to protect them from DNAse digestion (Durand *et al.*, 1987). One of these nuclear factors, NFIL-2A, which is present in both

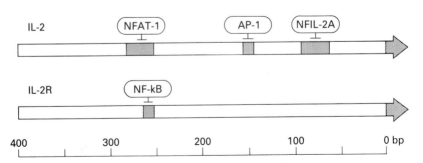

Fig. 6.2. IL-2 and IL-2R gene promotor sequences, showing the binding sites of nuclear regulatory proteins.

activated and non-activated T cells, binds to the regulatory site identified in the IL-2 enhancer between -93 and -63. This sequence is referred to as antigen receptor response element-1 (ARRE-1) (Fig. 6.2), since it can only be activated through the TCR/CD3 pathway and not by phorbol myristate acetate (PMA) which activates PKC. The IL-2 gene promoter is then activated by the sequence protected from DNAse digestion, once an activation signal is elicited in the TCR. In contrast, the constitutive activity of the IL-2 promoter when the NFIL-2A binding is disrupted by mutation implies that NFIL-2A exerts a negative signal in resting T cells (Nabel et al., 1988). Since NFIL-2A is present in both activated and non-activated cells, its presence and activity may not be influenced by immunosuppressive agents. A second antigen receptor response element (ARRE-2) present between -285 and -255 of the IL-2 enhancer is protected from DNAse by the nuclear factor of activated T cells-(NFAT) 1, which is only expressed in activated T cells (Shaw et al., 1988). There is evidence that deletion of the NFAT binding site significantly impairs activity of the IL-2 enhancer (Durand et al., 1987). Moreover, the increase in NFAT binding activity in nuclear extracts of activated T cells (Shaw et al., 1988) and the appearance of NFAT about 10 min before the earliest detectable IL-2 mRNA implies that activation of the IL-2 gene is dependent on prior activation of NFAT. Cooperation between NFAT and NFIL-2A results in full enhancer activity, though each binds to a different sequence. Recent studies by Granelli-Piperno et al. (1990) have shown that the binding of NFAT to the transcriptional element is suppressed by FK 506, thereby inhibiting IL-2 gene activation and consequently, lymphokine production.

A third sequence, the AP-1 binding site, which is responsible for IL-2 transcription in response to PMA, is identified at position -240. AP-1 is the cellular homologue of the protein product of the v-*jun* oncogene (Ryder et al., 1988). Binding of AP-1 to the AP-1 binding site makes a normally unresponsive promoter respond to agents that activate PKC. A functional AP-1 site in the IL-2 gene suggests a response to signals emanating from the TCR and to signals initiated by the activation of PKC. While the binding of AP-1 to its binding site has been shown to be markedly reduced by FK 506 in EL 4 lymphoma cells (Granelli-Piperno et al., 1990), its transcriptional enhancing activity is not affected by FK 506 in human synovial fibroblasts.

Activation of the IL-2R gene is also essential for commitment of T lymphocytes to cell division and immunological functions. A binding site for the PMA-responsive transcriptional factor NF-kB was localized between -255 and -268 of the IL-2R transcription initiation site. Granelli-Piperno et al. (1990) reported recently that FK 506 had only a slight inhibitory effect on NF-kB binding, which is consistent with the minimal effect of FK 506 on IL-2R mRNA expression discussed earlier.

Role of FKBP in immunosuppression

A novel class of cytosolic proteins of 'immunophilins' has become the focus of attention with regard to the mechanism of action of FK 506 and CsA. Two families of immunophilins have been identified, namely the cyclophilins (predominant member cyclophilin A) and the FK 506-binding proteins (FKBPs) (predominant member FKBP 12) which are believed to play essential roles in the immunosuppressive actions of CsA and FK 506 respectively (Harding *et al.*, 1989; Siekierka *et al.*, 1989; Maki *et al.*, 1990). Although their physiological role is unknown, both proteins possess peptidyl-prolyl *cis-trans* isomerase (PPIase) activity, that catalyses the slow *cis-trans* isomerization of ala-pro bonds in oligopeptides and accelerates slow, rate-limiting steps in the folding of several proteins (Fischer *et al.*, 1989). The PPIase activity of cyclophilin and FKBP is strongly inhibited by their respective ligands (Fischer *et al.*, 1989; Siekierka *et al.*, 1989b), suggesting that PPIase activity may play a role in lymphocyte activation.

FK 506 binds with high affinity to FKBP (Harding *et al.*, 1989; Siekierka *et al.*, 1989), a heat-stable cytosolic component with a molecular weight (10–12 kD) lower than cyclophilin (17 737 D) (Siekierka *et al.*, 1989; Palaszyncki *et al.*, 1991). No specific binding of FK 506 to purified calf thymus cyclophilin can be detected (Siekierka *et al.*, 1989) and anti-cyclophilin antibody does not cross-react with bovine or human FKBPs (Harding *et al.*, 1989). Cloning of FKBP (Standaert *et al.*, 1990; Tropschug *et al.*, 1990) has revealed that, despite their common enzymatic properties, FKBP and cyclophilin have dissimilar sequences.

The first 16 residues of human FKBP are identical to the corresponding bovine sequence (Harding *et al.*, 1989). cDNA of human lymphocyte FKBP has been synthesized and binds with mRNA species of 1.8 kb isolated from brain, lung, liver, placenta and leukocytes (Maki *et al.*, 1990; Standaert *et al.*, 1990), demonstrating the ubiquitous nature of this protein. The level of FKBP mRNA in (leukaemic) Jurkat T cells is, however, unaffected by cell activation stimulated through phorbol esters and ionomycin (Maki *et al.*, 1990). Inhibition of FKBP's PPIase activity is specific to the binding of FK 506 (or the structurally related macrolide rapamycin), while inhibition of cyclophilin's PPIase activity is specific to CsA (Siekierka *et al.*, 1989b; Dumont *et al.*, 1990a). Although binding of the drug by its receptor (or 'immunophilin') inhibits isomerase activity, recent results indicate that the immunosuppressive effects of FK 506 and CsA result from the formation of complexes between the drug and its respective isomerase (Liu *et al.*, 1991). Both FK 506–FKBP and CsA–cyclophilin complexes have been shown to bind specifically to three polypeptides — calmodulin and the two subunits of calcineurin (a Ca^{2+}-activated, serine-threonine protein phosphatase). In each case, the interaction of the immunophilin appears to be with calcineurin (Fig. 6.3). The drug–immun-ophilin complexes have been shown to block the Ca^{2+}-activated phospha-tase activity of calcineurin (Liu et al., 1991). Thus, calcineurin appears to be the target of the drug–immunophilin complexes.

A second, key observation in unravelling the molecular action of FK 506 is that the drug–immunophilin complexes block Ca^{2+}-dependent translocation of the pre-existing, cytoplasmic component of NFAT to the nucleus (Flanagan et al., 1991). The nuclear component of NFAT is transcriptionally inactive in all cells other than activated T lymphocytes (see above) and is induced by signals from the TCR. Its appearance is not blocked by FK 506 or CsA. Current thinking is that FK 506 and CsA block dephosphorylation of the cytoplasmic component of NFAT which is required for its translocation to the nucleus (Fig. 6.4). In the absence of both nuclear and cytoplasmic components, binding of NFAT to DNA and transcriptional activation of the IL-2 gene is suppressed.

Conclusion

It is now clear that FK 506 and CsA are pro-drugs and that their pharmacological action, resulting in immunosuppression, is dependent on binding to the appropriate immunophilin (FKBP or cyclophilin, respec-tively). This results in modulation of the enzymic activity of the protein phosphatase calcineurin which, in turn, may impair translocation of the cytosolic component of the IL-2 gene transcription factor NFAT to the T-cell nucleus. Several key issues remain to be resolved, including the physiological role of calcineurin. Elucidation of these and related molecu-lar events underlying T-cell activation will play an important role in the design of future clinical immunosuppressive agents.

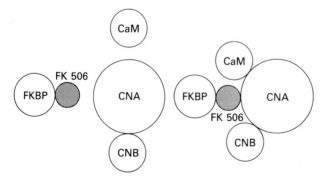

Fig. 6.3. Within the T lymphocyte, the FK 506–FKBP (FK 506 binding protein) complex binds with high affinity to calcineurin–calmodulin to form a pentameric complex which interferes with Ca^{2+}-dependent signalling pathways. Recent observa-tions indicate that calcineurin (a protein phosphatase) is the target of the FK 506–FKBP complex. CaM, calmodulin; CNA, calcineurin A; CNB, calcineurin B.

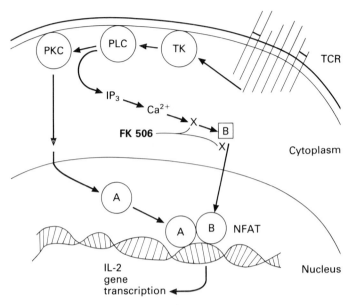

Fig. 6.4. Influence of FK 506 on signal transduction within T cells. FK 506 blocks translocation of the pre-existing cytoplasmic component of NFAT (B) to the nucleus by acting either on a Ca^{2+} signalling pathway or on translocation following the action of this pathway. Both components of NFAT are required for DNA binding and activation of the IL-2 gene. TCR, T-cell receptor; TK, tyrosine kinase; PLC, phospholipase C; PKC, protein kinase C; A, induced nuclear component of NFAT; B, existing cytoplasmic component of NFAT.

References

Abu-Elmagd, K., Fung, J. J., Alessiani, M., Jain, A., Venkataramanan, R. & Warty, V. S. (1991a). The effect of graft function on FK 506 plasma levels, doses and renal function: with particular reference to the liver. *Transplantation* **52**, 71.

Abu-Elmagd, K., Fung, J. J., Draviam, R., Shannon, W., Jain, A., Alessiani, M., Takaya, S., Venkataramanan, R., Warty, V., Tzakis, A., Todo, S. & Starzl, T. E. (1991b). Four hour versus 24 hour intravenous infusion of FK 506 in liver transplantation. *Transplantation Proceedings* **23**, 2767-2770.

Armitage, J. M., Kormos, R. L., Fung, J., Lavee, J., Fricker, F. J., Griffith, B. P. *et al* (1991). Preliminary experience with FK 506 in thoracic transplantation. *Transplantation* **52**, 164-167.

Bierer, B. E., Schreiber, S. L. & Burakoff, S. J. (1990). Mechanism of immunosuppression by FK 506 — preservation of T cell transmembrane signal transduction. *Transplantation* **49**, 1168-1202.

Bierer, B. E., Schreiber, S. L. & Burakoff, S. J. (1991). The effect of the immunosuppressant FK 506 on alternate pathways of T cell activation. *European Journal of Immunology* **21**, 439-445.

Burke, M. D., Omar, G., Thomson, A. W. & Whiting, P. H. (1990). Inhibition of the metabolism of cyclosporine by human liver microsomes by FK 506. *Transplantation* **50**, 901-902.

Cadoff, E. M., Venkataramanan, R., Krajack, A., Jain, A. S., Fung, J. J., Todo, S. & Starzl, T. E. (1990). Assay of FK 506 in plasma. *Transplantation Proceedings* **22**, 50-51.

Cooper, M. H., Gregory, S. H., Thomson, A. W., Fung, J. J., Starzl, T. E. & Wing, E. J. (1991). Evaluation of the influence of FK 506, rapamycin, and cyclosporine on processing and presentation of particulate antigens by macrophages: assessment of a drug 'carryover' effect. *Transplantation Proceedings* **23**, 2957-2958.

Dumont, F. J., Melino, M. R., Staruch, M. J., Koprak, S. L., Fischer, P. A. & Sigal, N. H. (1990a). The immunosuppressive macrolides FK 506 and rapamycin act as reciprocal antagonists in mature T cells. *Journal of Immunology* **144**, 1418-1424.

Dumont, F. J., Staruch, M. J., Koprak, S. L., Melino, M. R. & Sigal, N. H. (1990b). Distinct mechanisms of suppression of murine T cell activation by the related macrolides FK 506 and rapamycin. *Journal of Immunology* **144**, 251-258.

Durand, D. B., Bush, M. R., Morgan, J. G., Weiss, A. & Crabtree, G. R. (1987). A 275 basepair fragment at the 5' end of the interleukin 2 gene enhances expression from a heterologous promoter in response to signals from the T cell antigen receptor. *Journal of Experimental Medicine* **165**, 395.

Fischer, G., Wittmann-Liebold, B., Lang, K., Kiefhaber, T. & Schmid, F. X. (1989). Cyclophilin and peptidyl-prolyl *cis-trans* isomerase are probably identical proteins. *Nature* **337**, 476-478.

Flanagan, W. M., Corthesy, B., Bram, R. J. & Crabtree, G. R. (1991). Nuclear association of a T-cell transcription factor blocked by FK 506 and cyclosporin A. *Nature* **352**, 803-807.

Fujii, Y., Fujii, S. & Kaneko, T. (1989). Effect of a novel immunosuppressive agent, FK 506, on mitogen-induced inositol phospholipid degradation in rat thymocytes. *Transplantation* **47**, 1081-1082.

Goto, T., Kino, T., Hatanaka, H., Nishiyama, M., Okuhara, M., Kohsaka, M., Aoki, H. & Imanaka, H. (1987). Discovery of FK 506, a novel immunosuppressant isolated from *Streptomyces tsukubaenis*. *Transplantation Proceedings* **19** (suppl. 6), 4-8.

Granelli-Piperno, A., Nolan, P., Inaba, K. & Steinman, R. M. (1990). The effect of immunosuppressive agents on the induction of nuclear factors that bind to sites on the interleukin-2 promoter. *Journal of Experimental Medicine* **172**, 1869-1872.

Grevel, J. & Kahan, B. D. (1989). Pharmacokinetics of cyclosporin A. In Thomson, A. W. (ed.) *Cyclosporin, Mode of Action and Clinical Application*, pp. 252-266. Kluwer Academic Publisher, London.

Gschwendt, M., Kittstein, W. & Marks, F. (1989). The immunosuppressant FK 506, like cyclosporins and didemnin B, inhibits calmodulin-dependent phosphorylation of the elongation factor 2 *in vitro* and biological effects of phorbol ester TPA on mouse skin *in vivo*. *Immunobiology* **179**, 1-7.

Harding, M. W., Galat, A., Uehling, D. E. & Schreiber, S. L. (1989). A receptor for the immunosuppressant FK 506 is a *cis-trans* peptidyl-prolyl isomerase. *Nature* **341**, 758-760.

Jain, A. B., Venkataramanan, R., Cadoff, E., Fung, J. J., Todo, S., Krajack, A. & Starzl, T. E. (1990). Effect of hepatic dysfunction and T tube clamping on FK 506 pharmacokinetics and trough concentrations. *Transplantation Proceedings* **22**, 57-59.

Kay, J. E. & Benzie, C. R. (1990). T lymphocyte activation through the CD28 pathway is insensitive to inhibition by the immunosuppressive drug FK 506. *Immunology Letters* **23**, 155-160.

Kay, J. E., Benzie, C. R., Goodier, M. R., Wick, C. J. & Doe, S. E. A. (1989). Inhibition of T-lymphocyte activation by the immunosuppressive drug FK 506. *Immunology* **67**, 473-477.

Kino, T., Hatanaka, H., Hashimoto, M., Nishiyama, M., Goto, T., Okuhara, M., Kohsaka, M., Aoki, H. & Imanaka, H. (1987a). FK 506, a novel immunosuppressant isolated from a *Streptomyces*. I. Fermentation, isolation and physiochemical and biological characteristics. *Journal of Antibiotics* **40**, 1249–1255.

Kino, T., Hatanaka, H., Miyata, S., Inamura, N., Nishiyama, M., Yajima, T., Goto, T., Okuhara, M., Kohsaka, M., Aoki, H. & Ochiai, T. (1987b). FK 506, a novel immunosuppressant isolated from a *Streptomyces*. II. Immunosuppressive effect of FK 506 *in vitro*. *Journal of Antibiotics* **40**, 1256–1265.

Liu, J., Farmer, J. D., Lane, W. S., Friedman, J., Weissman, I. & Schreiber, S. L. (1991). Calcineurin is a common target of cyclophilin — cyclosporin A and FKBP–FK506 complexes. *Cell* **66**, 807–815.

Maki, N., Sekiguchi, F., Nishimaki, J., Miwa, K., Hayano, T., Takahashi, N. & Suzuki, M. (1990). Complementary DNA encoding the human T-cell FK 506-binding protein, a peptidylprolyl *cis-trans* isomerase distinct from cyclophilin. *Proceedings of the National Academy of Sciences USA* **87**, 5440–5443.

Markus, P. M., Van Den Brink, M. R. M., Luchs, B. A., Fung, J. J., Starzl, T. E. & Hiserodt, J. C. (1991). Effects of *in vitro* treatment with FK 506 on natural killer cells in rats. *Transplantation* **51**, 913–915.

Metcalfe, S. M. & Richards, F. M. (1990). Cyclosporine, FK 506, and rapamycin. Some effects on early activation events in serum-free, mitogen-stimulated mouse spleen cells. *Transplantation* **49**, 798–802.

Morris, R. E., Hoyt, E. G., Murphy, M. P. & Shorthouse, R. (1989). Immunopharmacology of FK 506. *Transplantation Proceedings* **21**, 1042–1044.

Muegge, K. & Durum, S. K. (1990). Cytokines and transcription factors. *Cytokines* **2**, 1–8.

Murase, N., Todo, S., Lee, P. H., Lai, H. S., Chapman, F., Nalesnik, M. A., Makowka, L. & Starzl, T. E. (1987). Heterotopic heart transplantation in the rat receiving FK 506 alone or with cyclosporine. *Transplantation Proceedings* **19** (suppl. 6), 71–75.

Nabel, G. J., Gorka, C. & Baltimore, D. (1988). T-cell-specific expression of interleukin 2, evidence for a negative regulatory site. *Proceedings of the National Academy of Sciences USA* **85**, 2934–2938.

Ochiai, T., Gunji, Y., Sakamoto, K., Suzuki, T., Isegawa, N., Asano, T. & Isono, K. (1989). Optimum serum trough levels of FK 506 in renal allotransplantation of the beagle dog. *Transplantation* **48**, 189–193.

Ochiai, T., Nakajima, K., Nagata, M., Suzuki, T., Asano, T., Uematsu, T., Goto, T., Hori, S., Kenmach, T., Nakagori, T. & Isono, K. (1987). Effect of a new immunosuppressive agent, FK 506, on heterotopic allotransplantation in the rat. *Transplantation Proceedings* **19**, 1284–1286.

Palaszynski, E. W., Donnelly, J. G. & Soldin, S. J. (1991). Purification and characterization of cyclosporine and FK 506 binding proteins from a human T-helper cell line. *Clinical Biochemistry* **24**, 63–70.

Propper, D. J., Woo, J., Thomson, A. W., Catto, G. R. D. & Macleod, A. M. (1990). FK 506-influence on anti-class I MHC alloantibody responses to blood transfusions. *Transplantation* **50**, 267–271.

Ryder, K., Lau, L. F. & Nathans, D. (1988). A gene activated by growth factors is related to the oncogene v-*jun*. *Proceedings of the National Academy of Sciences of the USA*, **85**, 1487.

Sawada, S., Suzuki, G., Kawase, Y. & Takaku, F. (1987). Novel immunosuppressive agent, FK 506. *In vitro* effects on the cloned T cell activation. *Journal of Immunology* **139**, 1797–1803.

Schreiber, S. L. (1991). Chemistry and biology of the immunophilins and their immunosuppressive ligands. *Science* **251**, 283–287.

Schreiber, S. L. & Crabtree, G. R. (1992). The mechanism of action of cyclosporin A and FK 506. *Immunology Today* **13**, 136–142.

Shapiro, R., Jordan, M., Fung, J., McCauley, J., Johnston, J., Iwaki, Y. (1991). Kidney transplantation under FK 506 immunosuppression. *Transplantation Proceedings* **23**, 920–923.

Shaw, J., Utz, P., Durand, D., Toole, J., Emmel, E. & Crabtree, G. (1988). Identification of a putative regulator of early T-cell activation genes. *Science* **241**, 202.

Siekierka, J. J., Staruch, M. J., Hung, S. H. Y. & Sigal, N. H. (1989). FK-506, a potent novel immunosuppressive agent, binds to a cytosolic protein which is distinct from the cyclosporin A-binding protein, cyclophilin. *Journal of Immunology* **143**, 1580–1583.

Standaert, R. F., Galat, A., Verdine, G. L. & Schreiber, S. L. (1990). Molecular cloning and overexpression of the human FK-506-binding protein FKBP. *Nature* **346**, 671–674.

Starzl, T. E., Abu-Elmagd, K., Fung, J. J., Todo, S., Tzakis, A., McCauley, J. & Demetris, A. J. (1991a). Clinical experience with FK 506. *Presse Medicale* (in press).

Starzl, T. E., Fung, J., Jordan, M., Shapiro, R., Tzakis, A., McCauley, J., Johnston, J., Iwaki, Y., Jain, A., Alessiani, M. & Todo, S. (1990). Kidney transplantation under FK 506. *Journal of the American Medical Association* **264**, 63–67.

Starzl, T. E., Fung, J., Venkataramanan, R., Todo, S., Demetris, A. J. & Jain, A. (1989). FK 506 for liver, kidney and pancreas transplantation. *Lancet* **ii**, 1000–1004.

Starzl, T. E., Todo, S., Tzakis, A., Alessiani, M., Casavilla, A., Elmagd-Abu, K. & Fung, J. (1991b). The many faces of multivisceral transplantation. *Surgery, Gynecology and Obstetrics* **172**, 335–344.

Tamura, K., Kobayashi, M., Hashimoto, K., Kojima, K., Nagase, K., Iwasaki, K., Kaizu, T., Tanaka, H. & Niwa, M. (1987). A highly sensitive method to assay FK 506 in plasma. *Transplantation Proceedings* **19** (suppl. 6), 23–29.

Tanaka, H., Kuroda, A., Marusawa, H., Hashimoto, M., Hatanaka, H., Kino, T., Goto, T. & Okuhara, M. (1987). Physiochemical properties of FK 506, a novel immunosuppressant isolated from *Streptomyces tsukubaensis*. *Transplantation Proceedings* (suppl. 6), 11–16.

Thomas, J., Matthews, C., Carroll, R., Loreth, R. & Thomas, F. (1990). The immunosuppressive action of FK 506: *in vitro* induction of allogeneic unresponsiveness in human CTL precursors. *Transplantation* **49**, 390–396.

Thomson, A. W. (1989). FK 506. How much potential? *Immunology Today* **10**, 6–9.

Thomson, A. W. (1990). FK 506: Profile of an important new immunosuppressant. *Transplantation Reviews* **4**, 1–13.

Tocci, M. J., Matkovich, D. A., Collier, K. A., Kwok, P., Dumont, F., Lin, S., Degudicibus, S., Siekierka, J. J., Chin, J. & Hutchinson, N. I. (1989). The immunosuppressant FK 506 selectively inhibits expression of early T cell activation genes. *Journal of Immunology* **143**, 718–726.

Todo, S., Demetris, A., Ueda, Y., Imventarza, O., Okuda, K., *et al.* (1987). Canine kidney transplantation with FK 506 alone or in combination with cyclosporin and steroids. *Transplantation Proceedings* **19** (suppl. 6), 57–61.

Todo, S., Fung, J. J., Demetris, A. J., Jain, A., Venkataramanan, R. & Starzl, T. E. (1990a). Early trials with FK 506 as primary treatment in liver transplantation. *Transplantation Proceedings* **22**, 13–16.

Todo, S., Fung, J. J., Starzl, T. E., Tzakis, A., Demetris, A. J., Kormos, R., Jain, A., Alessiani, M. & Takaya, S. (1990b). Liver, kidney, and thoracic organ transplantation under FK 506. *Annals of Surgery* **212**, 295–307.

Todo, S., Ueda, Y., Demetris, A. J. *et al.* (1988). Immunosuppression of canine, monkey, and baboon allografts by FK 506: with special reference to synergism with other drugs and to tolerance induction. *Surgery* **104**, 239.

Tropschug, M., Wachter, E., Mayer, S., Schonbrunner, & Schmid, F. X. (1990). Isolation and sequence of an FK 506-binding protein from *N. crassa* which catalyses protein folding. *Nature* **346**, 674–677.

Venkataramanan, R., Jain, A., Cadoff, E., Warty, V., Iwasaki, K., Nagase, K., Krajack, A., Imventarza, O., Todo, S., Fung, J. J. & Starzl, T. E. (1990). Pharmacokinetics of FK 506: Preclinical and clinical studies. *Transplantation Proceedings* **22** (suppl. 1), 52–56.

Venkataramanan, R., Jain, A., Warty, V., Abu-Elmagd, K., Furukawa, H., Imventarza, O., Fung, J. J. Todo, S. & Starzl, T. E. (1991). Pharmacokinetics of FK 506 following oral administration. A comparison of FK 506 and cyclosporine. *Transplantation Proceedings* **23**, 931–933.

Wang, S. C., Zeevi, A., Tweardy, D. J., Jordan, M. L. & Simmons, R. L. (1991). FK 506, rapamycin, and cyclosporine: effects on IL-4 and IL-10 mRNA levels in a T helper 2 cell line. *Transplantation Proceedings* **23**, 2920–2922.

Wasik, M., Gorski, A., Stepien-Sopniewska, B. & Lagodzinski, Z. (1991). Effect of FK 506 versus cyclosporine on human natural and antibody-dependent cytotoxicity reactions *in vitro*. *Transplantation* **51**, 268–270.

Williams, T. M., Eisenberg, L., Burlein, J. E., Norris, C. A., Pancer, S., Yao, D., Burger, S., Kamoun, M. & Kant, J. A. (1988). Two regions within the human IL-2 gene promoter are important for inducible IL-2 expression. *Journal of Immunology* **141**, 662–666.

Woo, J., Propper, D. J. & Thomson, A. W. (1990a). Antigen presentation and HLA-DR expression by FK 506-treated human monocytes. *Immunology* **71**, 551–555.

Woo, J., Sewell, H. F. & Thomson, A. W. (1990b). The influence of FK 506 on the expression of IL-2 receptors and MHC class II antigens on T cells following mitogen- or alloantigen-induced stimulation: a flow cytometric analysis. *Scandinavian Journal of Immunology* **31**, 297–304.

Woo, J., Propper, D. J., Macleod, A. M. & Thomson, A. W. (1990c). Influence of FK 506 and cyclosporin A on alloantibody production and lymphocyte activation following blood transfusion. *Clinical and Experimental Immunology* **82**, 462–468.

Yoshimura, N., Matsui, S., Hamashima, T. & Oka, T. (1989a). Effect of a new immunosuppressive agent, FK 506, on human lymphocyte responses *in vitro*. I. Inhibition of expression of alloantigen-activated suppressor cells, as well as induction of alloreactivity. *Transplantation* **47**, 351–356.

Yoshimura, N., Matsui, S., Hamashima, T. & Oka, T. (1989b). Effect of a new immunosuppressive agent, FK 506, on human lymphocyte responses *in vitro*. II. Inhibition of the production of IL-2 and γ-IFN, but not B cell-stimulating factor 2. *Transplantation* **47**, 36–39.

Zeevi, A., Duquesnoy, R., Eiras, G., Rabinowich, H., Todo, S., Makowka, L. & Starzl, T. E. (1987). Immunosuppressive effect of FK 506 on *in vitro* lymphocyte alloactivation: synergism with cyclosporine A. *Transplantation Proceedings* **19**, 40–44.

Zeevi, A., Eiras, G., Bach, F. H., Fung, J. J., Todo, S., Starzl, T. & Duquesnoy, R. (1990). Functional differentiation of human cytotoxic T lymphocytes in the presence of FK 506 and CsA. *Transplantation Proceedings* **22**, 106–109.

Chapter 7
Overview of FK 506 in transplantation

John Fung, Angus W. Thomson and Thomas E. Starzl

Introduction

In 1987, Ochiai *et al.*, reported the immunosuppressive qualities of a new immunosuppressive agent, FK 506, isolated from the fermentation broth of a soil fungus, *Streptomyces tsukubaensis*. Extensive *in vitro* studies, demonstrated the effectiveness of FK 506 in suppressing mixed lymphocyte cultures, apparently by inhibiting IL-2 synthesis following alloactivation (Kino *et al.*, 1987). The receptor for FK 506 has been identified, and has been characterized as a peptidyl-proly *cis-trans* isomerase (Harding *et al.*, 1989).

The background for the clinical development of FK 506 was based on a number of animal models which have shown a marked ability of the drug to prevent rejection following various types of organ transplants (Starzl *et al.*, 1987; Todo *et al.*, 1988; Murase *et al.*, 1990a,b), as well as to prevent the development of graft-versus-host disease (GVHD) following bone marrow transplantation (Markus *et al.*, 1991a). More interestingly, FK 506 possesses the ability to reverse ongoing rejection in animal models, as well as established GVHD after bone marrow transplantation (Markus *et al.*, 1991b). These properties continue to be evident during clinical testing of FK 506 (Starzl *et al.*, 1989).

This chapter will attempt to summarize the results of all human transplantation models in which FK 506 has been utilized as either

138

'rescue' therapy and/or 'primary' therapy, including liver (Starzl *et al.*, 1989; Fung *et al.*, 1990; Todo *et al.*, 1990), kidney (Starzl *et al.*, 1990; Todo *et al.*, 1990; Shapiro *et al.*, 1991), heart (Armitage *et al.*, 1991) and bone marrow transplantation (Fung *et al.*, 1990), at the University of Pittsburgh.

Methods

Study design

The trials in liver, kidney, heart and bone marrow transplantation were conducted at the University of Pittsburgh, Presbyterian University Hospital, Children's Hospital of Pittsburgh and the Veterans Administration Medical Center, with the approval of the respective Institutional Review Boards. Informed consent was obtained from patients or their appointed guardians.

Patient profiles

In the liver study, patients were treated with FK 506 as part of three studies, one being the rescue study, in which 57 patients were entered for the diagnosis of acute rejection, while 116 patients were converted from cyclosporin A (CsA) to FK 506 for chronic rejection. In the primary liver transplant group, 110 patients were treated with FK 506 and low-dose steroids, as the baseline immunosuppression following liver transplantation. A subsequent study involved a total of 81 patients, prospectively randomized to either FK 506 or CsA as the baseline immunosuppression following liver transplantation.

In the kidney study, patients were treated with FK 506 as part of two studies, one being the rescue study, in which 21 patients were entered for the diagnosis of rejection. In the primary kidney transplant group, 202 patients were treated with FK 506 and low-dose steroids, as the baseline immunosuppression following kidney transplantation. A randomized trial comparing FK 506 and CsA primary kidney transplantation included 26 patients in both arms.

In the heart study, patients were also divided into two groups. In the first group, 30 patients were treated with FK 506 for primary immunosuppression, while in the second group, ten patients were converted to FK 506 because of persistent rejection.

In the bone marrow study, patients were entered as part of a rescue study, in which 14 patients were treated with FK 506 for evidence of persistent manifestations of graft-versus-host disease, unresponsive to conventional treatment protocols.

Diagnostic evaluations

For patients who were experiencing organ dysfunction, the final categorization of dysfunction was based upon clinical, biochemical and/or histopathological findings. For all patients, either as primary or as rescue therapy, cause(s) or organ dysfunction were carefully sought, the workup being customized to the organ or tissue transplanted. Ultrasonic determination of vessel patency and radiographical evaluation of the biliary or urinary system were used to rule out a technical or mechanical defect. Angiography was performed when indicated. Appropriate viral cultures and stains were used to detect viral infections.

Protocol biopsies were utilized in the evaluation of efficacy of FK 506 therapy. All biopsies were blinded and interpreted by a single experienced transplant pathologist (A.J.D.). Biopsy specimens were fixed in neutral buffered formalin and stained routinely with haematoxylin and eosin, trichrome and reticulin stains. The criteria used for pathological diagnosis have been defined in previous reports (Billingham *et al.*, 1979; Demetris *et al.*, 1990).

Timing and details of therapy

Initiation of treatment with FK 506 was done in the hospital and was given initially as a parenteral dose, followed by conversion to an oral dose. The initial parenteral dose of FK 506 was 0.075–0.15 mg/kg, given intravenously. This was continued until the patient was able to ingest the oral form of FK 506. Generally, oral dosages of FK 506 were given at 0.30 mg/kg/day, in two divided doses. Dose adjustments of FK 506 were based upon monitoring of serum trough levels by enzyme linked immunosorbant assay (ELISA) (Tamura *et al.*, 1987) to achieve a 12-h trough level between 1.0–2.0 ng/ml, and also by adjustment according to clinical or biochemical parameters.

Evaluation of response

Periodic determinations of liver and kidney functions, including total bilirubin (TBIL), serum glutamic transaminases, SGOT and SGPT, alkaline phosphatase, blood urea nitrogen (BUN) and serum creatinine were performed. All values are expressed as the value ± 1 s.d. Protocol biopsies were obtained after initiation of FK 506 therapy.

Liver transplantation

Rescue therapy

In this population of 173 patients, of whom many were critically ill at the time of FK 506 conversion, there were 14 deaths (8.1%). The causes of death were numerous, but the incidence of mortality was directly corre-lated with the medical condition of the patient at the time or FK 506 conversion. Sepsis was the cause of death in four patients. Three patients died of haemorrhagic complications. Three patients died of metastatic carcinoma following transplantation. In two patients, retransplantation was not considered an option for the failing liver allograft. One patient was started on FK 506 with pathological findings of late chronic rejection, and died of technical causes during an attempted retransplantation. In one death no cause of death could be determined. This patient died at home and had been off FK 506 for 4 months when she died. She had renal failure and was on dialysis prior to and after discontinuation of FK 506 therapy.

The biochemical response of the liver allografts to FK 506 was analysed by classifying patients either into acute or chronic rejection, dependent upon the principal histopathological findings. For the 57 patients who were treated for acute rejection, documented on liver biopsy or as judged by biochemical and clinical parameters, the TBIL, SGOT, and SGPT values prior to FK 506 were: 4.68 ± 5.91 mg/dl, 240 ± 431 iu/l, and 292 ± 383 iu/l, respectively. These values fell, by the sixth month to: 0.76 ± 1.41 mg/dl, 98 ± 163 iu/l, and 90 ± 128 iu/l, respectively.

Patients with an entrance diagnosis of chronic rejection also had a beneficial response to FK 506. For the 116 patients treated for this specific indication, the total bilirubin fell to normal values (pre-FK 506, 5.07 ± 8.16 mg/dl; 6 months, 0.99 ± 1.47 mg/dl) while the average transaminase values were still slightly elevated above normal values (pre-FK 506, SGOT/SGPT, 200 ± 175 iu/l/275 ± 223 iu/l; 6 months, SGOT/SGPT, 44 ± 72 iu/l/101 ± 68 iu/l).

A clinicopathological study of the results of conversion of liver allografts from CsA to FK 506 immunosuppression revealed that the biochemical improvement seen above was correlated with histopathologi-cal improvement (Demetris et al., 1991). With both acute and chronic rejection, the biochemical improvement occurred earlier and in greater proportion than the pathological findings. Those patients with acute rejection fared better than those with chronic rejection, with a higher response rate. In those patients with chronic rejection, the liver function studies and the degree of bile ductular injury was significantly worse among those who failed than among those patients who responded.

Primary therapy

Of the original 110 primary liver transplant patients in the series, a total of 99 (90%) were alive at 12 months. These results were statistically better than those of the 325 CsA-treated control group, which had a 1-year patient survival of only 77%. The corresponding graft survival was also statistically better, with 83% of the FK 506 grafts surviving at 1 year, compared with 68% for the CsA group. The rate of retransplantation was only 6%, over one-half less than the 15% retransplant rate seen with the CsA control group. The 60-day mortality figure for FK 506-treated patients (6.7%) was statistically less than that of CsA (16.5%).

During the follow-up period, 50% of all recipients were taken off steroids and were maintained on single drug immunosuppression with FK 506. Yet 52.8% of all patients were rejection free during the entire period of study. The majority of rejection episodes were mild and easily controlled with a single dose of bolus steroids (either methylprednisolone or hydro-cortisone). Only 17.8% of the rejection episodes required further steroid treatment in the form of a steroid taper or additional steroid boluses. In addition, only 11.2% of the patients required anti-human CD3 (OKT3).

The incidence of serious infections, in spite of the potency of FK 506, does not appear to be alarming. The incidence of serious infections was about 50% less than that seen with a historical group of patients given CsA. Of note, is that the incidence of cytomegalovirus infections did not appear to be increased, when compared to patients on CsA.

Prospective randomized study

Based upon the encouraging results of the preliminary FK 506 experience, a study was started, comparing the use of FK 506 and CsA, along with steroids, in a prospective, randomized fashion, in patients undergoing primary liver transplantation. Eighty-one liver transplant recipients were randomized to either FK 506 (41 patients) or CsA (40 patients), following completion of the liver transplant. A single bolus of 1 g methylprednisolone followed by a daily dose of 20 mg methylprednisolone was the baseline steroid therapy for both groups of patients. Biochemical and histopathological parameters were monitored in order to determine the effectiveness of either therapy in preventing rejection. Rejection episodes were treated with a single bolus of 1 g methylprednisolone. If this treatment failed to reverse the rejection episode, a total of 50 mg OKT3 was administered. Those CsA patients who failed to respond to therapy were converted to FK 506, in an attempt to rescue the dysfunctional graft. With the ability to rescue CsA randomized dysfunctional grafts with FK 506, the patient and graft survival were essentially the same.

The median follow-up for both the CsA and FK 506 groups was 345 days (range 256–446 days). The 6-month-patient survival rate was 95% for the FK 506-treated group, while the corresponding value for the CsA-treated group was 89%. The corresponding graft survival was 93% for the FK 506-treated group, while the corresponding value for CsA-treated group was 81%. The 12-month-graft survival rate was 90% for FK 506, and 70% for CsA. Two patients in the FK 506-treated group and seven patients in the CsA-treated groups were retransplanted. The mortality associated with retransplantation was 50% in both groups. The total percentage of patients in the FK 506 group who were rejection-free during the entire length of follow-up was 53.7%, while that for CsA was 13.3%. The mean days to the first rejection was 21.5 days for the FK 506-treated group, and 9.9 days for the CsA-treated group. OKT3 for treatment of the original allograft was used in 30% of CsA-treated patients, compared with 20% of FK 506-treated patients. Steroid boluses averaged 0.99 times in the CsA-treated group, while this figure was 0.50 times in the FK 506-treated group. 72.6% of the CsA-treated patients were converted to FK 506, an average of 20 days after liver transplantation. The reasons for conversion were: persistent ischemic injury (5), patient dropout (1), Rh incompatibility with haemolysis (1), and steroid resistant or OKT3-resistant rejections (21).

Renal function in both groups of patients was assessed by the requirement for haemodialysis and the serum creatinine at monthly determinations. Haemodialysis was initiated in six CsA patients while still on CsA, while three other CsA patients required haemodialysis during the period of conversion to FK 506. In the FK 506-randomized group, four patients were placed on haemodialysis during the post-transplant period. The comparative incidence for haemodialysis requirement between the FK 506 and CsA groups was 10% and 21.6%, respectively. Long-term haemodialysis (after 3 months post-transplant) was required by one patient in each group.

The incidence of opportunistic infections was essentially the same for both groups. Patients who were randomized to CsA had a 22.5% incidence of cytomegalovirus (CMV) infections. This compared to a 22.0% incidence for patients on FK 506. In the 13 CsA patients who were not switched to FK 506, the incidence of CMV was 23% (3/13), and only one of the three patients received OKT3. In FK 506 patients, three of a total of nine cases of CMV occurred in patients who had previously received OKT3.

The severity of hypertension was assessed by the need for antihypertensive medications following transplantation. The incidence of hypertension in the overall CsA-randomized group was 52.9% versus 26.9% for the FK 506-treated group ($P < 0.01$), at 3 months post-transplant. This figure did not change appreciably over the follow-up period; at the 12-month-follow-up period, the corresponding hypertensive incidence was 48% for CsA and 33.3% for FK 506. The incidence of hypertension in the 14 patients, who were on CsA at the 3 month post-transplant period was 64.2%. The 12-month figure was 72.7% for those patients still on CsA, while the conversion group had an incidence similar to those given FK 506 from the start (36.4%).

The need for insulin therapy was evaluated by determining those patients who required insulin at the 3-month period following transplantation. There were no statistically significant differences between the two groups of patients. 17% of the patents in the FK 506 group required insulin at 3 months post-transplant. For the CsA group, 17.5% of the patients required insulin at the same time point.

Both FK 506 and CsA administration have been associated with side-effects, many of which are similar. The percentages and severity of patients experiencing treatment-related adverse reactions were recorded. This included evidence of neurotoxicity: trembling, paresthesias, insomnia, irritability, hyperkinetic behaviour, dysarthria, seizures, and coma. The incidence of side-effects was essentially the same in both groups.

The results of the current randomized study compare favourably with previously reported results using FK 506, and therefore do not appear to represent a bias in the performance of the study. It is important that the results of the current ongoing randomized trial are comparable to those results obtained in the historical series. The current results of patient and graft survival are as good, if not better, than those figures obtained in the past. One would expect that both graft and patient survival would be better in the randomized trial since high-risk patients are removed from randomization. The randomized FK 506 liver patients were compared to the survival curves of 271 non-randomized FK 506 recipients and 813 CsA recipients during the period of time corresponding to the utilization of Viaspan (Dupont). The 1-year patient survival for the high-risk FK 506 liver recipients not entered in the randomized trial approaches 82%, while graft survival is 76%. This compares to our historic CsA patient and graft survival of 77% and 68%, respectively. The improvement of the current randomized CsA group over the historic group may, in part, be, related to the ability to convert patients on CsA to FK 506.

Kidney transplantation

Rescue therapy

A total of 21 patients were converted from CsA-based immunosuppression to FK 506-based immunosuppression for persistent kidney rejection. One death was encountered. Of the 21 patients, ten were classified into late rejection episodes (> 60 days), while 11 were treated early in the post-transplant course (< 60 days). Seven of the 11 early rescues were successful, in contrast to only four of ten late rescues. Most of the failures of FK 506-rescue therapy in this group of patients were in patients who had chronic glomerulosclerosis and chronic rejection on biopsy, prior to FK 506 rescue. In those patients with acute cellular rejection, the results were better. The serum creatinine at the time of conversion, was also correlated with the success of therapy. Four of five (80%) patients with a serum creatinine < 3.0 mg/dl have good renal function, while only seven of 16

(44%) patients with a pre-conversion serum creatinine > 3.0 mg/dl have a functioning kidney. The overall serum creatinine prior to FK 506 conversion in the 11 successful switches was 3.70 ± 2.15 mg/dl, excluding the serum creatinine values of four patients who were on dialysis at the time of FK 506 conversion. The average creatinine after FK 506 switch was 2.84 ± 1.40 mg/dl, with all 11 grafts functioning.

Primary therapy

On March 27, 1989, a trial utilizing FK 506 and low-dose steroids was introduced at the University of Pittsburgh. A total of 411 kidney transplants have been performed during the period between 3/27/89 and 1/31/91. Twenty-nine kidneys were transplanted into patients who were recipients of other organ transplants. The results of these patients were limited by other factors such as patient survival and graft function of other organs, primarily that of the liver, and were excluded from further analysis. A study of the remaining 382 kidney transplant patients included 202 patients given FK 506 and low-dose steroids and 180 patients given CsA, low-dose steroids and azathioprine.

The average age of the recipients was 39 years; 11.3% of recipients were over 60-years old and 8.4% were in the paediatric age range. Approximately two-thirds of the patients in both groups were receiving their first kidney transplant. Fifteen per cent of patients were considered high antibody status (panel reactive antibodies (PRA) > 40%), placing them in a high-risk category for kidney transplantation. A slightly higher percentage of patients with living related transplants were given CsA (14% CsA versus 5% FK 506), while paediatric donors accounted for a higher percentage of the organs used in the FK 506 group (22% FK 506 versus 15% CsA). The mean follow-up was 11.3 ± 7.5 months. The overall patient survival at 1 year was 94.3% for the CsA group and 90.6% for the FK 506 group. The causes of death were similar between both groups, with cardiac causes accounting for 30% of deaths, sepsis for 26% of deaths and gastrointestinal complications for 22% of deaths.

For those patients receiving their first kidney transplant, the patient survival was essentially the same (92.8% CsA versus 92.7% FK 506). The graft survival at 1 year for these patients was 81.5% for the CsA group and 75.3% for FK 506. For the low immunological risk patients (PRA < 40%), the patient survival was 94.1% for CsA and 91.1% for FK 506, while the corresponding graft survival for the CsA was 81% versus 76% for FK 506.

Prospective randomized study

A randomized trial of FK 506 with low-dose steroids versus CsA with low-dose steroids was initiated in April, 1990. At this time, patients who were considered as low-risk candidates for kidney transplantation, i.e. receiving their first kidney transplant without significant known medical problems, and with low PRA, were randomized to either FK 506 or CsA with low-dose steroids. Patients who did not fulfill these criteria were considered high-risk patients and received FK 506 and low-dose steroids as part of a non-randomized protocol. When the results of patient and graft survival were examined, breaking down the randomized from the non-randomized patients, the effect of the non-randomized group on the FK 506 statistics could be seen. The patient and graft survival of the randomized patients were essentially the same (see Figs 7.1 and 7.2). The 1 year patient survival in the randomized CsA group was 92% and 96% for the FK 506 group. The corresponding graft survival was 79% and 81%. By shifting the high-risk patients into the FK 506 non-randomized trial, the overall patient and graft survival were lower in the FK 506 group. The 1-year patient and graft survival for the FK 506 non-randomized group was 90% while that for the CsA was 95%. More importantly, because of higher numbers of retransplant cases in the FK 506 group (32% for FK 506 versus 21% for CsA), the

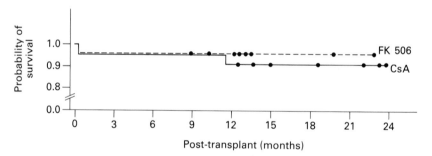

Fig. 7.1. Patient survival curves for FK 506 and CsA kidney transplant randomized patients are shown. Dots denote censored times.

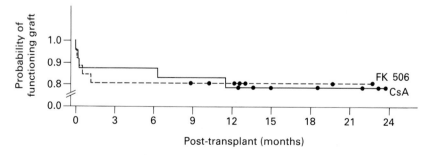

Fig. 7.2. The corresponding graft survival curves for the FK 506 and CsA kidney transplant randomized patients are shown. Dots denote censored times.

overall graft survival were somewhat less in the FK 506 group (74%) when compared to the CsA group (82%). The rates of rejection in the overall groups were similar, 57% in the FK 506 group and 54% in the CsA group.

The randomized trial was designed to evaluate not only patient and graft survival, but also to assess the effect of either FK 506 or CsA on other parameters such as the incidence of hypertension, infection, requirement for augmented immunosuppression, rates of rejection, and steroid requirements. Fifty-two patients were enrolled in the study, 26 randomized to both arms. The incidence of biopsy documented rejection was 73% in the CsA group and 46% in the FK 506 group ($P < 0.05$). Moreover, the requirement for OKT3 was 50% in the CsA group and 19% for the FK 506 group ($P < 0.03$). Thirty-five per cent of the CsA group required conversion to FK 506, while 4% of the FK 506 were considered treatment failures and required addition of azathioprine to control rejection. The rates of CMV infection were essentially the same, 15% for CsA and 12% for FK 506. The overall renal function was similar in both groups, with a mean serum creatinine of 1.9 mg/dl, and a mean blood urea nitrogen of 28 mg/dl for CsA and 26 mg/dl for FK 506. While over one-third of FK 506 patients were off steroids at the time of analysis, no CsA patient was steroid free ($P < 0.01$). While only 29% of patients on CsA were given no antihypertensive medications, over one-half (52%) of patients on FK 506 were free of antihypertensive medications ($P < 0.05$).

Heart transplantation

Rescue therapy

Ten patients were converted from CsA to FK 506 between 3 and 50 months post-transplant. The findings of persistent heart rejection defined by a $> 2 +$ grading of the endomyocardial biopsy by the Billingham criteria (Billingham *et al.*, 1979), included mononuclear cell infiltration, arteritis and in some instances, interstitial fibrosis. All patients had failed conventional immunotherapy, including at least two courses of antilymphocyte preparations, and two courses of augmented steroids during the preceding 6 months. The grading of endomyocardial biopsies, prior to conversion of FK 506, was 2.70 ± 0.48. Using the same criteria, the mean value of the follow-up biopsies after FK 506 was graded at 0.70 ± 0.67 ($P < 0.01$). The mean prednisone dose prior to FK 506 conversion was 14 mg/day, after FK 506 conversion this fell to 5.5 mg/day. One death occurred during the period of follow-up in a patient with disseminated aspergillosis.

Primary therapy

Thirty patients received FK 506 from the outset following heart transplantation. Eight patients were on circulatory assist devices prior to heart transplantation. Follow-up ranged from 1 to 10 months. Four patients have died, with an actual patient and graft survival of 87%. One patient with known pulmonary hypertension died on the third post-transplant day from right heart failure. One patient, with pre-existing lung disease and bronchiectasis, died from pulmonary infection, while two other patients died of sudden deaths, without a known cause. The rejection-free rate within the first 90 days was 60%. Only one patient required OKT3. Heart function was excellent in all patients. The average left ventricular rejection fraction, determined by gated nuclear scans or echocardiography, was 70% (range 58–75%).

Bone marrow transplantation

Rescue therapy

Fourteen patients with manifestations of chronic GVHD following bone marrow transplantation were placed on FK 506. All patients were on or had been on high doses of CsA and steroids. Seven patients had an original diagnosis of chronic myelogenous leukaemia, three were given bone marrow transplants for acute lymphoblastic leukaemias, one had aplastic anaemia, one for Burkitt's lymphoma and two had acute myelogenous leukaemias. All grafts were taken from human leukocyte antigen (HLA) identical siblings. The most common sites of involvement are skin and liver, followed by lung, gastrointestinal and musculoskeletal. The most objective parameters to evaluate response to FK 506 have been those with liver and skin involvement. The mean time after bone marrow transplantation to the time of FK 506 therapy was 17.7 months, and the mean follow-up was 5.8 months.

Of the 11 patients with liver involvement, five were referred for consideration for liver transplantation. Two of these eventually required liver transplantation, but both died. One died from sepsis following liver transplantation, while the other patient failed to awaken after transplantation, having been in stage IV coma prior to transplantation. Two other patients died, one of unknown causes at home, and the other from respiratory failure from pre-existing severe bronchiolitis obliterans. The other six patients had a marked response to FK 506-rescue therapy.

In the 11 patients with skin involvement, five have improved, while three with scleroderma like involvement have stable skin lesions. One of the patients dropped out of the study while two other patients died, one from pulmonary aspergillosis and the other of unknown causes.

Of the six patients with moderate to severe obliterative bronchiolitis, two patients died from worsening lung disease. The remaining four patients have stable or slightly improved pulmonary function. The remaining organ system involvement of musculoskeletal and the gastrointestinal tract have not shown progression during FK 506 therapy.

Limitations

Adverse reactions requiring treatment or adjustment of FK doses can be catagorized into four primary areas. These are (i) alterations in kidney functions; (ii) alterations in glucose metabolism; (iii) neurotoxicity; and (iv) susceptibility to infection or malignancy.

Alterations in kidney function are manifested by electrolyte abnormalities and changes in glomerular filtration, as evidenced by changes in serum creatinine. Hyperkalaemia is seen in 35% of patients, following administration of FK 506. Treatment of hyperkalaemia is generally with potassium-binding resins and potassium-restricted diets. Addition of a synthetic mineralocorticoid, Florinef, relieves the hyperkalaemia, by increasing potassium excretion by the kidney. Decrements in renal blood flow have been documented by nuclear medicine studies. The filtration fraction generally remains the same. Causes of altered renal function in transplant patients are multifactorial, and include: peri-operative hypotension, use of nephrotoxic antibiotics and a degree of pre-existing renal dysfunction. The alteration in renal function seen in patients on FK 506 is similar to that seen in patients on CsA. These changes are responsive to reduction in doses of FK 506. The incidence of renal failure requiring chronic haemodialysis is of the order of 4%, based on studies of liver transplant patients, although no patients have required maintenance haemodialysis following heart transplantation. The progression of chronic renal failure to dialysis-requiring renal failure is not known.

Alterations in glucose metabolism are the result of changes in peripheral sensitivity to insulin and/or changes in the response of the islet cells to hyperglycaemia. The incidence of new onset diabetes, i.e. those patients requiring insulin, is approximately 15% in FK 506 transplant patients. The incidence of new onset diabetes in other immunosuppressive regimens, incorporating CsA or azathioprine, is approximately 20%. The long-term consequence of insulin requirement in transplant patients, towards the development of diabetic complications is not known.

Rare but severe instances of neurotoxicity have been reported following FK 506 administration. Expressive aphasia has been seen in four liver transplant patients, although this has not been seen in any other types of FK 506-treated individuals. New onset seizures have also been reported in liver transplant patients, especially during the peri-operative transplant period. The susceptibility of such patients to changes in serum electrolytes has been previously reported. New onset seizures have not been reported in other patients treated with FK 506.

Post-transplant lymphoproliferative disease (PTLD) is an abnormality of lymphocyte proliferation in a setting of an immunosuppressed patient. The spectrum of PTLD can range from a benign lymphoid proliferation such as a mononucleosis syndrome to a frankly malignant lymphoid tumour. PTLD has been associated with all types of immunosuppressive therapy. The incidence of PTLD in the cyclosporin era is generally estimated between 2 and 4%. The median time following transplantation to the development of PTLD is 6 months; the majority of these tumours occur within 12 months following transplantation.

A total of 16 patients have developed *de novo* PTLD lesions while on FK 506 therapy. Seven of these patients died, although PTLD was associated with death in only five cases. The remaining nine patients had relatively mild forms of PTLD, three of these had a mononucleosis syndrome, and presented with sore throat and tonsillar enlargement. Treatment with lowering immunosuppression and intravenous acyclovir proved to cure all of them. In the remaining six patients, three required operative procedures (two small bowel resection, one liver resection) which were directly related to PTLD, while the other three were treated by a reduction of immunosuppression only. The incidence of *de novo* PTLD following initiation of FK 506 therapy is 1.4%. All of the cases of PTLD occurred within the first year following initiation of FK 506, with the median time from FK 506 therapy to onset of disease being 4 months. FK 506 shows no evidence of any increase in the risk of developing or succumbing to PTLD, when compared to previously quoted figures on the incidence of PTLD, based on other immunosuppressive regimens. No patients treated with FK 506 for non-transplant indications have developed any malignancies.

Cytomegalovirus infections are considered the most common opportunistic infection in the transplant patient. Several factors determine the severity and development of CMV infections. The seronegativity and use of intensive immunosuppression are considered major contributing factors. The incidence of CMV infections in the FK 506-treated transplant patients is 20%. This figure is similar to that seen in transplanted patients on CsA. No patients treated with FK 506 for non-transplant indications have developed CMV infections.

Discussion

Cyclosporin-based immunosuppression significantly enhanced both patient and graft survival in all solid organ transplants, when compared to the era of azthioprine and steroids (Starzl *et al.*, 1990). Its use in bone marrow transplantation has decreased the incidence and severity of

GVHD (Sullivan *et al.*, 1988). Nevertheless, most centres experience an unacceptably high complication rate related to ongoing GVHD or rejection. These immunologically related complications occur in over 70% of all cyclosporin-treated patients. In addition, the sequela of over-immunosuppression in attempts to treat rejection or GVHD, such as the use of excessive steroids and antilymphocyte preparations, are fraught with a high incidence of infectious complications. It stands to reason that a baseline immunosuppressive agent which allows for less incidence of rejection or GVHD, and easier treatment, would decrease both graft and patient loss. From the results of our studies presented here, the use of FK 506 in transplantation has these advantages. FK 506 appears to not only decrease the absolute incidence of rejection episodes, but makes the treatment of rejection simpler.

The ability of a new immunosuppressive agent to be dose adjustable for treatment of acute rejection, chronic rejection or GVHD, would represent an important asset; this ability has only been ascribed to steroids in the past. FK 506 can be used in this manner. In fact, the first response to a developing rejection, is to increase the dose of baseline FK 506. In rescue therapy, the marked ability of FK 506 to reverse acute rejection in both kidney and heart rejection, and both acute and chronic rejection in liver transplantation, and with chronic GVHD in bone marrow transplantation has not been seen with any immunosuppressive agent in the past. While the mechanism by which FK 506 is able to do this, is not known, it would appear that it would entail mechanisms other than simply inhibition of IL-2 synthesis.

The limitations of FK 506 have been defined. In chronic rejection, the ability of an organ to reverse the stigmata of chronic inflammation appears to determine the effectiveness of FK 506 rescue therapy. With the development of obliterative arteriopathy, or the absence of epithelial structures, e.g. biliary structures or kidney tubules, the ability of FK 506 to reverse organ dysfunction is limited. On the other hand, acute cellular rejection appears to respond well to initiation or adjustment of FK 506 therapy.

Prospective, randomized trials comparing FK 506 therapy with cyclosporin-based immunosuppression are currently underway. The preliminary results of the study being performed at the University of Pittsburgh in liver transplantation, are encouraging. Multicentre trials are also underway, and preliminary reports are also encouraging. A well defined endpoint, other than patient or graft loss, should be utilized, since the data presented here also suggests that a conversion to FK 506, will allow for allografts in danger of being lost to rejection, to be salvaged.

Other randomized trials in kidney, heart and bone marrow transplantation are also underway. The results of the randomized kidney transplant trial at the University of Pittsburgh has demonstrated a benefit of FK 506 in several important secondary endpoints, e.g. incidence of hypertension, although the primary endpoints of patient and graft survival are similar. One other centre, in Japan, has had some early experience with FK 506 for primary kidney transplantation. Between July and September 1990, 37 patients (32 living related and five cadaveric allografts) were enrolled in a study utilizing a fixed dose of 0.15 mg/kg/day intravenously followed by a fixed oral dose of 0.30 mg/kg/day. No attempts to adjust FK 506 doses to levels were made until an adverse event occurred. With follow-up of 5–8 months, all patients were alive, and all grafts functioning. Twenty-five per cent of patients were converted to other immunosuppressive drugs because of adverse events. Rejection was noted in 32% of the patients although no patients required OKT3. Nephrotoxicity was seen in 30% of patients, and responded in 92% of patients to a decrease in FK 506 dose. Adverse reactions to the drug were proportional to high levels of FK 506.

The toxicity profile of FK 506 is proportional to the efficacy of the drug. The major side-effects of the drug are similar to cyclosporin, with dose-related nephrotoxicity and neurotoxicity. Other known complications of immunosuppression, including diabetogenesis, infectious and malignant complications, are no greater with FK 506 than with other immunosuppressive therapies. As with any new agent, details regarding nuances of dose administration and adjustments, are continuing to be refined. In fact, it has been recently reported that FK 506 dosing must be adjusted to liver function and that attention to drug levels may be helpful in avoiding overdosing (Abu-Elmagd *et al.*, 1991; Starzl *et al.*, 1991).

References

Abu-Elmagd, K., Fung., J. J., Alessiani, M., Jain, Venkataramanan, R., Warty, V. S., Takaya, S., Todo, S., Day, R. & Starzl, T. E. (1991). The effect of graft function on FK 506 plasma levels, doses, and renal function: with particular reference to the liver. *Transplantation* **52**, 71–77.

Armitage, J. M., Kormos, R. L., Griffith, B. P., Hardesty, R. L., Fricker, F. J., Stuart, R. S., Marrone, G. C., Todo, S., Fung, J. & Starzl, T. E. (1991). The clinical trial of FK 506 as primary and rescue immunosuppression in cardiac transplantation. *Transplantation Proceedings* **23**, 1149–1152.

Billingham, M. (1979). Some recent advances in cardiac pathology. *Human Pathology* **10**, 367–386.

Demetris, A. J., Fung, J. J., Todo, S., Banner, B., Zerbe, T. Sysyn, G. & Starzl, T. E. (1990). Pathologic observations in human allograft recipients treated wtih FK 506. *Transplantation Proceedings* **23**, 25–36.

Demetris, A. J., Fung, J. J. Todo, S., Jain, A., Takaya, S., Alessiani, M., Abu-Elmagd, K., Van Thiel, D. H. & Starzl, T. E. (1991). Conversion of liver allograft recipients from cyclosporine to FK 506 immunosuppressive therapy: a clinicopathologic study of 96 patients. *Transplantation* (in press).

Fung, J. J., Todo, S., Jain, A., McCauley, J., Alessiani, M., Scotti, C. & Starzl, T. E. (1990). Conversion from cyclosporine to FK 506 in liver allograft recipients with cyclosporine-related complications. *Transplantation Proceedings* **22**, 6–12.

Harding, M. W., Galat, A., Uehling, D. E. & Schreiber, S. (1989). A receptor for the immunosuppressant FK 506 is a *cis-trans* peptidyl-proly isomerase. *Nature* **341**, 758-760.

Kino, T., Hatanaka, H., Miyata, S., Inamura, N., Nishiyama, M., Yajima, T., Goto, T., Okuhara, M., Kohsaka, M., Aoki, H. & Ochiai, T. (1987). FK 506, a novel immunosuppressant isolated from a streptomyces. II. Immunosuppressive effect of FK 506 *in vitro*. *Journal of Antibiotics* **40**, 1256-1260.

Markus, P. M., Cai, X., Ming, W., Demetris, A. J., Fung, J. J. & Starzl, T. E. (1991a). Prevention of graft-versus-host disease following allogeneic bone marrow transplantation in rats using FK 506. *Transplantation* **52**, 590-594.

Markus, P. M., Cai, X., Ming, W., Demetris, A. J., Fung, J. J. & Starzl, T. E. (1991b). FK 506 reverses acute graft-versus-host disease following allogeneic bone marrow transplantation in rats. *Surgery*, (in press).

Murase, N., Kim, D. G., Todo, S., Cramer, D. V., Fung, J. & Starzl, T. E. (1990a). Suppression of allograft rejection with FK 506. I. Prolonged cardiac and liver survival in rats following short-course therapy. *Transplantation* **50**, 186-189.

Murase, N., Kim, D. G., Todo, S., Cramer, D. V., Fung, J. & Starzl, T. E. (1990b). Induction of liver, heart, and multivisceral graft acceptance with a short course of FK 506. *Transplantation Proceedings* **22**, 74-75.

Ochiai, T., Nakajima, K., Nagata, M., Suzuki, T., Asano, T., Uematsu, T., Goto, T., Hori, S., Kenmochi, T., Nakagouri, T. & Isono, K. (1987). Effect of a new immunosuppressive agent, FK 506, on heterotopic cardiac allotransplantation in the rat. *Transplantation Proceedings* **19**, 1284-1286.

Shapiro, R., Jordan, M., Fung, J. J., McCauley, J., Johnston, J., Iwaki, Y. Tzakis, A., Hakala, T., Todo, S. & Starzl, T. E. (1991). Kidney transplantation under FK 506 immunosuppression. *Transplantation Proceedings* **23**, 920-923.

Starzl, T. E., Abu-Elmagd, K., Tzakis, A., Fung, J. J., Porter, K. A. & Todo, S. (1991). Selected topics on FK 506: with special references to rescue of extrahepatic whole organ grafts, transplantation of 'forbidden organs', side effects, mechanisms, and practical pharmacokinetics. *Transplantation Proceedings* **23**, 914-919.

Starzl, T. E., Demetris, A. J. & Van Thiel, D. (1998). Liver transplantation: a 31 year perspective. *Current Problems in Surgery* **28**, 51-240.

Starzl, T. E., Fung, J., Jordan, M., Shapiro, R., Tzakis, A., McCauley, J. Johnston, J. Iwaki, Y., Jain, A., Alessiani, M. & Todo, S. (1990). Kidney transplantation under FK 506. *Journal of the American Medical Association* **264**, 63-67.

Starzl, T. E., Makowka, L. & Todo, S. (1987). A potential breakthrough in immunosuppression. *Transplantation Proceedings* **19** (suppl. 6), 1-104.

Starzl, T. E., Todo, S., Fung, J., Demetris, A. J., Venkataramanan, R. & Jain, A. (1989). FK 506 for human liver, kidney, and pancreas transplantation. *Lancet* **ii**, 1000-1004.

Sullivan, K. M., Witherspoon, R. P., Storb, R., Deeg, H. J., Dahlberg, S., Sanders, J. E., Appelbaum, F. R., Doney, K. C., Weiden, P., Anasetti, C., Loughran, T. P., Hill, R., Shields, A., Yee, G., Shulman, H., Nims, J., Strom, S. & Thomas, E. D. (1988). Alternating-day cyclosporine and prednisone for treatment of high-risk chronic graft-v-host disease. *Blood* **2**, 555-561.

Tamura, K., Kobayashi, M., Hashimoto, K., Kojima, K., Nagase, K., Iwasaki, K., Kaize, T., Tanaka, H. & Niwa, M. (1987). A highly sensitive method to assay FK 506 levels in plasma. *Transplantation Proceedings* **19** (suppl. 6), 23-29.

Todo, S., Fung, J. J., Starzl, T. E., Tzakis, A., Demetris, A. J., Kormos, R., Jain, A., Alessiani, M. & Takaya, S. (1990). Liver, kidney, and thoracic organ transplantation under FK 506. *Annals of Surgery* **212**, 295-307.

Todo, S., Ueda, Y., Demetris, A. J., Imventarza, O., Nalesnik, M., Venkataramanan, R., Makowka, L. & Starzl, T. E. (1988). Immunosuppression of canine, monkey, and baboon allografts by FK 506 with special reference to synergism with other drugs and to tolerance induction. *Surgery* **104**, 239-240.

Part 3
Anti-T cell
monoclonal antibodies

Chapter 8
Anti-CD3 and anti-TCR monoclonal antibodies

Lucienne Chatenoud

Introduction

Depending on their fine specificity and the treatment protocol used, anti-T cell monoclonal antibodies (MoAb) can mediate either specific or selective immunosuppression *in vivo*.

Specific immunosuppression, i.e. the induction of tolerance towards autoantigens or alloantigens, can be achieved in two different ways. The first is the use of MoAb exclusively targeting clonotypic T cells via the variable portion of the $\alpha\beta$ heterodimer, while the second is the combined administration of the antigen with MoAb directed against precise cell subsets such as anti-CD4. The two strategies, addressed in detail elsewhere in this volume, are both very promising but are still at the experimental stage.

Selective immunosuppression is induced by the administration of MoAb targeting key molecules expressed by defined T-cell populations. The intensity of the immunosuppression is directly dependent on two distinct, non-exclusive elements — the functional relevance of the target receptor and the involvement of the target T-cell population in the pathological immune response. Non-specific, selective immunosuppression with anti-T cell MoAb should facilitate the adaptation of immunointervention to given pathological situations and help to avoid severe side-effects due to oversuppression, and common with polyclonal anti-T cell sera or conventional chemical immunosuppressants. Monoclonal antibodies to CD3 and T-cell receptor (TCR) are well suited to selective immunosuppression because of their direct interaction with monomorphic determinants of the TCR complex involved in antigen recognition and signal transduction.

The aim of this chapter is to review the salient features of anti-CD3 and anti-TCR MoAb administration *in vivo*, and to compare both their therapeutic potency and their capacity to induce not only short-term immunosuppression but also, under certain conditions, long-term immunoregulatory phenomena.

Certain characteristics of the CD3/TCR molecule must first be recalled since they account for some of the *in vivo* effects of specific MoAb. The CD3/TCR complex includes the antigen specific subunits α and β — transmembrane proteins with short (5–12 amino acid) hydrophylic cytoplasmic tails (Meuer *et al.*, 1983b; Oettgen *et al.*, 1984). Non-covalently associated to TCR $\alpha\beta$ are the three additional transmembrane CD3 polypeptide chains (γ(21 kDa), δ(25 kDa) and ε(25 kDa)) that regulate assembly and expression of TCR and are responsible for transduction of signals after ligand binding to $\alpha\beta$ (Clevers *et al.*, 1988; Borst *et al.*, 1984; Pessano *et al.*, 1985). A disulphide-linked homodimer $\zeta\zeta(\zeta$, 16 kDa) and heterodimer $\zeta\eta(\eta$, 22 kDa), originally considered as components of CD3, appear in fact to be subunits independently associated to TCR (Samelson *et al.*, 1985; Weissman *et al.*, 1985; Clevers *et al.*, 1988; Baniyash *et al.*, 1989).

All the polypeptide components of the complex are required for the expression of a functional CD3/TCR receptor at the T-cell surface; as a result, incomplete receptors are not generally expressed (Weiss & Stobo, 1984; McCleod *et al.*, 1986; Clevers *et al.*, 1988). Mutants lacking one of the TCR or CD3 chains cannot recognize antigens (Weiss & Stobo, 1984; McCleod *et al.*, 1986; Clevers *et al.*, 1988), and rare cases of aberrant CD3 expression associated with immunodeficiency have also been described in man (Regueiro *et al.*, 1986).

Some experimental evidence suggests that transient association of the CD3/TCR complex with other well-defined lymphocyte molecules such as CD4 and CD8 may be crucial to trigger T-cell functions correctly (Emmrich *et al.*, 1986; Saizawa *et al.*, 1987).

In vitro, anti-CD3 and anti-TCR MoAb have two distinct, potent and totally antagonistic effects: on the one hand, they strongly inhibit T-cell mitogenesis and cytotoxic or delayed-type hypersensitivity responses of differentiated specific T cells (Reinherz *et al.*, 1980; Haskins *et al.*, 1983; Meuer *et al.*, 1983a, 1984) while, on the other hand, they promote T-cell activation and cytokine release (van Wauwe *et al.*, 1980; Chang *et al.*, 1981; Burns *et al.*, 1982; van Lier *et al.*, 1987). This activation is particularly marked with anti-CD3 MoAb and has important therapeutic implications.

Clinical use of anti-CD3 and anti-TCR MoAb

Anti-CD3

OKT3 (anti-human CD3) was the first murine MoAb introduced into clinical practice, in 1981 (Cosimi *et al.*, 1981a,b). No experimental models were available at that time since, contrary to other anti-T-cell antibodies such as anti-CD4 and anti-CD8, MoAb specific for human CD3 do not cross-react with T cells from the most commonly used primates (Rhesus and Cynomolgus monkeys). In addition, MoAb recognizing murine CD3 were not available.

OKT3 has primarily been used to reverse rejection episodes, but has also been employed in the prevention of acute rejection (Cosimi *et al.*, 1981a,b; Ortho Multicenter Transplant Study Group, 1985; Debure *et al.*, 1988; Kreis *et al.*, 1989). Both single-centre and randomized multicentre studies (Goldstein *et al.*, 1986; Hirsch *et al.*, 1987; Norman *et al.*, 1988; Widmar *et al.*, 1988) have shown that OKT3 is highly effective both as a first-line anti-rejection agent, and in patients with rejection unresponsive to conventional high-dose steroids as so-called 'rescue' therapy. OKT3 is still the only commercially available MoAb and, in many transplantation centres, has now replaced conventional therapy with polyclonal antisera. The efficacy of OKT3 for rescue in kidney rejection resistant to high-dose steroids and/or polyclonal anti-T-cell antibodies has been documented in both prospective and retrospective studies. Unfortunately, differences in both the protocols used and the patient selection criteria (Goldstein *et al.*, 1986; Hirsch *et al.*, 1987; Norman *et al.*, 1988; Widmar *et al.*, 1988) have led to some discrepancies, and the results of randomized trials are so far unavailable.

Recent studies of liver and heart allograft recipients have shown that OKT3 significantly improves the rate of rejection reversal (Starzl & Fung, 1986; Collonna *et al.*, 1987; Fung *et al.*, 1987; Kremer *et al.*, 1987; Gordon *et al.*, 1988; First *et al.*, 1989).

The other indication for OKT3 is in the prophylaxis of allograft rejection. OKT3 lowers the frequency of delayed graft function and acute rejection, the latter appearing later than in control patients (Debure *et al.*, 1988; Kreis *et al.*, 1989). Similar data have been reported for liver allografts (Millis *et al.*, 1989).

In both treatment and prophylaxis of rejection, OKT3 is administered at 5 mg/day for 10–14 consecutive days. The dose was initially based on the results of Scatchard analysis of T-cell CD3 molecules and early trials showing that in the vast majority of patients it effectively reverses clinical and histopathological signs of rejection. Doses higher than 5 mg must be avoided since they increase the severity of the first-dose cytokine-related syndrome and the risk of excessive immunosuppression. Indeed, an increased incidence of severe viral infections may occur if OKT3 is administered at cumulative doses higher than 75 mg (Swinnen *et al.*, 1990). Published protocols have associated OKT3 with corticosteroids, azathioprine and, occasionally, cyclosporin A (CyA) which is usually added by the end of the OKT3 course to avoid overimmunosuppression.

Attempts have been made to use OKT3 in other settings such as autoimmune diseases. A small number of patients with multiple sclerosis or autoimmune type I diabetes were treated (Chatenoud *et al.*, 1989a; Weinshenker *et al.*, 1991) but the protocol was interrupted in both cases because of a very severe OKT3-induced cytokine-related acute syndrome (described below).

Anti-TCR

Of the anti-TCR MoAbs available, BMA-031 was the first used most intensively in the clinical setting (Schlitt *et al.*, 1989). Only about 100 patients have received BMA-031, but randomized trials now underway should provide more sound data on the clinical effectiveness of this MoAb.

BMA-031 was highly effective in an early pilot trial conducted by Land *et al.* (1988) which included ten patients with steroid-resistant renal allograft rejection episodes unresponsive to conventional therapy. Unfortunately, the authors were unable to reproduce these results in a larger series of patients. However, other groups confirmed the effectiveness of BMA-031 for rescue treatment, provided that high doses were used (50 mg/day for 7 days) (Pfeffer *et al.*, 1991). In contrast to OKT3, high doses of BMA-031 can be used safely since cell activation *in vivo* is minor and does not trigger massive cytokine release (see below).

Encouraging results were also reported with BMA-031 in the treatment of acute graft-versus-host disease (GVHD) (Beelen *et al.*, 1988), but randomized trials have not been conducted.

The results of a small pilot trial in our centre with BMA-031 for the prevention of acute renal allograft rejection pointed to a dose-related problem calling for adequate pharmacokinetic studies. BMA-031 (5 or 20 mg/day for 14 days) was inadequate for rejection prophylaxis since it was quickly cleared from the circulation by neutralizing antibodies following rapid and intense xenosensitization. Although its mode of action is apparently close to that of OKT3, BMA-031 undergoes faster elimination, this is linked to a different handling of the MoAb bound to the cell receptor.

All the data suggest that BMA-031 should be administered at higher doses than OKT3 and for shorter periods. Very encouraging results were recently obtained using another anti-TCR MoAb, TIOBg (mouse IgM) to treat biopsy-proven acute cellular renal allograft rejection (Waid *et al.*, 1992).

Experimental models

Anti-CD3

Like most MoAbs specific for T-cell antigens, anti-CD3 are highly species specific. A murine IgG1 MoAb (FN18) developed by Nooij & Jonker (1987) defines an antigen homologous to human CD3 in Rhesus monkeys. FN18 is highly effective in preventing allograft rejection (Nooij et al., 1986). In contrast to human CD3, RhT3 expresses an allotypic poly-morphism of the FN18-defined epitope: T cells negative for FN18 are present in c. 3% of Rhesus monkeys (Nooij et al., 1986; Nooij & Jonker, 1987). Anti-CD3 MoAb have now also been raised in mice, and various authors have used an MoAb (145 2C11) specifically directed at the murine CD3 e chain (Leo et al., 1987). Its effects in vitro and in vivo have been extensively dissected by several groups, including our own (Leo et al., 1987; Hirsch et al., 1988, 1989; Alegre et al., 1990; Ferran et al., 1990b). A single high dose of 145 2C11 (400 µg/mouse, compared to the 5 mg/day of OKT3 usually administered to humans) given within 24–48 h after trans-plantation significantly prolongs the survival of completely mismatched skin allografts in animals (33 days versus 13 days in controls) (Hirsch et al., 1988). Similar results have been obtained with consecutive injections of the MoAb at much lower doses (5–10 µg/day for 7 days). Very high doses can only be used in adult animals bred in germ-free conditions; in adult mice pathogen-free, but non-axenic, they cause a high mortality rate (in our experiments, 100% of animals in 24–48 h), this is due to the cytokine release syndrome described below (Hirsch et al., 1989; Alegre et al., 1990; Ferran et al., 1990b). 145 2C11 F(ab)'2 fragments are also effective in prolonging skin graft survival but the only relevant study has shown a need for consecutive high-dose injections (Hirsch et al., 1990).

145 2C11 has also been used to prevent and treat type I diabetes in the non-obese diabetic (NOD) mouse model (Hayward & Shreiber, 1989; and our unpublished data). NOD mice spontaneously develop a T-cell-mediated autoimmune disease leading to total destruction of insulin-producing pancreatic β cells. They show significant mononuclear cell infiltration of the islets of Langherans by 6–8 weeks of age and develop overt glycosuria and hyperglycaemia by 24–30 weeks.

Using NOD neonates, Hayward and Shreiber (1989) induced sub-stantial and durable protection from the disease by injecting a single high dose (250 µg) of anti-CD3. At 10 weeks of age only 8% of treated animals had developed insulitis (versus 80% of controls) and less than 10% showed overt diabetes at 8 months (versus 50% of controls). Perturbations of the T-cell repertoire inducing long-lasting specific tolerance, but not asso-ciated with visible signs of global immunosuppression, are probably involved in this particular model; anti-CD3 can penetrate into the thymus and interfere with thymocyte binding to cortical epithelial cells and further lymphocyte maturation. This is not the case in adult animals in which depletion, coating and antigenic modulation of medullary single-positive $CD3^+$ thymocytes do not occur. Indeed, the thymus rapidly eliminates double-positive $CD3^-$ cortical thymocytes due to endogenous cortico-steroid production associated with anti-CD3-induced cytokine release (Ferran *et al.*, 1990a).

For our part, we have concentrated on adult NOD mice. Injection of low doses (5 µg/day, for 5 consecutive days) of anti-CD3 to 10–12-week-old NOD females reversed established insulitis; the same effect was observed using higher dosages of F(ab′)2 fragments of anti-CD3 (50 µg/day for 5 days). In both cases the mononuclear cell infiltrate reappeared within 10–15 days of stopping the treatment.

We have also studied the effect of anti-CD3 on the incidence of diabetes in the cyclophosphamide-induction model, in which autoimmune attack can be accelerated and its incidence increased by two injections of cyclophosphamide (200 mg/kg) at a 15-day interval. Ten to 15% of 8-week-old NOD males and females develop the disease 10 days after the first administration and 60–100% of the animals are overtly diabetic 2–3 weeks after the second injection. Anti-CD3 (5 µg/day for 5 consecutive days) started on day 13 (1 day before the second cyclophosphamide injection) had a marked preventive effect; only 14% of treated animals developed diabetes, compared to 90% of controls receiving normal ham-ster immunoglobulins (unpublished data). As was the case with insulitis, F(ab′)2 fragments showed a similar effect.

These results suggest that a more general blockade of T-cell-mediated immune functions, as in the case of the skin graft model, takes place in adult NOD mice however, in contrast to the neonate model, this promotes long-term but not permanent T-cell unresponsiveness.

Anti-TCR

MoAb recognizing monomorphic determinants in the mouse and rat TCR have been used *in vivo*. In the DA-LEW rat strain combination. MoAb R73 significantly prolonged skin allograft survival (24.2 versus 9.4 days) if applied twice at day −1 and +1 at high doses (1 mg) (Kurrle *et al.*, 1991). Identical results were obtained with F(ab′)2 fragments (Kurrle *et al.*, 1991). In mice, preliminary results using MoAb H57-597 were less clearcut; some authors described a significant prolongation of completely mismatched skin allograft survival, while others only found a mild effect (Kurrle *et al.*, 1991; Sempe *et al.*, 1991).

Anti-TCR treatment is effective for the prevention and treatment of autoimmune diseases. BDF1 hybrid mice develop a chronic form of graft-versus-host disease when injected with parental spleen cells (Kurrle *et al.*,

1991). This autoimmune disease starts 5–6 weeks after spleen cell injection and resembles human systemic lupus erythematosus. Almost all the mice develop glomerulonephritis and proteinuria, and usually die within 12 weeks. Two injections of MoAb H57-597 after the onset of the disease (days 57 and 60) significantly delayed the appearance of proteinuria and prolonged survival (55% survival at 300 days after spleen cell injection versus 0% in controls) (Kurrle et al., 1991).

In NOD mice, H57-597 MoAb treatment prevented the onset of both spontaneous and cyclophosphamide-induced diabetes (Sempe et al., 1991). The MoAb reversed not only established insulitis but also the first signs of metabolic disturbances (glucosuria and hyperglycaemia) which appear spontaneously in females. The therapeutic effect of the MoAb was fully reversible at the end of treatment (Sempe et al., 1991).

Mode of action of anti-CD3 and anti-TCR MoAb

Anti-CD3 and anti-TCR fall into the category of cell-depleting MoAb, although this is not their exclusive mode of action. In man, all peripheral T cells disappear rapidly (30–60 min) following the first OKT3 injection (5 mg) (Cosimi et al., 1981a; Chatenoud et al., 1982, 1983, 1986a). This extremely rapid effect, also seen in the murine model, is difficult to explain solely on the basis of cell lysis and is probably related to cell marginalization secondary to anti-CD3-induced expression of adhesion molecules on the vascular endothelium (M. Goldman, personal communication). Anti-CD3-induced opsonization and phagocytosis by reticuloendothelial cells seems to be a late phenomenon; evocative histopathological aspects are seen in the spleen of treated animals 48 h after the first injection. Another possible mechanism involves cell conjugate formation through binding of bivalent anti-CD3 to two distinct lymphocytes (Wong & Colvin, 1991). In vitro data show that if one of the cells is a $CD8^+$ cytotoxic precursor, the non-specific activation induced by anti-CD3 binding may drive it to kill the $CD3^+$ bystander (Wong & Colvin, 1991).

The peripheral depletion observed with anti-TCR in both clinical and experimental settings is also profound and rapid. The only difference is that some circulating, BMA-031-coated cells persist, while this is very rare with anti-CD3.

With both anti-CD3 and anti-TCR, small but significant numbers of T cells reappear in the circulation by the second to the fifth day of consecutive treatment (Chatenoud et al., 1982, 1983, 1986a; Chatenoud & Bach, 1984; Wonigeit et al., 1989). These T cells show antigenic modulation of the CD3/TCR complex, being either $CD3-TCR-CD4^+$ or $CD3-TCR-CD8^+$. The absence of circulating $CD3^+TCR^+$ cells is a useful parameter for monitoring the effectiveness of OKT3. Demodulation occurs within 8–12 h *in vitro* when the cells are incubated in the absence of MoAb, and *in vivo* when MoAb serum levels decline (due to immunization or cessation of treatment) (Chatenoud *et al.*, 1982, 1983, 1986a; Chatenoud & Bach, 1984). One interesting observation is that when used at the same dosage (5 mg/day) and independently of ongoing sensitization, BMA-031 is consumed more rapidly than OKT3; BMA-031 is undetectable in serum 24 h after injection, while OKT3 levels range from 500–1500 ng/ml. This suggests a more rapid turnover of the CD3–TCR/BMA-031 complex than the CD3–TCR/OKT3 complex and implies different internalization and re-expression. This has pharmacokinetic implications and may explain why higher BMA-031 doses are apparently required for therapeutic efficacy.

OKT3-modulated cells from patients receiving the MoAb in the absence of any other immunosuppressive treatment are totally unresponsive to mitogens and alloantigens (Chatenoud *et al.*, 1982, 1983, 1986a; Chatenoud & Bach, 1984). This corresponds to the profound immunosuppression exhibited by these patients; no allograft rejection is observed while CD3 cells are detectable in the circulation (Debure *et al.*, 1988; Chatenoud *et al.*, 1982, 1983, 1986a).

More studies of deep organ T cells in patients have involved OKT3. Ellenhorn *et al.* (1990) studied the cell phenotypes of lymph nodes from ten OKT3-treated patients prior to and within the first 2–8 h of the first injection. the most prominent feature was T-cell activation evidenced by the expression of specific interleukin 2 receptors (IL-2R), associated with OKT3 T-cell coating and minor signs of antigenic modulation. Caillat-Zucman *et al.* (1990) performed a longitudinal study on renal biopsies from patients receiving a 10-day course of OKT3 for allograft rejection. Although significant clearing of $CD3^+$ infiltrating T cells was seen in specimens taken at day 10, residual lymphocytes showed antigenic modulation (Caillat-Zucman *et al.*, 1990). It is therefore important to emphasize that complete clearance of infiltrating T cells is not a prerequisite for a durable clinical effect of OKT3.

More detailed results have been obtained with murine models. A single 145 2C11 administration within a very wide dose range (10–400 µg/mouse i.v.) very rapidly cleared all $CD3^+$ cells from the peripheral blood (Hirsch *et al.*, 1988). In contrast, a single high dose (70–400 µg) did not lead to complete T-cell elimination from spleen and lymph nodes; maximal depletion (*c.* 80–90%) occurred by the 10th day post-injection and the remaining T cells showed antigenic modulation of the CD3/TCR complex (Hirsch *et al.*, 1988). A normal T-cell pattern was only recovered after several weeks, and this occurred faster for $CD4^+$ than for $CD8^+$ cells. Mice receiving single low doses (5–20 µg) of anti-CD3 showed less depletion (*c.* 20–30%), but antigenic modulation of CD3/TCR on remnant

T cells was again observed (our unpublished data). Protocols similar to those used clinically, i.e. consecutive injections of low anti-CD3 doses (5–10 μg) induce significant cell depletion by the end of treatment, the only difference with the single high-dose administration being faster recovery (within 1 week) (our unpublished data).

As in the clinical setting, IL-2 receptors appear on T cells independently of the dose; expression is transient, peaking at 18–20 h after the first injection and then totally disappearing, even in the case of daily treatment (Hirsch et al., 1989). Histological examination has shown firm evidence of cell lysis and reticuloendothelial cell destruction, particularly in the spleen, liver and lymph nodes (Hirsch et al., 1988; Ferran et al., 1990b).

Results with anti-TCR in mice are similar; antigenic modulation and cell coating are more marked than depletion in spleen and lymph nodes, contrasting with almost complete disappearance of TCR$^+$ cells from peripheral blood.

Finally, it is important to stress that the mode of action of anti-CD3 and anti-TCR is not restricted to cellular depletion and antigenic modulation. The delivery of inhibitory or activating intracellular signals as a consequence of anti-CD3/TCR cell binding and antigenic modulation may trigger T-cell-mediated immunoregulatory circuits that could turn out to be a major mode of action (Feldmann et al., 1985; Pantaleo et al., 1987). Unfortunately, the fine characterization of both the intracellular triggering signals and subsequent immunoregulatory mechanisms is incomplete.

Anti-CD3 and anti-TCR-induced T-cell activation *in vivo*

A systemic reaction is invariably observed when anti-CD3 MoAbs are injected (Cosimi et al., 1981a,b; Ortho Multicenter Transplant Study Group, 1985; Chatenoud et al., 1989b). An acute clinical syndrome occurs only after the first OKT3 injection and is associated with high fever, chills, headaches, vomiting, diarrhoea and, occasionally, more severe reactions such as pulmonary oedema, aseptic meningitis and hypotension (Cosimi et al., 1981a,b; Ortho Multicenter Transplant Study Group, 1985; Abramowicz et al., 1989; Chatenoud et al., 1989b, 1990). Although spontaneously reversible and seldom life-threatening at a dose of 5 mg, the syndrome precludes the use of OKT3 in settings other than transplantation. In mice, a similar transient reaction is characterized by somnolence, hypomotility, diarrhoea, hypothermia and piloerection (Alegre et al., 1990; Ferran et al., 1990b).

This syndrome corresponds to the monocyte-dependent anti-CD3-mediated lymphokine release observed *in vitro* (van Wauwe et al., 1980;

Chang *et al.*, 1981; Burns *et al.*, 1982; van Lier *et al.*, 1987). The first anti-CD3 injection causes a dramatic release of several cytokines into the systemic circulation, both in clinical and experimental conditions (Abramowicz *et al.*, 1989; Chatenoud *et al.*, 1989b, 1990; Alegre *et al.*, 1990; Ferran *et al.*, 1990a,b). Tumour necrosis factor (TNF), interferon (IFN)γ, IL-2, IL-3, IL-4, IL-6 and granulocyte-macrophage-colony-stimulating factor (GM-CSF) are all detectable in the circulation. In contrast, no IL-1β or IFNα is detected. In mice, histological studies show lesions involving not only lymphoid organs but also the lung and liver (inflammatory cell infiltration and diffuse vascular congestion), two well-known targets for cytokines (Ferran *et al.*, 1990b). This activation is monocyte-dependent and probably occurs via opsonization of anti-CD3-coated lymphocytes; anti-CD3 F(ab')$_2$ fragments do not promote cytokine release and are well tolerated (Hirsch *et al.*, 1990). However, detailed studies of mice have demonstrated that the vast majority of the cytokines released, including TNF, are of T-cell origin.

Comparative experience with anti-TCR MoAb further stresses the importance of the epitope recognized on the CD3/TCR complex in massive T-cell activation. Anti-TCR MoAb (BMA-031 in particular) are very well tolerated when injected *in vivo* — only mild fever and moderate gastrointestinal symptoms have been reported. After the first BMA-031 injection, only TNF is released in the circulation. These results support our findings in anti-CD3-treated mice, i.e. that synergism between cytokines is required to induce the characteristic clinical syndrome; TNF alone, even when released in large amounts, is insufficient (Ferran *et al.*, 1991a). Several *in vitro* data support the view that BMA-031 and OKT3 induce distinct cell activation pathways. Antibodies to CD28 exert little if any co-stimulatory effect with anti-CD3 on peripheral lymphocytes; in contrast, the effect is highly significant with BMA-031, especially on purified T cells (Kurrle *et al.*, 1991). Moreover, it has been proposed that BMA-031 preferentially activates certain T-cell subsets, namely CD45RA$^+$ cells (Schwinzer *et al.*, 1992).

Other evidence supporting the cause–effect relationship between cytokine release and the anti-CD3-induced syndrome include the observations that other opsonizing and/or depleting MoAb (e.g. anti-CD4 and anti-CD8) that do not induce cell activation and cytokine release are perfectly well tolerated and that effective prevention of the anti-CD3-induced syndrome is achieved in mice and patients by pre-treatment with anti-TNF antibodies (Ferran *et al.*, 1991b; Charpentier *et al.*, 1992). Importantly, the beneficial effect of anti-TNF is not only due to the neutralization of TNF biological activity but also to a pre-transcriptional modulation of other anti-CD3-induced cytokines (upregulation of IFNγ and downregulation of IL-3 and IL-6) (Ferran *et al.*, submitted).

Xenosensitization

Immunization against the murine immunoglobulin molecule was one of the first drawbacks in early trials of anti-CD3 MoAb. With the antibody alone (no conventional immunosuppressants) all patients showed very significant titres of anti-OKT3 IgM and IgG antibodies by day 5–7 of consecutive treatment (Chatenoud *et al.*, 1982, 1983, 1986a). Sensitization is seen with all types of xenogeneic MoAb recognizing cell surface receptors used in both clinical and experimental settings, independently of their fine specificity (Baudrihaye *et al.*, 1984; Benjamin *et al.*, 1986; Chatenoud *et al.*, 1986a; Villemain *et al.*, 1986; Jonker & den Brok, 1987; Hafler *et al.*, 1988). Anti-TCR MoAb also trigger an immune response, which is more intense than that observed with OKT3; it regularly occurs within the first 5 days of consecutive treatment and is associated with very high titres of IgG and IgM antibodies.

This humoral response is important given its potent neutralizing effect, essentially due to IgG antibodies. Contrary to polyclonal antisera, sensitization to MoAb never leads to clinically evident immune complex disease (serum sickness).

These peculiarities of the response are related to its restriction in terms of both specificity and clonality. Contrary to polyclonal anti-T-cell immunoglobulins, anti-T-cell MoAb induce a response that does not exhibit broad 'anti-mouse' specificity but selectively recognizes the in-jected xenogeneic immunoglobulin. This was shown for the first time with affinity chromatography-purified serum fractions from patients immun-ized against OKT3 (Baudrihaye *et al.*, 1984; Chatenoud, 1986; Chatenoud *et al.*, 1986a). Only two sorts of anti-OKT3 antibody were detected, recognizing either isotypic (IgG2) or idiotypic determinants of OKT3 (Baudrihaye *et al.*, 1984; Chatenoud, 1986; Chatenoud *et al.*, 1986a). Only anti-idiotypic antibodies competed with OKT3 for binding to the T-cell receptor, thereby neutralizing the therapeutic effect. The restriction is more evident in the case of anti-BMA-031 antibodies — an exclusive anti-idiotypic response is seen in the vast majority of patients (Chatenoud *et al.*, submitted). The restriction of the response implies that even if sensitization against a given MoAb occurs, a second course using an MoAb showing different specificity (implying expression of distinct idiotypes) or the same specificity but different idiotypes may be effective. For example, consecu-tive use of BMA-031 and OKT3 is successful, since anti-BMA-031 antibodies never cross-react with OKT3 and vice-versa. Jonker and Den Brok (1987) showed that the same was true for the consecutive use of different anti-CD4 with distinct idiotypes in monkeys.

Further pointing to the restriction of B-cell clones committed to the anti-MoAb response, isoelectrofocusing experiments with sera from patients receiving OKT3 and BMA-031, and from monkeys treated with anti-CD4 and anti-CD8 MoAb, revealed that the response is oligoclonal (Chatenoud *et al.*, 1986b).

It thus appears that the neutralizing potential of the anti-MoAb response is more dependent on its specificity than on the overall amount of antibodies produced, since only a few specific clones are recruited. Thus, immune complexes do form in insufficient amounts to cause a generalized reaction.

Why the administration of relatively small amounts of homogeneous xenogeneic proteins via a non-immunogenic route (i.v.) should provoke such a powerful anti-idiotypic humoral response is not fully understood. An appealing hypothesis is that MoAb recognizing cell surface structures follow a particular pathway for antigen presentation relative to those recognizing circulating molecules, which favours the generation of anti-idiotypic antibodies (Benjamin *et al.*, 1986). This indirectly attributes a key role to the variable portion of the MoAb in determining immunogenicity. However, recent data showing that humanized chimeric MoAb do not provoke an anti-idiotypic response underline the importance of the carrier effect of the constant portion.

In clinical practice, the association of appropriate dosages of chemical immunosuppressants with most MoAb (BMA-031 is an exception) may significantly decrease the frequency and intensity of sensitization. In the case of OKT3, adding corticosteroids and azathioprine at adequate doses decreases the frequency of sensitization from 90–95% to 40–60% (Chatenoud *et al.*, 1986a; Cosimi, 1987; Hricik *et al.*, 1990). Cyclosporin A association further decreases the rate to 15–25% depending on the report. In most cases antibodies appear only at or after the end of the OKT3 treatment course and do not affect efficacy.

Sensitization to BMA-031 seems more difficult to control by the simple addition of other immunosuppressants. From the limited data available at present we can only deduce that with BMA-031 corticosteroids + azathioprine do not prevent the onset of a rapid and intense response. More extensive controlled trials are required (especially with CsA) to draw firm conclusions.

Needless to say, major efforts and hopes are being placed on the development of chimeric or reshaped humanized MoAb (Riechmann *et al.*, 1988). With the various clinical studies already in progress with humanized anti-T-cell MoAb of different specificities we should soon know whether the very encouraging results initially reported are valid on a larger scale.

Conclusion

The potent immunosuppressive activity of anti-CD3 is well established. This MoAb should no doubt find new applications in autoimmune diseases once its two major side-effects, xenosensitization and the first-dose acute syndrome, have been circumvented. Direct proof of the clinical immunosuppressive potency of anti-TCR is still awaited. Clinical trials now in progress are aimed at extending promising preliminary data.

For these two MoAbs, it remains to be determined whether, in addition to selective short-term immunosuppression, they might in some way be able to mediate permanent specific unresponsiveness. Although it is possible to induce long-term disease remission following neonatal treatment of NOD mice with anti-CD3 (Hayward & Shreiber, 1989), this is a special situation in which anti-CD3 directly interferes with T-cell maturation.

Interestingly, data obtained both *in vitro* and *in vivo* show that low-dose anti-CD3 is unique in its ability to trigger T-cell-mediated regulatory processes. *In vitro*, Delfraissy *et al.* (1985) showed that low doses of soluble OKT3 induce T-suppressor cells specific for the 2,4,6-trinitrophenyl-polyacrylamide (TNP-PAA) antibody response. In contrast with the mitogenic effect of OKT3, suppressor T cells induction was independent of the presence of monocytes, since it could also be induced in highly monocyte-depleted cultures. Moreover, this effect was also induced by non-mitogenic F(ab')2 OKT3 fragments (Delfraissy *et al.*, 1985).

In vivo, Ellenhorn *et al.* (1988) showed that single low doses of anti-CD3 (4 μg/mouse) induced specific immune responses. In a C3H fibrosarcoma model, none of the mice injected with a single low dose (4 μg) of 145 2C11 developed tumours. Moreover these animals were also resistant to a second tumour inoculum 2 months later, in the absence of additional MoAb therapy, showing that they had developed active immunity mediated by specific cytotoxic T cells (Ellenhorn *et al.*, 1988).

All these findings are highly encouraging for further experimental work and, in the near future, clinical protocols.

References

Abramowicz, D., Schandenne, L., Goldman, M., Crusiaux, A., Vereestraeten, P., De Pauw, L., Wybran, J., Kinnaert, P., Dupont, E. & Toussaint, C. (1989). Release of tumor necrosis factor, interleukin 2, and gamma-interferon in serum after injection of OKT3 monoclonal antibody in kidney transplant recipients. *Transplantation* **47**, 606–613.

Alegre, M., Vandenabeele, P., Flamand, V., Moser, M., Leo, O., Abramowicz, D., Urbain, J., Fiers, W. & Goldman, M. (1990). Hypothermia and hypoglycemia induced by anti-CD3 monoclonal antibody in mice; role of tumor necrosis factor. *European Journal of Immunology* **20**, 707–710.

Baniyash, M., Hsu, V. W., Seldin, M. F. & Klausner, R. D. (1989). The isolation and characterization of the murine T cell antigen receptor δ-chain gene. *Journal of Biological Chemistry* **264**, 13252–13257.

Baudrihaye, M. F., Chatenoud, L., Kreis, H., Goldstein, G. & Bach, J. F. (1984). Unusually restricted anti-isotype human immune response to OKT3 monoclonal antibody. *European Journal of Immunology* **14**, 686–691.

Beelen, D. W., Graeven, U., Schulz, G., Grosse-Wilde, H., Doxiadis, I., Schaefer, U. W., Quabeck, K., Sayer, H. & Schmidt, C. G. (1988). Treatment of acute graft-versus-host disease after HLA-partially matched marrow transplantation with a monoclonal antibody (BMA-031) against the T cell receptor. First results of a phase-I/II trial. *Onkologie* **11**, 56–58.

Benjamin, R. J., Cobbold, S. P., Clark, M. R. & Waldmann, H. (1986). Tolerance to rat monoclonal antibodies. *Journal of Experimental Medicine* **163**, 1539–1552.

Borst, J., Colligan, J. E., Oettgen, H., Pessano, S., Malin, R. & Terhorst, C. (1984). The gamma and epsilon chains of the human T3/T cell receptor complex are distinct polypeptides. *Nature* **312**, 455–458.

Burns, G. F., Boyd, A. W. & Beverley, P. C. L. (1982). Two monoclonal anti-human T lymphocyte antibodies have similar biologic effects and recognize the same cell surface antigen. *Journal of Immunology* **129**, 1451–1457.

Caillat-Zucman, S., Blumenfeld, N., Legendre, C., Noël, L. H., Bach, J. F., Kreis, H. & Chatenoud, L. (1990). The OKT3 immunosuppressive effect. *In situ* antigenic modulation of human graft-infiltrating T cells. *Transplantation* **49**, 156–160.

Chang, T. W., Kung, P. C., Gingras, S. P. & Goldstein, G. (1981). Does OKT3 monoclonal antibody react with an antigen-recognition structure on human T cells? *Proceedings of the National Academy of Sciences of the United States of America* **78**, 1805–1808.

Charpentier, B., Hiesse, L., Lantz, O., Ferran, C., Stephens, S., O'Shaugnessy, D., Bodmer, M., Fries, D., Bach, J. F. & Chatenoud, L. (1992). Anti-human tumor necrosis factor monoclonal antibody prevents OKT3-induced acute syndrome. *Transplantation* (in press).

Chatenoud, L. (1986). The immune response against therapeutic monoclonal antibodies. *Immunology Today* **7**, 367–368.

Chatenoud, L. & Bach, J. F. (1984). Antigenic modulation. A major mechanism of antibody action. *Immunology Today* **5**, 20–25.

Chatenoud, L., Baudrihaye, M. F., Chkoff, N., Kreis, H. & Bach, J. F. (1983). Immunologic follow-up of renal allograft recipients treated prophylactically by OKT3 alone. *Transplantation Proceedings* **15**, 643–645.

Chatenoud, L., Baudrihaye, M. F., Chkoff, N., Kreis, H., Goldstein, G. & Bach, J. F. (1986a). Restriction of the human in vivo immune response against the mouse monoclonal antibody OKT3. *Journal of Immunology* **137**, 830–838.

Chatenoud, L., Baudrihaye, M. F., Kreis, H., Goldstein, G., Schindler, J. & Bach, J. F. (1982). Human *in vivo* antigenic modulation induced by the anti-T cell OKT3 monoclonal antibody. *European Journal of Immunology* **12**, 979–982.

Chatenoud, L., Ferran, C. & Bach, J. F. (1989a). *In vivo* anti-CD3 treatment of autoimmune patients (Letter). *Lancet* **ii**, 164.

Chatenoud, L., Ferran, C., Legendre, C., Thourard, I., Merite, S., Reuter, A., Gevaert, Y., Kreis, H., Franchimont, P. & Bach, J. F. (1990). *In vivo* cell activation following OKT3 administration; systemic cytokine release and modulation by corticosteroids. *Transplantation* **49**, 697–702.

Chatenoud, L., Ferran, C., Reuter, A., Legendre, C., Gevaert, Y., Kreis, H., Franchimont, P. & Bach, J. F. (1989b). Systemic reaction to the monoclonal antibody OKT3 in relation to serum levels of tumor necrosis factor and interferon γ. *New England Journal of Medicine* **320**, 1420–1421.

Chatenoud, L., Jonker, M., Villemain, F., Goldstein, G. & Bach, J. F. (1986b). The human immune response to the OKT3 monoclonal antibody is oligoclonal. *Science* **232**, 1406–1408.

Clevers, H., Alarcon, B., Wileman, T. & Terhorst, C. (1988). The T cell receptor/CD3 complex: a dynamic protein ensemble. *Annual Review of Immunology* **6**, 629–662.

Colonna, J. O., Goldstein, L. I., Brems, J. J., Vargas, J. H. & Brill, J. E. (1987). A prospective study on the use of monoclonal anti-T3-cell antibody (OKT3) to treat steroid-resistant liver transplant rejection. *Archives of Surgery* **122**, 1120–1123.

Cosimi, B. (1987). Clinical development of Orthoclone OKT3. *Transplantation Proceedings* **14** (suppl 1), 7–16.

Cosimi, A. B., Burton, R. C., Colvin, R. B., Goldstein, G., Delmonico, F. L., La Quaglia, M. P., Tolkoff-Rubin, N., Rubin, R. H., Herrin, J. T. & Russel, P. (1981a). Treatment of acute renal allograft rejection with OKT3 monoclonal antibody. *Transplantation* **32**, 535–539.

Cosimi, A. B., Colvin, R. B., Burton, R. C., Rubin, R. H., Goldstein, G., Kung, P. C., Hansen, P., Delmonico, F. L. & Russel, P. S. (1981b). Use of monoclonal antibodies to T-cell subsets for immunologic monitoring and treatment in recipients of renal allografts. *New England Journal of Medicine* **305**, 308–314.

Debure, A., Chkoff, N., Chatenoud, L., Lacombe, M., Campos, H., Noel, L. H., Goldstein, G., Bach, J. F. & Kreis, H. (1988). One month prophylactic use of OKT3 in cadaver kidney transplant recipients. *Transplantation* **45**, 546–553.

Delfraissy, J. F., Wallon, C., Boue, F., Vazquez, A. & Galanaud, P. (1985). Suppressor T cell induction by soluble OKT3 antibody does not require cross-linking of the T3 molecule. *European Journal of Immunology* **15**, 433–438.

Ellenhorn, J. D. I., Hirsch, R., Schreiber, H. & Bluestone, J. A. (1988). Administration of anti-CD3 prevents malignant progressor tumor growth. *Science* **242**, 569–571.

Ellenhorn, J. D. I., Woodle, E. S., Ghobreal, I., Thistlethwaite, J. R. & Bluestone, J. (1990). Activation of human T cells *in vivo* following treatment of transplant recipients with OKT3. *Transplantation* **50**, 608–612.

Emmrich, F., Strittmatter, U. & Eichmann, K. (1986). Synergism in the activation of human CD8 T cells by cross-linking the T cell receptor complex with the CD8 differentiation antigen. *Proceedings of the National Academy of Sciences of America* **83**, 8298–8302.

Feldmann, M., Zanders, E. D. & Lamb, J. R. (1985). Tolerance in T-cell clones. *Immunology Today* **6**, 58–62.

Ferran, C., Dy, M., Merite, S., Sheehan, K., Schreiber, R., Leboulanger, F., Landais, P., Bluestone, J. A., Bach, J. F. & Chatenoud, L. (1990a). Corticosteroids reduce morbidity and cytokine release in anti-CD3 MoAb treated mice. *Transplantation* **50**, 642–648.

Ferran, C., Dy, M., Sheehan, K., Merite, S., Schreiber, R., Landais, P., Grau, G., Bluestone, J. A., Bach, J. F. & Chatenoud, L. (1991a). Inter-mouse strain differences in the *in vivo* anti-CD3 induced cytokine release. *Clinical and Experimental Immunology* **86**, 537–543.

Ferran, C., Dy, M., Sheehan, K., Schreiber, R., Grau, G., Bluestone, J. A., Bach, J. F. & Chatenoud, L. (1991b). Cascade modulation by anti-tumor necrosis factor monoclonal antibody on interferon γ interleukin 3 and interleukin 6 release after triggering of the CD3/T cell receptor activation pathway. *European Journal of Immunology* **21**, 2349–2353.

Ferran, C., Sheehan, C., Dy, M., Schreiber, R., Merite, S., Landais, P., Noel, L. H., Grau, G., Bluestone, J. A., Bach, J. F. & Chatenoud, L. (1990b). Cytokine related syndrome following injection of anti-CD3 monoclonal antibody: further evidence for transient *in vivo* T cell activation. *European Journal of Immunology* **20**, 509–515.

First, M. R., Schroeder, T. J., Hurtubise, P. E., Mansour, M. E., Penn, I., Munda, R., Balistreri, W. F., Alexander, J. W., Melvin, D. B., Fidler, J. P., Ryckman, F. C. & Brunson, M. E. (1989). Successful retreatment of allograft rejection with OKT3. *Transplantation* **47**, 88–91.

Fung, J. J., Markus, B. H., Gordon, R. D., Esquivel, C. O. & Makowka, L. (1987). Impact of Orthoclone OKT3 on liver transplantation. *Transplantation Proceedings* **19** (suppl. 1), 37–44.

Goldstein, G., Norman, D. J., Shield, C. F., Kreis, H. & Burdick, J. (1986). OKT3 monoclonal antibody reversal of acute renal allograft rejection unresponsive to conventional immunosuppressive treatments. In Meryman H. T. (ed), *Transplantation: Approaches to Graft Rejection*, pp. 329–249. Alan R. Liss Inc, New York.

Gordon, R. D., Tazkis, A. G., Iwatsuki, S., Todo, S., Esquivel, C. O., Marsh, J. W., Stieber, A., Makowka, L. & Starzl, T. E. (1988). Experience with Orthoclone OKT3 in liver transplantation. *American Journal of Kidney Diseases* **11**, 141–144.

Hafler, D. A., Ritz, J., Schlossmann, S. F. & Weiner, H. L. (1988). Anti-CD4 and anti-CD2 monoclonal antibody infusions in subjects with multiple sclerosis. Immunosuppressive effect and anti-mouse immune response. *Journal of Immunology* **141**, 131–138.

Haskins, K., Kubo, R., White, J., Pigeon, M., Kappler, J. & Marrack, P. (1983). The major histocompatibility complex-restricted antigen receptor on T cells. I. Isolation with a monoclonal antibody. *Journal of Experimental Medicine* **157**, 1149–1169.

Haywad, A. R. & Shreiber, M. (1989). Neonatal injection of CD3 antibody into nonobese diabetic mice reduces the incidence of insulitis and diabetes. *Journal of Immunology* **143**, 1555–1559.

Hirsch, R., Bluestone, J. A., DeNenno, L. & Gress, R. E. (1990). Anti-CD3 F(ab′)2 fragments are immunosuppressive *in vivo* without evoking either the strong humoral response or morbidity associated with whole mAb. *Transplantation* **49**, 1117–1123.

Hirsch, R., Eckhaus, M., Auchincloss, H. Jr., Sachs, D. H. & Bluestone, J. A. (1988). Effects of *in vivo* administration of anti-T3 monoclonal antibody on T cell function in mice. I. Immunosuppression of transplantation responses. *Journal of Immunology* **140**, 3766–3772.

Hirsch, R., Gress, R. E., Pluznik, D. H., Eckhaus, M. & Bluestone, J. A. (1989). Effects of *in vivo* administration of anti-T3 monoclonal antibody on T cell function in mice. II. *In vivo* activation of T cells. *Journal of Immunology* **142**, 737–743.

Hirsch, R. L., Layton, P. C., Barnes, L. A., Kremer, A. B. & Goldstein, G. (1987). Orthoclone OKT3 treatment of acute renal allograft rejection in patients receiving maintenance cyclosporine therapy. *Transplantation Proceedings* **19** (suppl. 1), 32–36.

Hricik, D. E., Mayes, J. T. & Schulak, J. A. (1990). Inhibition of anti-OKT3 antibody generation by cyclosporine. Results of a prospective randomized trial. *Transplantation* **50**, 237–240.

Jonker, M. & Den Brok, J. H. A. M. (1987). Idiotype switching of CD4-specific monoclonal antibodies can prolong the therapeutic effectiveness in spite of host anti mouse IgG antibodies. *European Journal of Immunology* **17**, 1547–1553.

Kreis, H., Chkoff, N., Chatenoud, L., Debure, A., Lacombe, M., Chrétien, Y., Legendre, C., Caillat-Zucman, S. & Bach, J. F. (1989). A randomized trial comparing the efficacy of OKT3 used to prevent or to treat rejection. *Transplantation Proceedings* **21**, 1741–1745.

Kremer, A. B., Barnes, L., Hirsch, R. & Goldstein, G. (1987). Orthoclone OKT3 monoclonal antibody reversal of hepatic and cardiac allograft rejection unresponsive to conventional immunosuppressive treatments. *Transplantation Proceedings* **19** (suppl. 1), 54–57.

Kurrle, R., Schorlemmer, H. U., Shearman, C., Lauffer, L., Frank, K., Kanzy, E. J. & Seiler, F. R. (1991). Analysis of the immunoregulatory capacity of anti-α/β-TCR and anti-CD3 monoclonal antibodies. *Transplantation Proceedings* **23**, 272–276.

Land, W., Hillebrand, G., Illner, W. D., Abendroth, D., Hancke, E., Schleibner, S., Hammer, C. & Racenberg, J. (1988). First clinical experience with a new TCR/CD3-

monoclonal antibody (BMA-031) in kidney transplant patients. *Transplantation Proceedings* **1**, 116–117.

Leo, O., Foo, M., Sachs, D. H., Samelson, L. E. & Bluestone, J. A. (1987). Identification of a monoclonal antibody specific for a murine T3 polypeptide. *Proceedings of the National Academy of Sciences of the United States of America* **84**, 1374–1378.

McCleod, C., Mining, L., Gold, D., Terhorst, C. & Wilkinson, M. (1986). Negative transregulation of T-cell antigen receptor/T3 complex mRNA expression in murine T lymphoma somatic cell hybrids. *Proceedings of the National Academy of Sciences of the United States of America* **83**, 6989–6993.

Meuer, S. C., Acuto, O., Hercend, T., Schlossman, S. F. & Reinherz, E. (1984). The human T cell receptor. *Annual Review of Immunology* **2**, 23–50.

Meuer, S. C., Cooper, D. A., Hodgdon, J. C., Hussey, R. E., Fitzgerald, K. A., Schlossman, S. F. & Reinherz, E. L. (1983a). Identification of the receptor for antigen and major histocompatibility complex on human inducer T lymphocytes. *Science* **222**, 1239–1241.

Meuer, S. C., Fitzgerald, K. A., Hussey, R. E., Hodgdon, J. C., Schlossman, S. F. & Reinherz, E. L. (1983b). Clonotypic structures involved in antigen specific human T cell function. Relationship to the T3 molecular complex. *Journal of Experimental Medicine* **157**, 705–719.

Millis, J. M., McDiarmid, S. V., Hiatt, J. R., Brems, J. J., Colonna II, J. O., Klein, A. S., Ashizawa, T., Hart, J., Lewin, K., Goldstein, L. I., Levy, P. & Busuttil, R. W. (1989). Randomized prospective trial of OKT3 for early prophylaxis of rejection after liver transplantation. *Transplantation* **47**, 82–88.

Nooij, F. J. M. & Jonker, M. (1987). The effect on skin allograft survival of a monoclonal antibody specific for a polymorphic CD3-like cell surface molecule in rhesus monkeys. *European Journal of Immunology* **17**, 1089–1093.

Nooij, F. J. M., Jonker, M. & Balner, H. (1986). Differentiation antigens on rhesus monkey lymphocytes. II. Characterization of RhT3, a CD3-like antigen on T cells. *European Journal of Immunology* **16**, 981–984.

Norman, D. J., Barry, J. M., Bennett, W. M., Leone, M., Henell, K., Funnell, B. & Hubert, B. (1988). The use of OKT3 in cadaveric renal transplantation for rejection that is unresponsive to conventional anti-rejection therapy. *American Journal of Kidney Diseases* **11**, 90–93.

Oettgen, H., Kappler, J., Tax, W. J. M. & Terhorst, C. (1984). Characterization of the two heavy chains of the T3 complex on the surface of human T lymphocytes. *Journal of Biological Chemistry* **259**, 12039–12048.

Ortho Multicenter Transplant Study Group (1985). A randomized clinical trial of OKT3 monoclonal antibody for acute rejection of cadaveric renal transplants. *New England Journal of Medicine* **313**, 337–342.

Pantaleo, G., Olive, D., Poggi, A., Pozzan, T., Moretta, L. & Moretta, A. (1987). Antibody-induced modulation of the CD3/T cell receptor complex causes T cell refractoriness by inhibiting the early metabolic steps involved in T cell activation. *Journal of Experimental Medicine* **166**, 619–624.

Pessano, S., Oettgen, H., Bhan, A. K. & Terhorst, C. (1985). The T3/T cell receptor complex: antigenic distinction between the 20-kD T3 (T3-δ and T3-ε) subunits. *EMBO Journal* **4**, 337–344.

Pfeffer, P. F., Jakobsen, A., Albrechtsen, D., Sodal, G., Brekke, I., Bentdal, O., Leivestadn, T., Fauchald, P. & Flatmark, A. (1991). BMA-031 effectively reverses steroid-resistant rejection in renal transplants. *Transplantation Proceedings* **23**, 1099–1100.

Regueiro, J. R., Arnaiz-Villera, Ortiz de Landazuri, M., Martin-Vella, J. M., Vicario, J. L., Pascual-Ruiz, V., Guerra-Garciz, F., Alcarni, J., Lopez-Botet, M. & Manzanares,

J. (1986). Familial defect of CD3 (T3-) expression by T cells associated with rare gut epithelial cell autoantibodies. *Lancet* **i**, 1274–1275.

Reinherz, E. L., Hussey, R. E. & Schlossman, S. F. (1980). A monoclonal antibody blocking human T cell function. *European Journal of Immunology* **10**, 758–762.

Riechmann, L., Clark, M., Waldmann, H. & Winter, G. (1988). Reshaping human antibodies for therapy. *Nature* **332**, 323–327.

Saizawa, K., Rojo, J. & Janeway, C. A. Jr. (1987). Evidence for a physical association of CD4 and the CD3:α:β:T cell receptor. *Nature* **328**, 260–263.

Samelson, L. E., Harford, J. B. & Klausner, R. D. (1985). Identification of the components of the murine T cell antigen receptor complex. *Cell* **43**, 223–231.

Schlitt, H. J., Kurrle, R. & Wonigeit, K. (1989). T cell activation by monoclonal antibodies directed to different epitopes on the human T cell receptor/CD3 complex: evidence for two different modes of activation. *European Journal of Immunology* **19**, 1649–1655.

Schwinzer, R., Schlitt, H. J. & Wonigeit, K. (1992). Monoclonal antibodies to common epitopes of the human α/β T-cell receptor preferentially activate CD45RA + T-cells. *Cellular Immunology* **140**, 31–41.

Sempe, P., Bedossa, P., Richard, M. F., Villa, M. C., Bach, J. F. & Boitard, C. (1991). Anti-α/β T cell receptor monoclonal antibody provides an efficient therapy for autoimmune diabetes in diabetic (NOD) mice. *European Journal of Immunology* **21**, 1163–1169.

Starzl, T. E. & Fung, J. J. (1986). Orthoclone OKT3 in treatment of allografts rejected under cyclosporin-steroid therapy. *Transplantation Proceedings* **18**, 937–941.

Swinnen, L. J., Costanzo-Nordin, M. R., Fisher, S. G., O'Sullivan, E. J., Johnson, M. R., Heroux, A. L., Dizikes, G. J., Pifarre, R. & Fisher, R. I. (1990). Increased incidence of lymphoproliferative disorder after immunosuppression with the monoclonal antibody OKT3 in cardiac transplant recipients. *New England Journal of Medicine* **323**, 1723–1728.

Van Lier, R. A. W., Boot, J. H. A., De Groot, E. R. & Aarden, L. A. (1987). Induction of T cell proliferation with anti-CD3 switch-variant monoclonal antibodies; effects of heavy chain isotype in monocyte dependent systems. *European Journal of Immunology* **17**, 1599–1604.

Van Wauwe, J. P., De May, J. R. & Goossens, J. G. (1980). OKT3: a monoclonal anti-human T lymphocyte antibody with potent mitogenic properties. *Journal of Immunology* **124**, 2708–2713.

Villemain, F., Jonker, M., Bach, J. F. & Chatenoud, L. (1986). Fine specificity of antibodies produced in rhesus monkeys following *in vivo* treatment with anti-T cell murine monoclonal antibodies. *European Journal of Immunology* **16**, 945–949.

Waid, T. H., Lucas, B. A., Thompson, J. S., Brown, S. A., Munch, L., Prebeck, R. J. & Jezek, D. (1992). Treatment of acute cellular rejection with T10B9.1A-31 or OKT3 in renal allograft recipients. *Transplantation* **53**, 80–96.

Weinshenker, B. G., Bass, B., Karlik, S., Ebers, G. C. & Rice, G. P. A. (1991). An open trial of OKT3 in patients with multiple sclerosis. *Neurology* **41**, 1047–1052.

Weiss, A. & Stobo, J. D. (1984). Requirement for the coexpression of T3 an the T cell antigen receptor on a malignant human T cell. *Journal of Experimental Medicine* **160**, 1284–1299.

Weissman, A. M., Samelson, L. E. & Clausner, R. D. (1986). A new subunit of the human T cell antigen receptor. *Nature* **324**, 480–482.

Widmer, U., Frei, D., Keusch, G., Burger, H. R. & Larglader, F. (1988). OKT3 treatment of steroid- and/or anti-thymocyte globulin-resistant renal allograft rejection occurring on triple baseline immunosuppression including cyclosporine A. *Transplantation Proceedings* **20** (suppl. 6), 90–95.

Wong, J. T. & Colvin, R. B. (1991). Selective reduction and proliferation of the CD4$^+$ and CD8$^+$ T cell subsets with bispecific monoclonal antibodies: evidence for inter-T cell-mediated cytolysis. *Clinical Immunology and Immunopathology* **58**, 236–250.

Wonigeit, K., Nashan, B., Schwinzer, R., Schlitt, H. J., Kurrle, R., Racenberg, J., Seiler, F., Ringe, B. & Pichlmayr, R. (1989). Use of a monoclonal antibody (BMA-031) against the T cell receptor for prophylactic immunosuppressive treatment after liver transplantation. *Transplantation Proceedings* **21**, 2258–2259.

Chapter 9
Therapeutic anti-CD4 antibodies

Frank Emmrich and Jean-François Bach

The CD4 molecule: structure and function

The mature CD4 molecule is a 55 kDa monomeric glycoprotein which was found first on a subset of T lymphocytes (Reinherz & Schlossman, 1980; Maddon *et al.*, 1985). It consists of an extracellular region (*c.* 370 amino acid residues), a hydrophobic transmembrane domain (26 amino acid residues), and a highly charged cytoplasmic domain of 38 amino acid residues (Maddon *et al.*, 1985; Littman, 1987). Its cytoplasmic domain is strongly conserved across mammalian species, with nearly 80% homology between human and mouse sequences, whereas the extracellular and transmembrane region show overall homologies of only 55% between human and mouse (Maddon *et al.*, 1987). The molecule has four extracellular immunoglobulin-like domains, denoted V1–V4, with a homology of the outer domain to human VLk of 30% (Reinherz & Schlossman, 1980; Littman *et al.*, 1988). It has therefore been classified as a member of the immunogloblin gene family (Clark *et al.*, 1987). Crystallographic studies of soluble CD4 derivatives have revealed a rod-like structure of 125 Å length with a diameter of 25–30 Å (Davis *et al.*, 1990; Kwong *et al.*, 1990). The three-dimensional structure has been described for the first two domains. As predicted, both resemble immunogloblin (Ig) domains with a β-strand sandwich structure (Ruy *et al.*, 1990; Wang *et al.*, 1990). The V1 structure is very similar to Ig V regions with the disulphide bond linking strands B

176

and F. However, the CD4 gene locus found on the short arm of chromosome 12 and consisting of a single gene is not linked to any known Ig gene family (Isobe et al., 1986).

Meanwhile, CD4 was also found on monocytes, macrophages and Langerhans' cells (Wood et al., 1983) as well as on eosinophils (Lucey et al., 1989) and endothelial cells of the hepatic sinusoids (Scoazec & Feldmann, 1990). CD4 epitopes were also described in sperm cells (Gobert et al., 1990) and in the brain (Tourveille et al., 1986). It is interesting to note, that rat brain lacks CD4 while CD4 was found on some dendritic cells in the rat (Steiniger et al., 1984; Tourveille et al., 1986). The best known and probably functionally most important physiological ligands for CD4 are major histocompatibility complex (MHC) class II encoded molecules. Direct evidence for CD4 binding to MHC class II molecules comes from experiments showing that fibroblasts transfected with a CD4 expression vector adhere specifically to cells expressing MHC class II molecules (Doyle & Strominger, 1987). Of special importance was the finding that $CD4^+$ T cells are restricted to recognize antigen only in the context of MHC class II molecules (Dialynas et al., 1983; Swain, 1983; Emmrich, 1988). When purified MHC class II molecules were incorporated into artificial lipid membranes and used in conjunction with peptide antigen to stimulate lymphokine-producing antigen-specific T cell hybridomas, not only anti-MHC class II but also anti-CD4 antibodies could block activation (Watts et al., 1984) whereas other anti-T-cell antibodies failed to inhibit. One might envisage that CD4 acts as an adhesion molecule increasing the probability of aggregate formation (i.e. the avidity) between T cell and accessory cell.

However, several experiments have shown that CD4 in T cells is more than a simple adhesion molecule. In addition, it seems to act as a coreceptor for the T-cell receptor (TCR)/CD3 complex, contributing to its signalling function. Several studies have provided evidence for a physical interaction between CD4 and TCR/CD3 by showing the comodulation of CD4 and CD3 molecules (Saizawa et al., 1987; Anderson et al., 1988) as well as coclustering of CD4 and CD3 to the cell–cell interface upon T-cell activation (Kupfer et al., 1987). This may be interpreted as the formation of microclusters within the phospholipid-bilayer consisting of CD4 and TCR/CD3 as soon as the T cell becomes activated via TCR/CD3. In this model, MHC class II molecules act as a physiological 'clamp' (see Fig. 9.1). According to this model, microclusters can be formed artificially by bispecific antibody constructs (Emmrich, 1988; Emmrich et al., 1988) capable of cross-linking CD4 and TCR/CD3 (reviewed in Emmrich, 1988) on the cell membrane thereby providing a strong activation signal. The synergism was demonstrated by using a special anti-CD3 antibody which is unable to activate resting T cells under limited conditions even if cross-linked (Emmrich et al., 1988). In conjunction with anti-CD4, however,

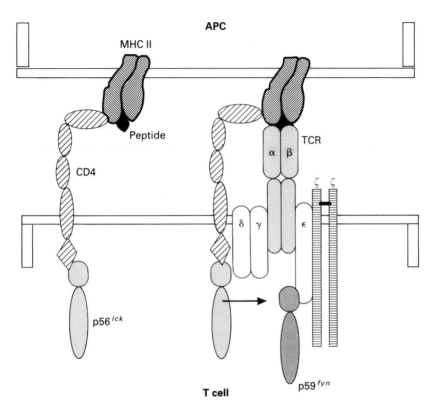

Fig. 9.1. Interaction of CD4 with MHC class II molecule on a potential antigen-presenting cell (APC). The MHC class II molecule is depicted as ligand for both TCR and CD4, thus acting as physiological 'clamp' that brings together CD4 and the CD4-associated tyrosine-kinase p56^{lck} with TCR/CD3. CD3ζ can be phosphorylated upon T cell triggering possibly by p56^{lck} or the CD3-associated tyrosine-kinase p59^{fyn}.

expression of functional IL-2 receptors could be induced (Emmrich *et al.*, 1986, 1987). Other anti-CD3 antibodies can activate T cells on their own provided they are crosslinked. Such an anti-CD3 antibody may cause association between CD4 and the TCR/CD3 complex as demonstrated recently by fluorescence resonance energy transfer experiments (Mittler *et al.*, 1989).

Interestingly, the association did not occur when a truncated CD4 protein lacking the cytoplasmic domain was used instead of complete CD4 (Sleckman *et al.*, 1988). This finding stresses the importance of the carboxyterminal cytoplasmic domain of CD4 which is required for signal transduction. A transfected cell containing only the truncated CD4 could not be stimulated by using MHC class II molecules incorporated into liposomes in contrast to the complete wild-type CD4^{+} hybridoma cell (Sleckman *et al.*, 1988). Recently, a non-covalent association between CD4 and the protein tyrosine kinase p56^{lck} has been described (Rudd et al., 1988; Veillette et al., 1988) which depends on the presence of the 28 membrane-proximal residues of the cytoplasmic domain of CD4 (Turner et al., 1990). p56^{lck} is a T-cell-specific member of the src family of protein-tyrosine kinases (Marth et al., 1985) which becomes phosphory-lated on tyrosine residues upon stimulation (Veillette et al., 1988) and, in turn, may phosphorylate the zeta-subunit of the TCR/CD3 complex (Veillette et al., 1989), a polypeptide which is thought to be critical for TCR/CD3-mediated signal transduction. Moreover, there is a large vari-ety of membrane-bound or cytoplasmic substrates for the tyrosine kinase and its activation or deactivation upon CD4-triggering may transmit signals independent of TCR/CD3.

It should be noted that besides MHC class II molecules, other ligands for CD4 have also been described. Well known is the gp120 of the human immunodeficiency virus (HIV) with a binding site close to and partially overlapping but not identical to the MHC class II interaction site (Clayton et al., 1989; Lamarre et al., 1989). Recently, a cytokine — the lymphocyte chemoattractant factor (Rand et al., 1991) — and immunoglobulin molecules (Lederman et al., 1990; Lenert et al., 1990) were described as potential ligands for CD4. One laboratory has defined amino acid residues 21–38 of the first extracellular domain of CD4 as interaction site, homologous to the interaction site of V_L and V_H immunoglobulin do-mains. In contrast, the other group has reported on CD4-binding by Fc fragments but not F(ab')$_2$ of IgG (Like et al., 1986). Whether or not the alternative ligands are able to transmit signals as suggested for gp120 (Kornfeld et al., 1988) and the lymphocyte chemoattractant factor (Rand et al., 1991) remains to be established.

In conclusion, the data concerning the physiological role of CD4 have revealed a dual function of the molecule. It seems to act as a low-affinity adhesion molecule for MHC class II bearing cells and as a coreceptor for antigen recognition by the TCR/CD3 complex enhancing TCR/CD3-mediated signals. However, as demonstrated by several groups, triggering of the CD4 molecule may also provide negative signals which will be one of the subjects in the following section.

In vitro properties of anti-CD4 antibodies

Before going into details, it should be mentioned that evaluation of the numerous reports on anti-CD4 effects *in vitro* is a difficult task. According to a rough estimate based on phylogenetic differences of primate CD4 molecules at least 25 different CD4 epitopes were postulated (Jonker et al., 1989). It is known from other cell surface molecules and has been found with CD4 as well that binding to a certain epitope might elicit a response quite different from triggering a distinct epitope. Consequently, the capability of a monoclonal antibody (MoAb) to CD4 differs with regard to mobilization of intracellular calcium when crosslinked, or to synergistic activation in co-crosslinking experiments with TCR/CD3, or to inhibition of anti-CD3 mediated stimulation (Bank & Chess, 1985). The diversity is best illustrated by B66, a unique anti-CD4 MoAb able to stimulate a proliferative response on its own presumably by mediating an association to TCR/CD3 (Carrel et al., 1989).

Another feature that differs among anti-CD4 MoAbs is their capacity to induce modulation, i.e. disappearance of the target antigen from the membrane upon antibody binding. As described for CD3, the presence of Fc-receptor-bearing monocytes is required for the initiation of CD4 modulation (Horneff et al., 1992). It was interesting to note that stimulation via CD3 was not reduced but rather enhanced in CD4-modulated cells (Schrezenmeier & Fleischer, 1988). On the other hand, reduction of CD4 density together with masking of the target molecule hampers aggregate formation with MHC class II$^+$ accessory cells and may exert a negative effect in antigen-induced T cell stimulation. Other adhesion molecules seem to be affected indirectly (Mazerolles et al., 1991), thus reducing adhesion of activated T cells. A marked influence on their homing pattern is quite likely and may account for the redistribution of cells after antibody binding in vivo.

In the foregoing section, the co-receptor function of CD4 when CD4 and TCR/CD3 are co-ligated leading to a synergistic positive signal has been discussed. However, if both receptors are ligated separately by using soluble anti-CD4 antibodies the physiological stimulation of resting T cells by nominal antigen is inhibited in vitro resulting in a considerably reduced proliferative response (Biddison et al., 1982) and lymphokine secretion (Swain et al., 1983; Wilde et al., 1983). Ease of inhibition by anti-CD4 seems to be inversely related to the avidity of the T-cell receptor (Portoles & Janeway, 1989). It does not matter whether soluble or cellular antigens are used; allogeneic and most intensely, autologous mixed lymphocyte reactions can also be inhibited by anti-CD4 (Engleman et al., 1981; Wilde et al., 1983).

However, anti-CD4 MoAbs inhibit T-cell functions stimulated by lectins also in the presence of MHC class II negative accessory cells (Bekoff et al., 1985). Even stimulation by anti-receptor antibodies without any accessory cells can be inhibited irrespective of whether it is achieved by co-crosslinking of CD4 with CD3 (Emmrich et al., 1987) or by crosslinking a stimulatory anti-CD3 MoAb alone (Bank & Chess, 1985). Blocking of adhesion to MHC class II molecules obviously cannot account for this effect. One might assume that anti-CD4 binding hinders the physical proximity between CD4 and TCR/CD3 which seems to be required for optimal activation. But, there are anti-CD4 MoAbs that inhibit T-cell stimulation not involving the TCR/CD3 complex. It appears as if a direct negative signal can be transmitted by anti-CD4 independent of TCR/CD3 ligation. This view is further supported by the notion that pre-treatment of CD4$^+$ T cells with anti-CD4 significantly reduces intracellular Ca^{2+} mobilization and the proliferative response to subsequent stimulation by anti-CD3 induced TCR/CD3 crosslinking (Tsygankov *et al.*, 1992). Pre-treatment with anti-CD4 for a similar time interval (45 min) prepares some T cells to undergo apoptosis, i.e. programmed cell death, when stimulated with an anti-TCRβ antibody (Newell & Haughn, 1990). Taken together, anti-CD4 antibodies seem to be able to block an antigen-stimulated T-cell activation by: (i) inhibiting adhesion to accessory cells; (ii) preventing formation of microclusters between TCR/CD3 and CD4; and (iii) exerting a negative signal whose molecular basis and duration remains to be defined.

It will be very difficult to evaluate which of the inhibition mechanisms is most relevant in a complex T-cell response. It is a general experience, that initiation of T-cell activation in resting T cells is more easily inhibited by anti-CD4 than functions in activated T cells. The CD4$^+$ and CD29$^+$ T-cell subpopulation (memory T cells) seems to be preferentially affected (Takeuchi *et al.*, 1987).

In vivo effects of anti-CD4 monoclonal antibodies in mice

Antibodies used

Anti-CD4 MoAbs have been extensively used in mice. Most studies were performed by using the same antibody GK1.5 which is a cell-depleting rat IgG2b antibody. The majority of other antibodies used in mice have been produced by H. Waldmann's group. Two of these antibodies are also depleting: YTS 191.1, a rat IgG2b and YTA 3.1. Others are non-depleting such as YTS 177.9, a rat IgG2a (Qin *et al.*, 1990). Interestingly, YTS 191.1 and YTA 3.1 antibodies react with two distinct non-overlapping epitopes of the CD4 molecule and show synergy for depletion and immunosuppression when they are used together (Qin *et al.*, 1987).

Effects on lymphocytes

Most of the antibodies used experimentally are depleting. They induce a profound CD4-selective lymphocyte depletion in blood, spleen and lymph nodes (but not the thymus) after a single antibody injection of 0.2–5 mg. The depletion is quasi-immediate and complete ($> 90\%$) and persists for approximately 10 days, recovery starting thereafter and reaching completion after 4–6 weeks. In the case of non-depleting antibodies, rat Ig-coated CD4 cells are detected in peripheral blood and lymphoid organs.

Effects on antibody response

Anti-CD4 MoAbs inhibit IgM and IgG primary and secondary antibody responses to thymus-dependent antigens such as bovine serum albumin or chicken ovalbumin (Wofsy et al., 1985), sperm whale myoglobin and to a lesser degree KLH (Goronzy et al., 1986), human and rat immunoglobulin (Coulie et al., 1985; Wofsy et al., 1985; Qin et al., 1990).

The immunosuppressive effect is lost when treatment is started after day 3 but the antigen injection can be delayed up to 15 days after the first antibody injection (Goronzy et al., 1986). The CD4$^+$ cell depletion is not needed to get this effect since F(ab')2 fragments can also suppress antibody responses (Gutstein & Wofsy, 1986). Interestingly, the use of a low antibody dose (50 μg) which induces partial depletion is not any more suppressive and may, conversely, tend to enhance immune responsiveness as assessed by increased serum IgG level, particularly IgG1, and enhanced plaque-forming cell (PFC) response to sheep red blood cells (SRBC) (Cowdery et al., 1991). These results are reminiscent of several data indicating a suppressor function for a CD4 T-cell subset. However, tolerance could be induced by low antibody doses (60 ng/mouse) by using a pair of anti-CD4 MoAbs without CD4 cell depletion.

Effects on cell-mediated immunity

Anti-CD4 MoAbs suppress delayed-type hypersensitivity reactions (Kelley et al., 1987). The immunosuppressive effect is still observed in C5-deficient mice suggesting that complement is not required. Weekly treatment with 1 mg GK1.5 i.v., starting the first injection 3 days before skin grafting prolongs fully allogeneic skin graft survival for 9–18 days. Anti-CD4 also inhibits the appearance of CD8$^+$ cytotoxic T cells against allogeneic cells (Woodcock et al., 1986; Weyand et al., 1989a) and virus infected cells (Weyand et al., 1989b). Rejection occurs concomitantly with the appearance of cytotoxic T cells in spite of persisting CD4 cell depletion. Prolongation of skin allograft incompatible at minor non-H-2 antigens is obtained at lower antibody dose (Qin et al., 1987).

Only few data are available in other species than the mouse. Several groups have reported a prolongation of renal allograft survival in monkeys using murine and human CD4 monoclonals (Jonker et al., 1987; Cosimi et al., 1991) with interesting synergy between the two antibodies OKT4 and OKT4A both in pre-transfused and non-transfused monkey (Jonker et al., 1985).

Tolerance induction under the cover of anti-CD4

Anti-CD4 antibodies have the unique property of facilitating the induction of immunological tolerance to soluble or cellular antigens. Qin et al. (1990)

THERAPEUTIC ANTI-CD4 ANTIBODIES

using a non-depleting anti-CD4 antibody have induced tolerance in mice against human and rat immunoglobulins and allogeneic bone marrow and skin differing at multiple minor antigens. In the latter case, it was necessary to use anti-CD4 and anti-CD8 antibodies simultaneously.

Maintenance of the tolerance state to soluble antigens requires repeated injections of the antigen, a condition which is not necessary for skin allografts which are not cleared like soluble antigens. This necessity for continuous antigen exposure probably involves T cells recently emerged from the thymus since adult thymectomized mice remain tolerant to soluble antigens without reinforcement (Qin *et al.*, 1990). Anti-CD4 antibodies can induce tolerance to themselves as well as to simultaneously added MoAbs of other specificities, however there are some exception (Gutstein *et al.*, 1986).

A tolerance to fully H-2 incompatible islet and heart allografts was obtained with indefinite survival by Shizuru *et al.* (1990) when administering GK1.5 at the time of transplantation. Interestingly, in this model, induction of anti-CD4-mediated tolerance to I-E^k in IE$^-$ mice occurred in the absence of deletion of the potentially IE-reactive Vβ11$^+$ clones. Additionally, this tolerance state was associated with *in vitro* anergy of Vβ11$^+$ CD4$^+$ and CD8$^+$ cells as evaluated by the proliferative response and IL-2 production in response to anti-Vβ11 immobilized MoAb. Similar results have been reported by Qin *et al.* (1990): in anti-CD4 treated mice tolerant to M1s-1^a an anti-Vβ6 MoAb does not stimulate Mls-1^a reactive Vβ6$^+$CD4$^+$ cells (Qin *et al.*, 1990). This anergy could not be eliminated by *in vitro* addition of recombinant IL-2 (Alters *et al.*, 1991).

The mechanism of anti-CD4 antibody induced tolerance is unclear. CD4 cell depletion is not mandatory since tolerance can be obtained with both CD4 depleting and non-depleting antibodies although it cannot be excluded that the mechanisms of anti-CD4 mediated tolerance differs for depleting and non-depleting antibodies. The fact that it is not broken by injection of unprimed spleen (Qin *et al.*, 1990) would argue in favour of the involvement of a suppressor mechanism as well as the rupture of anti-CD4 induced allogeneic tolerance secondary to injection of an anti-CD8 MoAb (Seydel *et al.*, submitted). However, there has been no direct evidence of active transfer of tolerance. Alternatively, one may hypothesize that CD4 cells are made anergic as suggested by the unresponsiveness to alloantigen and to stimulation by anti-TCR antibodies.

Mouse sensitization against rat anti-CD4 monoclonal antibodies

Anti-CD4 MoAbs used in the experiments described above are all of rat origin and thus prone to elicit an antibody response, as has been observed for most MoAbs even when they show a clear immunosuppressive effect. However, when used at high dosage (5 mg) depleting anti-CD4 MoAbs do not sensitize (Cobbold *et al.*, 1984; Coulie *et al.*, 1985, Ranges *et al.*, 1985;

Wofsy & Seaman, 1985; Wofsy et al., 1985; Benjamin et al., 1986). This unresponsiveness is not only due to immunosuppression since it persisted 42 days after the injection of YTS 191.1 when the mice have already recovered immunocompetence (Benjamin & Waldmann, 1986) and extends to all IgG2b MoAbs but not to their idiotypes. It should be realized though that the capacity of tolerance induction is not a general feature of all anti-CD4 MoAbs at least when used at lower doses. Thus OKT4A, a mouse anti-human anti-CD4, sensitizes monkey (and humans) with all known features of anti-MoAb sensitization, notably coexistence of anti-isotype and anti-idiotype antibodies (Chatenoud et al., 1986).

Anti-CD4 monoclonal antibody therapy in autoimmune diseases

Anti-CD4 MoAbs, and particularly GK1.5 which was used in most experiments described below, inhibit the onset or can even stop the course of most experimental autoimmune diseases in which they have been evaluated.

Murine lupus erythematosus

Weekly injections of (NZB × NZW)F1 mice (B/W) with anti-CD4 MoAb starting at 4 months of age, prior to the onset of overt autoimmune disease, reduce the titre of anti-DNA antibodies and prevent the onset of glomerulonephritis and renal failure (Wofsy & Seaman, 1985) with a clearly prolonged survival time. Major CD4 cell depletion is observed over all the therapy period but this depletion is not mandatory to the effect of the antibody since $F(ab')_2$ fragments that do not deplete had similar favourable effects on disease course as the entire molecule (Tite et al., 1986). Importantly, because it is more directly relevant to therapeutic usage in man, anti-CD4 MoAb therapy is still efficacious when started after the time of disease onset when high anti-DNA antibody titres and proteinuria are observed (Wofsy & Seaman, 1987). Similar observations have been made in other models of murine lupus: MRL/lpr mice (Santoro et al., 1988) and BX5B mice (Wofsy, 1986). Only a minority of anti-CD4 treated BW mice develop an immune response against the MoAb and these mice which are no longer protected develop a full blown lupus syndrome.

Murine diabetes

The NOD mouse is the most studied spontaneous experimental model of insulin dependent diabetes mellitus (IDDM). Diabetes occurs in female mice at 4–6 months of age and is preceded by a long phase of clinically silent insulitis (T-cell infiltration of the islets). The disease can be transferred from diabetic animals to syngeneic healthy recipient by infusion of purified T cells derived from overtly diabetic mouse spleen. These transfer experiments have shown that diabetes pathogenesis involves both CD4 and CD8 cells, since *in vitro* elimination of either of these two subpopulations at the time of transfer prevents the disease transfer (Bendelac *et al.*, 1987). Additionally, a large proportion of diabetogenic T-cell clones (capable of transferring the disease) express the CD4 phenotype (Haskins *et al.*, 1989).

A number of investigations have evaluated the *in vivo* effect of anti-CD4 MoAB on diabetes onset in NOD mice (Koike *et al.*, 1987; Hayward *et al.*, 1988; Charlton & Mandel, 1989). Anti-CD4 MoAb prevents the onset of IDDM when the treatment is started at the age of 3 months (insulitis without clinically overt diabetes), provided that the injections are repeated weekly (a single three-course therapy does not protect). Prevention from disease is associated with clearing of the islets that appear free of lymphocytes at 9 months of age. Interestingly in the weeks following cessation of therapy reinfiltration of islets may occur without diabetes (hyperglycaemia). Charlton and Mandem (1989) using another anti-CD4 MoAb, H129-19, also observed the reappearance of insulitis several weeks after cessation of anti-CD4 therapy which was started at 35–100 days of age.

NOD mice treated before onset of insulitis at a young age (2 weeks) by giving high doses of GK1.5 twice weekly for 12 weeks, do not develop insulitis and diabetes (Koike *et al.*, 1987). Injecting a single antibody dose in young NOD mice at various ages (weeks 2, 4, 5 and 6), Hayward *et al.* (1988) only observed the prevention of insulitis when the treatment was given at week 5 (with partial effect at weeks 2–4) and in association with an anti-CD8 antibody suggesting that at these early stages either T-cell subset could induce insulitis, a conclusion at variance with studies made in older mice. Finally, Wang *et al.* (1988) have shown transient prevention of diabetes recurrence in fully diabetic NOD mice grafted with syngeneic islets. These data indicate that even at very late stages of the disease anti-CD4 may still be efficient although transiently.

In the same vein, Charlton and Mandel (1988) have shown that a non-depleting anti-CD4 MoAb (H129-19) prevents cyclophosphamide-induced diabetes, which indirectly indicates an effect of anti-CD4 MoAb on the late stages of the disease.

One should lastly note that anti-CD4 MoAb has also been shown to prevent low-dose streptozotocin-induced diabetes (Herold *et al.*, 1987; Shizuru & Fathman, submitted). Surprisingly anti-CD4 antibodies do not protect pre-diabetic BB rats from becoming diabetic while anti-CD8 antibodies do (Like *et al.*, 1986). However, none of the three antibodies tested depleted CD4 cells and one may wonder whether they had any immunosuppressive activity at the dosage used.

In conclusion, anti-CD4 MoAbs may have several effects in NOD mice. They significantly reduce the established insulitis when they are given at the time of disease onset. They may clear insulitis but the effect is then only transient although the protection from diabetes may persist for a long period of time. They may act on effector cells but also very transiently. Anti-CD4 MoAb may also affect suppressor cells as exemplified by the induction of sensitivity to diabetes transfer afforded by anti-CD4 in adult thymectomized NOD mice (Boitard et al., 1989).

Experimental allergic encephalomyelitis

Administration of anti-CD4 MoAb prevents the development of experimental allergic encephalomyelitis (EAE) in the mouse (Waldor et al., 1985) and the rat (Brostoff & Mason, 1984). At the paralytic stage, anti-CD4 MoAb still reverses EAE. The effect is associated in these experiments with CD4-cell depletion in the mouse but not in the rat.

Anti-CD4 MoAb has also been shown to prevent EAE when given to mouse recipients of encephalitogenic T-cell suspensions derived from mice immunized against mouse spinal cord homogenate. This effect is not observed using an anti-CD8 MoAb.

Several isotypic variants of anti-rat anti-CD4 MoAb recognizing the same epitope of the CD4 molecule have been evaluated by Steinman et al. (1992). The IgG1 and IgG2b antibodies have proved to be superior to the IgG2a antibodies in preventing EAE in rats although they are not depleting for CD4 cells. Similarly, Steinman (1992) studied a family of rat–mouse chimeric molecules using the GK1.5 V regions and the constant regions of mouse IgG1, IgG2b and IgG3 mutants showing that the chimeric antibodies were more efficient than the initial GK1.5 molecule in cytotoxicity. The IgG2a was slightly more effective than the initial GK1.5 molecule in preventing EAE. IgG1 had a similar efficacy as compared to GK1.5. In contrast, GK1.5 IgG3 was not effective in EAE at the dose of 100 μg.

Other experimental diseases

Anti-CD4 MoAb therapy has also been shown to inhibit experimental allergic myasthenia gravis (Christadoss & Dauphinee, 1986). Treatment with GK1.5 also resulted in a significant decrease in the incidence of collagen type II induced arthritis in DBA/1-mice and delayed onset of the disease. However, treatment beginning after a strong anti-collagen IgG response did not alter disease expression. Combined treatments with both, anti-Thy 1.2 and anti-CD4 MoAb prevented the further advancement of arthritis (Hom et al., 1988). Similarly, anti-rat CD4 (OX35) could only temporarily inhibit rat-collagen type II arthritis and adjuvant-induced arthritis when given in the established disease. However, when given at high doses after disease induction but before regular onset of arthritis it completely suppressed all symptoms of arthritis and made the rats resistant to further attempts to induce arthritis (Billingham *et al.*, 1989).

Anti-CD4 antibodies in clinical studies

A central role of CD4$^+$ T cells for initiation and perpetuation of various autoimmune diseases has been demonstrated in many experimental animal models. Prevention and successful treatment of these diseases by anti-CD4 antibodies have encouraged clinical studies. The first report on anti-CD4 treatment dates back to 1987 (Herzog *et al.*, 1987) and describes clinical improvement in patients with rheumatoid arthritis having received anti-CD4 (antibodies VIT4 and M-T151) for 7 consecutive days (10 mg/day). A more detailed report on the same study was published later (Herzog *et al.*, 1989; Walker *et al.*, 1989) demonstrating reduction of the number of swollen joints and of pain assessment and improvement in Ritchie's articular index within 7 days of treatment. However, the level of rheumatoid factor, immune complexes and other laboratory parameters did not change during or after treatment, even at doses of 20 mg/day (Herzog *et al.*, 1989). Another study with a different anti-CD4 antibody (MAX.16H5) demonstrated similar clinical efficacy but also a significant decrease in the erythrocyte sedimentation rate, total immunoglobulin levels and rheumatoid factor titre after anti-CD4 treatment (*c.* 20 mg/day) In this study, nine patients with severe intractable rheumatoid arthritis resistant to gold, were treated with D-penicillamine and methotrexate (Horneff *et al.*, 1991a). Using similar inclusion criteria, ten patients were treated with 20 mg/day of antibody B-F5 (Wendling *et al.*, 1991) and recently, another study was published with 20 mg/day of antibody M-T151 (Reiter *et al.*, 1991). Only limited information is available of a further study with MoAb B-F5 in another ten rheumatoid arthritis patients (Didry *et al.*, 1991).

Since anti-CD4 therapy has been investigated most extensively in the studies mentioned above using rather similar protocols, it seems reasonable to consider these experiences for a general discussion. Clinical response to the first course of treatment could be observed in 37 of 46 patients by an improvement of more than 25% of Ritchie's articular index together with an improvement of various other scoring systems. The clinical response in most cases started immediately during treatment and lasted from 3 weeks to 3 months, in some cases over 5 months. Although no long lasting complete remission could be induced, the results seem encouraging in view of the selection of severe intractable cases. In all studies the antibodies were well tolerated with only mild and short lasting side-effects like low-grade fever (seven cases) mostly at the first injection or urticaria (two cases). No increased rate of infectious diseases or alterations in organ function could be observed during or after treatment and no case of a malignancy has yet been reported since the beginning of anti-CD4 treatment in 1987.

Unexpectedly, a profound immunosuppression was not observed after anti-CD4 treatment in humans. Most notably, acquired immune deficiency syndrome (AIDS) patients who received 10–40 mg anti-CD4 (MoAb 13B8.2) daily for 10 days did not show any indication of increased susceptibility to infections, instead, an increased number of functional circulating $CD4^+$ T cells was found in two out of seven patients treated (Dhiver et al., 1989). In rheumatoid arthritis patients a transient reduction of skin test reactivity and the in vitro cellular response to recall antigens was found with M-T151 during treatment which recovered thereafter (Herzog et al., 1989). Human anti-mouse antibody responses developed albeit less frequently and with lower titres as compared to other murine MoAbs not directed to T cells (Horneff et al., 1991c). Together, there is no indication that the moderate and transient immunosuppression detected by laboratory parameters and observed in those patients who responded to therapy increases the risk of acquiring other diseases especially bacterial or viral infections.

Twenty-six of the 46 rheumatoid arthritis patients developed a low titre human anti-mouse antibody (HAMA) response. A more detailed analysis with MAX.16H5 revealed that the HAMA titres were only transiently elevated and primarily of the IgG isotype with about 25% of the activity directed against idiotypic determinants (Horneff et al., 1991c). Interestingly three patients with HAMA titres who received a second course of treatment after 3 months responded well clinically (Horneff et al., 1991a). This observation indicates that the HAMA response does not necessarily interfere with therapeutical efficacy. One possible reason could be the high affinity of MAX.16H5 ($K_D = 5 \times 10^{-10}$ M) which would allow it to compete effectively with blocking HAMAs (Emmrich et al., 1991a). Some observations suggest that HAMAs by cross-linking antibodies on the cell membrane may even augment anti-CD4-mediated effects (Jonker & den Brok; Veilette et al., 1989). A novel approach to reduce HAMAs is the production of hybrid molecules in which only the antibody recognition site is of mouse origin. A chimeric antibody containing the V region of a mouse anti-CD4 MoAb (cM-T412) is already being used in the treatment of rheumatoid arthritis and has been found to be effective (van der Lubbe et al., 1991b; Moreland et al., 1991). It is questionable whether further 'humanization', i.e. the use of the complementarity determining regions only, may be needed to prevent HAMA formation to common immunoglobulin determinants and to reduce significantly the anti-idiotypic response.

To explain the results of anti-CD4 treatment it is necessary to differentiate between immediate and long-term effects. Blocking of adhesion and T-cell recognition and transmission of a negative signal have been discussed above as possible immediate anti-CD4 effects. What do the clinical studies indicate? A common observation in all studies and with all antibodies was the immediate depletion of CD4$^+$ T cells from the circulation, for instance with MAX.16H5, down to about 100 cells/μl or less with a minimum at 1 h after antibody injection over 30 min (Horneff et al., 1991a). Earlier work in animal models led to the conclusion that CD4 T-cell depletion is required for effective therapy (Cobbold et al., 1984) and only depletory anti-CD4 antibodies were effective in the murine experimental allergic encephalitis (Alters et al., 1986). However, clinical studies have now revealed that all anti-CD4 antibodies are depletory although at varying degrees depending on the antibody or the individual patient without correlation to the clinical response. It seems as if CD29$^+$ cells are predominantly depleted (Herzog et al., 1989).

No indication was found for direct cytotoxicity or antibody-mediated cytotoxicity in vitro or for massive cell destruction in vivo with any of the antibodies used. A special feature of one MoAb (MAX.16H5) is the modulation of CD4 in vitro and in vivo in many recipients down to about 20–50% of the original antigen density (Christadoss & Dauphinee, 1986). Modulation was more persistent than depletion from circulation and recovered only after cessation of treatment during 1 to 2 weeks. Since non-modulatory anti-CD4 antibodies also show immediate clinical efficacy and because CD4 was also modulated on T cells of non-responders to the same extent, modulation too may not be sufficient to explain clinical efficacy.

There is no evidence that the antibody isotypes used did determine clinical response since mouse IgG2a (M-T151) as well as IgG1 (MAX.16H5, BF5) were equally effective. However, it is likely that VIT4, M-T 151 and MAX.16H5 recognize distinct epitopes (Waldor et al., 1985). It remains to be established whether binding to a certain epitope is critical for the obvious differences, e.g. in the capacity of different antibodies to reduce rheumatoid factor concentration and several laboratory parameters of acute inflammation.

Little is known about the anti-CD4 effects on cells other than T lymphocytes. A moderate depletion of circulating monocytes has been observed after treatment (Herzog et al., 1989; Horneff et al., 1991a) and in a few cases monocyte-derived cytokines were elevated immediately after injection of the antibody, but only for a few hours (Horneff et al., 1991b). It is unknown whether antibody binding to CD4$^+$ monocytes has a major influence on therapeutic response.

The value of anti-CD4 conditioning for graft survival in comparison to anti-CD8 treatment has been elegantly demonstrated by Cobbold et al. (1984) in a mouse skin graft model. However, little is known about the use of anti-CD4 in human tissue/organ transplantation (reviewed in Sablinski *et al.*, 1991). Preliminary experiences are available with kidney transplantation followed by anti-CD4 (MoAb BL4) in conjunction with azathioprine and prednisolone (Morel *et al.*, 1990). In this study, early rejection episodes were noted in four out of 12 patients which is comparable to patients treated with antilymphocyte globulins (ALG). Treatment was started 1 day after transplantation and was discontinued after 3–14 days. At present, MAX.16H5 is being tested in renal transplantation recipients to treat late rejection episodes occurring later than 1 year after transplantation (Reinke *et al.*, 1991). 0.6 mg/kg antibody was given on 3 consecutive days. A rapid fall in serum creatinine concentration, was observed in all five patients within 3 days, while 2 weeks were required to reach a significant decrease in serum creatinine in a control group of 6 patients who received a methylprednisolone bolus. Biopsies before and 20–22 days after therapy showed a reduction of interstitial infiltrates while parameters of severe acute rejection, (oedema or haemorrhages) disappeared completely. The results are encouraging for the further use of anti-CD4 in the management of rejection crises (Sablinski *et al.*, 1991).

Besides rheumatoid arthritis there is increasing experience with anti-CD4 therapy in other putative autoimmune diseases (Table 9.1). No significant clinical improvement was observed in four patients with multiple sclerosis treated with anti-CD4 (MoAb 19THY 5D7, IgG2a) (Hafler *et al.*, 1988) but, a few years later, the encouraging results obtained in rheumatoid arthritis obviously have stimulated recent pilot trials with different antibodies and similar protocols in Crohn's disease and ulcerative colitis (Emmrich *et al.*, 1991), systemic lupus erythematosus (Hiepe *et al.*, 1991), mycosis fungoides (Knox *et al.*, 1991), relapsing polychondritis (Choy *et al.*, 1991; van der Lubbe *et al.*, 1991a) and severe psoriasis (Dhiver *et al.*, 1989; Nicolas *et al.*, 1991; Prinz *et al.*, 1991) and even in multiple sclerosis where Steinman *et al.* (1992) have observed a very promising effect in an open trial of 29 patients using the MT412 depleting anti-CD4 showing immediate improvement in many cases. However, improvement was only transient with few exceptions. The first report on a long-lasting, perhaps permanent remission was in the treatment of severe vasculitis (Mathieson *et al.*, 1990).

More difficult to explain than the immediate effects of anti-CD4 treatment is improvement lasting longer than 3 weeks. A persistent but moderate reduction in circulating CD4 T cells observed in rare cases provide no sufficient explanation. The antibodies are cleared rapidly from the circulation within 8–12 h at an injected dose of 20 mg irrespective of whether they are of IgG1 or IgG2a isotype (Walker *et al.*, 1989; Horneff *et al.*, 1991a). It is not known how long they remain able to exert any direct

Table 9.1. Pilot studies with anti-CD4 antibodies in human diseases

Disease	Antibodies	Study/year of publication		Reference
Rheumatoid arthritis	MT151, VIT4	Basel, München	1987, 1989	Herzog et al., 1987, Herzog et al., 1989, Walker et al., 1989
	MAX.16H5	Erlangen	1991	Horneff et al., 1991a, Horneff et al., 1991b, Horneff et al., 1991c
	B-F5	Besancon	1991	Wendling et al., 1991
	cM T412	Birmingham, Ala.	1991	Moreland et al., 1991[1]
	cM T412	Leiden	1991	Van der Lubbe et al., 1991b[1]
Multiple sclerosis	19THY5D7	Boston	1988	Hafler et al., 1988
Severe vasculitis	YNB46.1.8SG2B1.19	Cambridge (UK)	1990	Mathieson et al., 1990[2]
Ulcerative colitis	MAX.16H5	Rostock	1991	Emmrich et al., 1991
Crohn's disease	MAX.16H5	Rostock	1991	Emmrich et al., 1991
Severe psoriasis	BB14	Lyon	1991	Nicolas et al., 1991
	MT151	München	1989/1991	Prinz et al., 1991[2]
Systemic lupus erythematosus	MAX.16H5	Berlin	1991	Hiepe et al., 1991[2]
Late kidney graft rejection	MAX.16H5	Berlin	1991	Reinke et al., 1991
Relapsing polychondritis	cM T412	Leiden	1991	Van der Lubbe et al., 1991a[2]
	cM T412	London	1991	Choy et al., 1991[2]
Mycosis fungoides	cSK3	Stanford	1991	Knox et al., 1991

[1] Meeting abstract; [2] case report.

function and it is hard to believe that they maintain their function for weeks and months. Moreover, some recent observations that may indicate the possibility of even longer and perhaps permanent remission of certain autoimmune diseases upon anti-CD4 treatment deserve attention. Matthieson et al. (1990) have reported on a case of severe vasculitis treated several times with an anti-CD52 antibody (Campath 1H) with significant but only transient improvement. However, permanent remission now lasting for more than 2 years has been induced by injecting an anti-CD4 antibody subsequent to anti-CD52 (Mathieson et al., 1990). Recently, two more cases, one patient with severe ulcerative colitis (Emmrich et al., 1991) and another patient with systemic lupus erythematosus (Hiepe et al., 1991) have developed long-term remission for more than 1 year after anti-CD4 treatment alone or anti-CD4 treatment followed by a methylprednisolone bolus later on. These observations are stimulating and call to mind animal experiments demonstrating tolerance induction under the umbrella of anti-CD4 to soluble protein antigens or to organ transplants (Cobbold et al., 1984; Benjamin & Waldmann, 1986). Cobbold et al. (1990) have called it 'reprogramming' of the immune system which can be induced by preventing cellular cooperation followed by a gradual release from blockade. There is some preliminary evidence to suggest that in autoimmune diseases where the antigen is unknown but always present, such reprogramming can be achieved. In NOD mice, which spontaneously develop diabetes mellitus later in life, outbreak of the disease can be prevented by long-term but limited treatment with anti-CD4 from birth (Shizuru et al., 1988).

The experience with anti-CD4 in clinical studies is limited and more extended and controlled studies are needed. However, even more important is the investigation of the molecular and/or cell biological mechanism that the effects are based on. It might well be that a combination of anti-CD4 antibodies against different epitopes or combination of antibodies against various T-cell surface antigens might be more effective by reducing the amount of antibody required or by introducing synergistic principles of inactivation. Timing of antibody treatment has been demonstrated to be important and needs further exploration.

What is the future prospect of anti-CD4 therapy? It can be anticipated that the number of clinical pilot trials and more extended studies will increase throughout the forthcoming years and will include even more autoimmune diseases in which the pathogenesis implicates helper T cells. Based on the stimulating experiments of Herman Waldmann's laboratory on tolerance induction by anti-T cell antibodies more refined clinical studies are likely to be performed for the induction of transplantation tolerance. However, one should not forget that even the many experiments in animal models have not yet fully clarified the mode of action of anti-CD4 antibodies and much further work needs to be done.

References

Alters, S. E., Shizuru, J. A., Ackerman, J., Grossman, D., Seydel, K. B. & Fathman, C. G. (1991). Anti-CD4 mediates clonal anergy during transplantation tolerance induction. *Journal of Experimental Medicine* **173**, 491-494.

Alters, S. E., Shizuru, J. A., Ackerman, J., Grossman, D., Seydel, K. B. & Fathman, C. G. (1991). Anti-CD4 mediates clonal anergy during transplantation tolerance induction. *Journal of Experimental Medicine* **173**, 491-494.

Anderson, P., Blue, M. L. & Schlossman, S. F. (1988). Comodulation of CD3 and CD4. Evidence for a specific association between CD4 and approximately 5% of the CD3: T cell receptor complexes on helper T lymphocytes. *Journal of Immunology* **140**, 1732-1737.

Bank, I. & Chess, L. (1985). Perturbation of the T4 molecule transmits a negative signal to T cells. *Journal of Experimental Medicine* **162**, 1294-1303.

Bekoff, M., Kakiuchi, T. & Grey, M. H. (1985). Accessory cell function in the Con A response: role of Ia-positive and Ia-negative accessory cells. *Journal of Immunology* **134**, 1337-1343.

Bendelac, A., Carnaud, C., Boitard, C. & Bach, J. F. (1987). Syngeneic transfer of autoimmune diabetes from diabetic NOD mice to healthy neonates. Requirement for both L3T4 + and Lyt-2 + T cells. *Journal of Experimental Medicine* **166**, 823-832.

Benjamin, R. J., Cobbold, S. P., Clark, M. R. & Waldmann, H. (1986). Tolerance to rat monoclonal antibodies. Implications for serotherapy. *Journal of Experimental Medicine* **163**, 1539-1552.

Benjamin, R. J. & Waldmann, H. (1986). Induction of tolerance by monoclonal antibody therapy. *Nature* **320**, 449-451.

Biddison, W. E., Rao, P. E., Talle, M. A., Goldstein, G. & Shaw, S. (1982). Possible involvement of the OKT4 molecule in T cell recognition of class II HLA antigens. Evidence from studies of cytotoxic T lymphocytes specific for SB antigens. *Journal of Experimental Medicine* **156**, 1065-1076.

Billingham, J. E. J., Fairchild, S., Griffin, E., Drayer, L. & Hicks, C. (1989). Monoclonal antibody therapy for arthritis. In Lewis, A. J., Doherty N. S. & Ackerman N. R. (eds), *Therapeutic Approaches to Inflammatory Diseases*, pp. 242-253. Elsevier Science Publishing, Amsterdam.

Boitard, C., Yasunami, R., Dardenne, M. & Bach, J. F. (1989). T-cell mediated inhibition of the transfer of autoimmune diabetes in NOD mice. *Journal of Experimental Medicine* **169**, 1669-1680.

Brostoff, S. W. & Mason, D. W. (1984). Experimental allergic encephalomyelitis: successful treatment *in vivo* with a monoclonal antibody that recognizes T helper cells. *Journal of Immunology* **133**, 1938-1942.

Carrel, S., Lamarre, D., Isler, P., Rapin, C., Fleury, S., Salvi, S., Sekaly, R. P. & Cerottini, J.-C. (1989). A positive signal is transducted via surface CD4 molecules. *Research in Immunology* **140**, 545-561.

Charlton, B. & Mandel, T. (1988). Progression from insulitis to beta cell destruction in NOD mice requires L3T4 + lymphocytes. *Diabetes* **37**, 1108-1112.

Charlton, B. & Mandel, T. E. (1989). Recurrence of insulitis in the NOD mouse after early prolonged anti-CD4 monoclonal antibody treatment. *Autoimmunity* **4**, 1-7.

Chatenoud, L., Jonker, M., Villemain, F., Golstein, G. & Bach, J. F. (1986). The human immune response against the OKT3 monoclonal antibody is oligoclonal. *Science* **232**, 1406-1408.

Choy, E. H., Chikanza, J. C., Kingsley, G. H. & Panayi, G. S. (1991). Chimaeric anti-CD4 monoclonal antibody for relapsing polychondritis. *Lancet* **338**, 450.

Christadoss, P. & Dauphinee, M. J. (1986). Immunotherapy for myasthenia gravis: a murine model. *Journal of Immunology* **136**, 2437-2440.

Clark, S., Jeffries, W., Barclay, N., Gagnon, J. & Williams, A. (1987). Peptide and nucleotide sequences of rat CD4 (W3/25) antigen: Evidence for derivation from a structure with four immunoglobulin-related domains. *Proceedings of the National Academy of Sciences of the United States of America* **84**, 1649–1653.

Clayton, L., Sieh, M., Poius, D. & Reinherz, E. (1989). Identification of human CD4 residues affecting class II MHC versus HIV-1 gp120 binding. *Nature* **339**, 548–551.

Cobbold, S. P., Jayaswiya, A., Nash, A., Prospero, T. D. & Waldmann, H. (1984). Therapy with monoclonal antibodies by elimination of T cell subsets *in vivo*. *Nature* **312**, 548–551.

Cobbold, S. P., Qin, S. & Waldmann, H. (1990). Reprogramming the immune system for tolerance with monoclonal antibodies. *Seminars in Immunology* **2**, 377–387.

Cosimi, A. B., Delmonico, F. L., Wright, J. K., Wee, S. L., Preffer, F. I., Bedel, M. & Colvin, R. B. (1991). OKT4A monoclonal antibody immunosuppression of cynomolgus renal allograft recipients. *Transplantation Proceedings* **23**, 501–503.

Coulie, P. G., Coutleir, J. P., Uttenhove, C., Lambotte, P. & van Snick, J. (1985). *In vivo* suppression of T-dependent antibody responses by treatment with a monoclonal anti-L3T4 antibody. *European Journal of Immunology* **15**, 638–640.

Cowdery, J. S., Tolaymat, N. & Weber, S. P. (1991). The effect of partial *in vivo* depletion of CD4 T cells by monoclonal antibody. Evidence that incomplete depletion increases IgG production and augments *in vitro* thymic-dependent antibody responses. *Transplantation* **51**, 1072–1075.

Davis, S. J., Brady, R., Barclay, N., Harlos, K., Dodson, G. & Williams, A. (1990). Crystallization of a soluble form of the rat T cell surface glycoprotein CD4 complexed with Fab from the W3/25 monoclonal antibody. *Journal of Molecular Biology* **213**, 7–10.

Dhiver, C., Olive, D., Rousseau, S., Tamalet, C., Lopez, M., Galindo, J.-R., Mourens, M., Hirn, M., Gastand, J. A. & Mawas, C. (1989). Pilot phase I study using zidovudine with a 10-day course of anti-CD4 monoclonal antibody in seven AIDS patients. *AIDS* **3**, 835–842.

Dialynas, D. P., Wilde, D. B., Marrack, P., Pierres, A., Wall, K. A., Havran, W., Otten, G., Loken, M. R., Pierres, M., Kappler, J. & Fitch, F. W. (1983). Characterization of the murine antigenic determinant, designated L3T4a, recognized by monoclonal antibody GK1.5: expression of L3T4a by functional T cell clones appears to correlate primarily with class II MHC antigen-reactivity. *Immunological Reviews* **74**, 29–56.

Didrey, C., Portoles, P., Andary, M., Brochier, J., Combe, B., Clot, J. & Sany, J. (1991). Treatment of rheumatoid arthritis (RA) with monoclonal anti-CD4 antibodies. Clinical results. (Abstract A 162). *Arthritis and Rheumatism* **34**, S 92.

Doyle, C. & Strominger, J. L. (1987). Interaction between CD4 and class II MHC molecules mediates cell adhesion. *Nature* **330**, 256–259.

Emmrich, F. (1988). Activation of T cells by crosslinking the T cell receptor complex with the differentiation antigens CD4 or CD8. Implications for the generation of MHC-restriction and for repertoire selection in the thymus. *Immunology Today* **9**, 296–300.

Emmrich, F., Horneff, G., Becker, W., Lüke, W., Potocnik, A., Kanzy, U., Kalden, J. R. & Burmester, G. (1991a). Anti-CD4 antibody for treatment of chronic inflammatory arthritis. *Agents and Actions* **S. 32**, 165–170.

Emmrich, F., Kanz, L. & Eichmann, K. (1987). Cross-linking of the T cell receptor complex with the subset-specific differentiation antigen stimulates interleukin 2 receptor expression in human CD4 and CD8 T cells. *European Journal of Immunology* **17**, 529–534.

Emmrich, F., Rieber, P., Kurrle, R. & Eichmann, K. (1988). Selective stimulation of human T lymphocyte subsets by hetero-conjugates of antibodies to the T cell receptor and to subset-specific differentiation antigens. *European Journal of Immunology* **18**, 645–648.

Emmrich, J., Seyfarth, M., Fleig, W. E. & Emmrich, F. (1991). Treatment of inflammatory bowel disease with anti-CD4 monoclonal antibody. *Lancet* **338**, 570–571.

Engleman, E. G., Benike, C. J., Grumet, F. C. & Evans, R. L. (1981). Activation of human T lymphocyte subsets: helper and suppressor/cytotoxic T cells recognize and respond to distinct histocompatibility antigens. *Journal of Immunology* **27**, 2124–2129.

Gobert, B., Amiel, C., Tang, J. Q., Barbarino, P., Bene, M. C. & Faure, G. (1990). CD4-like molecules in human sperm. *FEBS Letters* **261**, 339–342.

Goronzy, J., Weyand, C. M. & Fathman, C. G. (1986). Long-term humoral unresponsiveness in vivo induced by treatment with monoclonal antibody against L3T4. *Journal of Experimental Medicine* **164**, 911–925.

Gutstein, N. L. & Wofsy, D. (1986). Administration of F(ab')₂ fragments of monoclonal antibody to L3T4 inhibits humoral immunity in mice without depleting L3T4 + cells. *Journal of Immunology* **137**, 3414–3419.

Gutstein, N. L., Seaman, W. E., Scott, J. H. & Wofsy, D. (1986). Induction of immune tolerance by administration of monoclonal antibody to L3T4. *Journal of Immunology* **137**, 1127–1132.

Hafler, D. A., Ritz, J., Schlossman, S. F. & Weiner, H. L. (1988). Anti-CD4 and anti-CD2 monoclonal antibody infusions in subjects with multiple sclerosis. *Journal of Immunology* **141**, 131–138.

Haskins, K., Portas, M., Bergman, B., Lafferty, K. & Bradley, B. (1989). Pancreatic islet-specific T-cell clones from nonobese diabetic mice. *Proceedings of the National Academy of Sciences of the United States of America* **86**, 8000–8004.

Hayward, A. R., Cobbold, S. P., Waldmann, H., Cooke, A. & Simpson, E. (1988). Delay in onset of insulitis in NOD mice following a single injection of CD4 and CD8 antibodies. *Journal of Autoimmunity* **1**, 91–96.

Herold, K. C., Montag, A. B. & Fitch, F. W. (1987). Treatment with anti-T lymphocyte antibodies prevents induction of insulitis in mice given multiple doses of streptozotocin. *Diabetes* **36**, 796–801.

Herzog, C., Walker, C., Mueller, W., Rieber, P., Reiter, C., Riethmüller, G., Wassmer, P., Stockinger, H., Madic, O. & Pichler, W. J. (1989). Anti-CD4 antibody treatment of patients with rheumatoid arthritis. I. Effect on clinical course and circulating T cells. *Journal of Autoimmunity* **2**, 627–642.

Herzog, C., Walker, C., Pichloer, W., Aeschliman, A. & Wassmer, P. (1987). Monoclonal anti-CD4 in arthritis. *Lancet* **333**, 1461–1462.

Hiepe, F., Volk, H.-D., Apostoloff, E., von Baehr, R. & Emmrich, F. (1991). Treatment of severe systemic lupus erythematosus with an anti-CD4 monoclonal antibody. *Lancet* **338**, 1529–1530.

Hom, J. T., Butler, L. D., Riedl, P. E. & Bendele, A. M. (1988). The progression of the inflammation in established collagen-induced arthritis can be altered by treatments with immunological or pharmacological agents which inhibit T cell activities. *European Journal of Immunology* **18**, 881–888.

Horneff, G., Guse, A. H., Schulze-Koops, H., Kalden, J. R., Burmester, G. R. & Emmrich, F. (1992). Human CD4-modulation *in vivo* induced by antibody treatment. *Clinical Immunology and Immunopathology* (in press).

Horneff, G., Burmester, G. R., Emmrich, F. & Kalden, J. R. (1991a). Treatment of rheumatoid arthritis with an anti-CD4 monoclonal antibody. *Arthritis and Rheumatism* **34**, 129–140.

Horneff, G., Krause, A., Emmrich, F., Kalden, J. R. & Burmester, G. R. (1991b). Elevated levels of circulating tumor necrosis factor-α, interferon-γ and interleukin-2 in systemic reactions induced by anti-CD4 therapy in patients with rheumatoid arthritis. *Cytokine* **3**, 1–2.

Horneff, G., Winkler, T., Kalden, J. R., Emmrich, R. & Burmester, G. R. (1991c). Human anti-mouse antibody response induced by anti-CD4 monoclonal antibody therapy in patients with rheumatoid arthritis. *Clinical Immunology and Immunopathology* **59**, 89–103.

Isobe, M., Huebner, K., Maddon, P. J., Littman, D. R., Axel, R. & Croce, C. M. (1986). The gene encoding the T cell surface protein T4 is located on human chromosone 12. *Proceedings of the National Academy of Sciences of the United States of America* **83**, 4399–4402.

Jonker, M. & den Brok, J. H. A. M. (1987). Idiotype switching of CD4-specific monoclonal antibodies can prolong the therapeutic effectiveness inspite of host anti-mouse IgG antibodies. *European Journal of Immunology* **17**, 1547–1553.

Jonker, M., Neuhaus, P., Zurcher, C., Fucello, A.. & Goldstein, G. (1985). OKT4 and OKT4A antibody treatment as immunosuppression for kidney transplantation in rhesus monkeys. *Transplantation* **39**, 247–253.

Jonker, M., Nooij, F. J. M. & Steinhof, G. (1987). Effects of CD4 and CD8 specific monoclonal antibodies *in vitro* and *in vivo* on T cells and their relation to the allograft response in rhesus monkeys. *Transplantation Proceedings* **19**, 4308–4314.

Jonker, M., Slingerland, W., Niphuis, H., Solub, E. S., Thornton, G. B., Smit, L. & Gloudsmit, J. (1989). Epitope definition of CD4 by primate studies and the anti-ID response to CD4-specific mab: failure to induce anti-ID specific for HIV. In Knapp, W., Dörken, B., Gilks, W. R., Rieber, E. P., Schmidt, R. E., Stein, H. & von dem Borne, A. E. G. (eds) *Leucocyte typing IV*, pp. 319–322. Oxford University Press, Oxford.

Kelley, V. E., Gaulton, G. N. & Strom, T. B. (1987). Inhibitory effects of anti-interleukin 2 receptor and anti-L3T4 antibodies on delayed type hypersensitivity: the role of complement and epitope. *Journal of Immunology* **138**, 2771–2775.

Knox, S. J., Levey, R., Hodgkinson, S., Bell, R., Brown, S., Wood, G. S., Hoppe, R., Abel, E. A., Steinman, L., Berger, R. G., Gaiser, C., Young, G., Bindl, J., Hanham, A. & Reichert, T. (1991). Observations on the effect of chimeric anti-CD4 monoclonal antibody in patients with mycosis fungoides. *Blood* **77**, 20–30.

Koike, T., Itoh, Y., Ishii, T., Ito, I., Takabayashi, K., Muruyama, N., Tomoika, H. & Yoshida, S. (1987). Preventive effect of monoclonal anti-L3T4 antibody on development of diabetes in NOD mice. *Diabetes* **36**, 539–541.

Kornfeld, H., Cruikshank, W., Pyle, S., Berman, J. & Center, D. (1988). Lymphocyte activation by HIV-1 envelope glycoprotein. *Nature* **335**, 445–448.

Kupfer, A., Singer, S. J., Janeway Jr. C. A. & Swain, S. L. (1987). Coclustering of CD4 (L3T4) molecule with the T cell receptor is induced by specific direct interaction of helper T cells and antigen-presenting cells. *Proceedings of the National Academy of Sciences of the United States of America* **84**, 5888–5892.

Kwong, P. D., Ryu, S.-E., Hendrickson, W., Axel, R., Sweet, R., Folena-Wasserman, G., Hensley, P. & Sweet, R. (1990). Molecular characteristics of recombinant human CD4 as deduced from polymorphic crystals. *Proceedings of the National Academy of Sciences of the United States of America* **87**, 6423–6427.

Lamarre, D., Ashkenazi, A., Fleur, S., Smith, D., Sekaly, R.-P. & Capon, D. J. (1989). The MHC-binding and gp120-binding functions of CD4 are separable. *Science* **245**, 743–746.

Lederman, S., Yellin, M. J., Cleary, A. M., Gulick, R. & Chess, L. (1990). Recombinant, truncated CD4 molecule (rT4). *Journal of Immunology* **144**, 214–220.

Kenert, P., Kroon, D., Spiegelberg, H., Golub, E. S. & Zanetti, M. (1990). Human CD4 binds immunoglobulin. *Science* **248**, 1639–1643.

Like, A. A., Biron, C. A., Weringer, E. J., Byman, K., Sroczynski, E. & Guberski, D. L. (1986). Prevention of diabetes in biobreeding/worcester rats with monoclonal antibodies that recognize T lymphocytes or natural killer cells. *Journal of Experimental Medicine* **164**, 1145–1159.

Littman, D. R. (1987). The structure of the CD4 and CD8 genes. *Annual Review of Immunology* **5**, 561–584.

Littman, D. R., Maddon, P. J. & Axel, R. (1988). Altered repertoire of endogenous immunoglobulin gene expression in transgenic mice containing a rearranged μ heavy chain gene (letter with corrected CD4 sequence). *Cell* **55**, 541.

Lucey, D. R., Dorsky, D. I., Nicholson-Weller, A. & P. F. (1989). Human eosinophils express CD4 protein and bind human immunodeficiency virus 1 gp120. *Journal of Experimental Medicine* **169**, 327–321.

Maddon, P. J., Littman, D. R., Godfrey, M., Maddon, D. R., Chess, L. & Axel, R. (1985). The isolation and nucleotide sequences of cDNA encoding the T cell surface protein T4: a new member of the immunoglobulin gene family. *Cell* **42**, 93–104.

Maddon, P. J., Molineaux, S. M., Maddon, D. E., Zimmerman, K. A., Godfrey, M., Alt, F. W., Chess, L. & Axel, R. (1987). Structure and expression of the human and mouse T4 genes. *Proceedings of the National Academy of Sciences of the United States of America* **84**, 9155–9159.

Marth, J. D., Peet, R., Krebs, E. G. & Perlmutter, R. M. (1985). A lymphocyte-specific protein-tyrosine kinase gene is rearranged and overexpressed in the murine T cell lymphoma. *Cell* **43**, 393–404.

Mathieson, P. W., Cobbold, S. P., Hale, G., Clark, M. R., Oliveria, D. B. G., Lockwood, C. M. & Waldmann, H. (1990). Monoclonal antibody therapy in systemic vasculitis. *New England Journal of Medicine* **323**, 250–254.

Mazerolles, F., Hauss, P., Barbat, C., Figdor, C. D. & Fischer, A. (1991). Regulation of LFA-1 mediated T cell adhesion by CD4. *European Journal of Immunology* **21**, 887–894.

Mittler, R. S., Goldman, S. J., Spitalny, G. L. & Burakoff, S. J. (1989). T cell receptor-CD4 physical association in a murine T cell hybridoma: induction by antigen receptor ligation. *Proceedings of the National Academy of Sciences of the United States of America* **86**, 8531–8535.

Morel, P., Vincent, C., Cordier, G., Panaye, G., Carosella, E. & Revillard, J. P. (1990). Anti-CD4 monoclonal antibody administration in renal transplanted patients. *Clinical Immunology and Immunopathology* **56**, 311–322.

Moreland, L. W., Bucy, R. P., Pratt, P. W., Khazaeli, M. B., LoBuglio, A. F., Ghrayeb, J., Daddona, P., Sanders, M. E., Kilgariff, C., Riethmüller, G. & Koopman, W. J. (1991). Use of a chimeric anti-CD4 monoclonal antibody in refractory rheumatoid arthritis. (Abstract 97). *Arthritis and Rheumatism* **34**, S49.

Newell, K. M. & Haughn, L. J. (1990). Death of mature T cells by separate ligation of CD4 and the T cell receptor for antigen. *Nature* **347**, 286–289.

Nicolas, J. F., Chamchick, N., Thivolet, J., Wijdenes, J., Morel, P. & Revillard, J. P. (1991). CD4 antibody treatment of severe psoriasis. *Lancet* **338**, 321.

Portoles, P. & Janeway Jr., C. A. (1989). Inhibition of the response of a cloned CD4+ T-cell line to different class II major histocompatibility complex ligands by anti-CD4 and by anti-receptor Fab fragments are directly related. *European Journal of Immunology* **19**, 83–87.

Prinz, J., Braun-Falco, O., Meurer, M., Daddona, P., Reiter, C., Rieber, P. &

Riethmüller, G. (1991). Chimaeric CD4 monoclonal antibody in treatment of generalized pustular psoriasis. *Lancet* **338**, 320-321.

Qin, S., Cobbold, S., Tighe, H., Benjamin, R. & Waldmann, H. (1987). CD4 monoclonal antibody pairs for immunosuppression and tolerance induction. *European Journal of Immunology* **17**, 1159-1165.

Qin, S., Wise, M., Cobbold, S. P., Leong, L., Kong, Y-C. M., Parnes, J. R. & Waldmann, H. (1990). Induction of tolerance in peripheral T cells with monoclonal antibodies. *European Journal of Immunology* **20**, 2737-2745.

Rand, T. H., Cruikshank, W. W., Center, D. M. & Weller, P. F. (1991). CD4-mediated stimulation of human eosinophils: lymphocyte chemoattractant factor and other CD4-binding ligands elicit eosinophil migration. *Journal of Experimental Medicine* **173**, 1521-1528.

Ranges, G. E., Sriram, S. & Cooper, S. M. (1985). Prevention of type II collagen-induced arthritis by in vivo treatment with anti-L3T4. *Journal of Experimental Medicine* **162**, 1105-1110.

Reinherz, E. L. & Schlossman, S. F. (1980). The differentiation and function of human T lymphocytes. *Cell* **19**, 821-827.

Reinke, P., Volk, H. D., Miller, H., Neuhaus, K., Fietze, E., Herberger, J., Herberger, D., von Baehr, R. & Emmrich, F. (1991). Anti-CD4 therapy of acute rejection in long-term renal allograft recipients. *Lancet* **338**, 702-70.

Reiter, C., Kakavand, B., Rieber, E. P., Schattenkirchner, M., Riethmüller, G. & Krüger, K. (1991). Treatment of rheumatoid arthritis with monoclonal CD4 antibody M-T151. Clinical results and immunopharmacologic effects in an open study, including repeated administration. *Arthritis and Rheumatism* **4**, 525-536.

Rudd, C. E., Trevillyan, J. M., Dasgupta, J. V., Wong, L. L. & Schlossman, S. F. (1988). The CD4 receptor is complexed in detergent lysates to a protein-tyrosine kinase (pp58) from human T lymphocytes. *Proceedings of the National Academy of Sciences of the United States of America* **85**, 5190-5194.

Ruy, S.-E., Kwong, P. D., Truneh, A., Porter, T., Arthos, J., Rosenberg, M., Dai, X., Young, N., Axel, R., Sweet, R. & Hendrickson, W. (1990). Crystal structure of an HIV-binding recombinant fragment of human CD4. *Nature* **348**, 419-426.

Sablinski, T., Hancock, W. H., Tilney, N. L. & Kupiec-Weglinski, J. W. (1991). CD4 monoclonal antibodies in organ transplantation — a review of progress. *Transplantation* **52**, 579-589.

Saizawa, K., Rojo, J. & Janeway Jr., C. A. (1987). Evidence for a physical association of CD4 and the CD3:α:β T cell receptor. *Nature* **328**, 260-263.

Santoro, T. J., Portanova, J. P. & Kotzin, B. L. (1988). The contribution of L3T4+ T cells to lymphoproliferation and autoantibody production in MRL/lpr mice. *Journal of Experimental Medicine* **167**, 1713-1718.

Schrezenmeier, H. & Fleischer, B. (1988). A regulatory role for the CD4 and CD8 molecules in T cell activation. *Journal of Immunology* **141**, 398-403.

Scoazec, J. Y. & Feldmann, G. (1990). Both macrophages and endothelial cells of the human hepatic sinusoid express the CD4 molecules, a receptor for the human immunodeficiency virus. *Hepatology* **12**, 505-510.

Seydel, K., Shizuru, J., Grossman, D., Wu, A., Alters, S. & Fathman, C. G. (1992). Anti-CD8 abrogates the effect of anti-CD4 mediated islet allograft survival in rat model (submitted).

Shizuru, J. A. & Fathman, C. G. (1992). Anti-CD4 antibodies in experimental autoimmune diseases-diabetes (submitted).

Shizuru, J. A., Seydel, K. B., Flavin, T. F., Wu, A. P., Kong, C. C., Granthoyt, E., Fujimoto, N., Billingham, M. E., Starnes, V. A. & Fathman, C. G. (1990). Pre-transplant anti-CD4 monoclonal antibody therapy induces donor specific unresponsiveness to cardiac allografts in rat. *Transplantation* **50**, 366-373.

Shizuru, J. A., Taylor-Edwards, C., Banks, B. A., Gregory, A. K. & Fathman, C. G. (1988). Immunotherapy of the nonobese diabetic mouse: treatment with an antibody to T-helper lymphocytes. *Science* **240**, 659–662.

Sleckman, B. P., Peterson, A., Foran, J. A., Gorga, J. C., Kara, C. J., Strominger, J. L., Burakoff, S. J. & Greenstein, J. L. (1988). Functional analysis of a cytoplasmic domain-deleted mutant of the CD4 molecule. *Journal of Immunology* **141**, 49–54.

Steiniger, B., Klempnauer, J. & Wonigeit, K. (1984). Phenotype and histological distribution of interstitial dendritic cells in the rat pancreas. *Transplantation* **38**, 169–174.

Steinman, L., Lindsey, W., Alters, S. & Hodgkinson, S. (1992). Anti-CD4 therapy: from treatment of experimental allergic encephalomyelitis to clinical trials in multiple sclerosis. In Bach, J. F. (ed.) *Monoclonal Antibody and Peptide Therapy in Autoimmune Diseases*. Marcel Dekker, New York.

Swain, S. L. (1983). T cell subsets and the recognition of MHC class. *Immunological Reviews* **74**, 129–142.

Swain, S. L., Dutton, R. W., Schwab, R. & Yamamoto, J. (1983). Xenogeneic human anti-mouse T cell responses are due to the activity of the same functional T cell subsets responsible for allospecific and major histocompatibility complex-restricted responses. *Journal of Experimental Medicine* **157**, 720–729.

Takeuchi, T., Schlossman, S. F. & Morimoto, C. (1987). The T4 molecule differentially regulating the activation of subpopulations of T4$^+$ cells. *Journal of Immunology* **139**, 665–671.

Tite, J., Sloan, A. & Janeway, C. A. (1986). The role of L3T4 in T cell activation: L3T4 may be both an Ia-binding protein and a receptor that transduces a negative signal. *Journal of Molecular and Cellular Immunology* **2**, 179–190.

Tourveille, B., Gorman, S. D., Field, E. H., Hunkapillar, T. & Parnes, J. R. (1986). Isolation and sequence of L3T4 complementary cDNA clones: expression in T cells and brain. *Science* **234**, 610–614.

Tsygankov, A. Y., Broker, B. B., Guse, A. H., Meinke, U., Roth, E., Rossman, C. & Emmrich, F. (1992). Preincubation with anti-CD4 influences activation of human T cells by subsequent co-crosslinking with anti-CD3. (submitted).

Turner, J. M., Brodsky, M. H., Irving, B. A., Levin, S. D., Perlmutter, R. M. & Littman, D. R. (1990). Interaction of the unique N-terminal region of tyrosine kinase p56^{lck} with cytoplasmic domains of CD4 and CD8 is mediated by cysteine motifs. *Cell* **60**, 755–765.

van der Lubbe, P., Miltenburg, A. & Breedveld, F. (1991a). Anti-CD4 monoclonal antibody for relapsing polychondritis. *Lancet* **337**, 1349.

van der Lubbe, P. A., Reiter, C., Riethmüller, G., Sanders, M. E. & Breedveld, F. C. (1991b). Treatment of rheumatoid arthritis (RA) with chimeric CD4 monoclonal antibody. (Abstract A 143). *Arthritis and Rheumatism* **34**, S 89.

Veillette, A., Bookman, M. A., Horak, E. M. & Bolen, J. B. (1988). The CD4 and CD8 T cell surface antigens are associated with the internal membrane tyrosine-protein kinase p56^{lck}. *Cell* **55**, 301–308.

Veillette, A., Bookman, M. A., Horak, E. M., Samelson, L. E. & Bolen, J. B. (1989). Signal transduction through the CD4 receptor involves the activation of the internal membrane tyrosine-protein kinase p56^{lck}. *Nature* **338**, 257–259.

Waldor, M., Sriram, K. S., Hardy, R., Herzenberg, L. A., Herzenberg, L., Lanier, L., Lim, M. & Steinman, L. (1985). Reversal of experimental allergic encephalomyelitis with a monoclonal antibody to a T cell subset marker (L3T4). *Science* **227**, 415–417.

Walker, C., Herzog, C., Rieber, P., Mueller, W. & Pichler, W. J. (1989). Anti-CD4 antibody treatment of patients with rheumatoid arthritis: II Effect of *in vivo* treatment on *in vitro* proliferative response of CD4 cells. *Journal of Autoimmunity* **2**, 643–649.

Wang, J. H., Yan, Y. W., Garrett, T. P., Liu, J. H., Rodgers, D. W., Garlick, R. L., Tarr, G. E., Husain, Y., Reinherz, E. L. & Harrison, S. C. (1990). Atomic structure of a fragment of human CD4 containing two immunoglobulin-like domains. *Nature* **348**, 411–418.

Wang, Y., McDuffie, M., Nomikos, I. N., Hao, L. & Lafferty, K. J. (1988). TITRE. *Transplantation* **46**, 101–106.

Watts, T. H., Brian, A. A., Kappler, J. W., Marrack, P. & McConnell, H. M. (1984). Antigen presentation by supported planar membranes containing affinity-purified I-A^d. *Proceedings of the National Academy of Sciences of the United States of America* **81**, 7564–7568.

Wendling, D., Wijdenes, J., Racadot, E. & Morel-Fourrier, B. (1991). Therapeutic use of monoclonal anti-CD4 antibody in rheumatoid arthritis. *Journal of Rheumatology* **18**, 325–327.

Weyand, C. M., Goronzy, J., Swarztrauber, K. & Fathman, C. G. (1989a). Immunosuppression by anti-CD4 treatment *in vivo*: cellular and humoral responses to alloantigens. *Transplantation* **47**, 1039–1042.

Weyand, C. M., Goronzy, J., Swarztrauber, K. & Fathman, C. G. (1989b). Immunosuppression by anti-CD4 treatment *in vivo*: persistence of secondary antiviral immune response. *Transplantation* **47**, 1034–1039.

Wilde, D. B., Marrack, P., Kappler, J., Dialynas, D. P. & Fitch, F W. (1983). Evidence implicating L3T4 in class II MHC antigen reactivity: monoclonal antibody GK1.5 (anti-L3T4a) blocks class II MHC antigen-specific proliferation, release of lymphokines, and binding by cloned murine helper T lymphocyte lines. *Journal of Immunology* **131**, 2178–2183.

Wofsy, D. (1986). Administration of monoclonal anti-T cell antibodies retards murine lupus in BXSB mice. *Journal of Immunology* **136**, 4554–4560.

Wofsy, D., Mayes, D. C., Woodcock, J. & Seaman, W. E. (1985). Inhibition of humoral immunity *in vivo* by monoclonal antibody to L3T4: studies with soluble antigens in intact mice. *Journal of Immunology* **135**, 1698–1701.

Wofsy, D. & Seaman, W. E. (1985). Successful treatment of autoimmunity in NZB/NZW F$_1$ mice with monoclonal antibody to L3T4. *Journal of Experimental Medicine* **161**, 378–391.

Wofsy, D. & Seaman, W. E. (1987). Reversal of advanced murine lupus in NZB/NZW mice by treatment with monoclonal antibody to L3T4. *Journal of Immunology* **138**, 3247–3253.

Wood, G. S., Warner, N. L. & Warnke, R. A. (1983). Anti-Leu-3/T4 antibodies react with cells of monocytes/macrophages and Langerhans lineage. *Journal of Immunology* **131**, 212–216.

Woodcock, J., Wofsy, D., Eriksson, E., Scott, J. H. & Seaman, W. E. (1986). Rejection of skin grafts and generation of cytotoxic T cells by mice depleted of L3T4$^+$ cells. *Transplantation* **42**, 636–642.

Chapter 10
Anti-T-cell receptor V$_\beta$ antibodies for treatment of autoimmune diseases

Hans Acha-Orbea

Introduction

Central to the induction of an immune or an autoimmune response is the formation of a trimolecular complex between antigenic peptide fragments, major histocompatibility complex (MHC) class I and class II molecules and the T-cell receptor (for review see Acha-Orbea *et al.*, 1989). Many different accessory molecules help to intensify this specific interaction. The T lymphocytes restricted to MHC class II molecules express CD4 molecules, the other major T-cell subpopulation recognizes peptides bound to class I molecules and expresses CD8 molecules. For the initiation of the majority of immune and autoimmune responses CD4$^+$ T cells are required.

The discrimination between own and foreign or altered antigens (self–non-self discrimination) is a key element of the immune system. On one side, the immune system can attack invading organisms or destroy cancerous cells, on the other side the healthy cells of the body are spared from immune attack. Several levels of tolerance allow this distinction. During maturation of T lymphocytes in the thymus, T cells which are strongly reactive with self components are eliminated (negative selection) (Kappler *et al.*, 1987, 1988; Kisielow *et al.*, 1988; MacDonald *et al.*, 1988) and T cells which have a weak affinity for ones own MHC antigens are positively selected. In healthy individuals autoreactive T lymphocytes can be easily found in the peripheral repertoire after stimulation *in vitro* (Hohlfeld *et al.*, 1984; Martin *et al.*, 1990; Pette *et al.*, 1990; Wucherpfenning *et al.*, 1990; Liblau *et al.*, 1991; Sun *et al.*, 1991). But these autoreactive T cells are kept silent by peripheral tolerance mechanisms (Rammensee *et al.*, 1989; Jones *et al.*, 1990; Webb *et al.*, 1990). Failure at any of these self-protective mechanisms could lead to autoimmune conditions.

The T-cell receptor (TCR) is a highly polymorphic antigen recognition structure. Each T-cell clone expresses one type of these heterodimeric receptors which are composed of an α and a β chain. In the order of 10^{10} different receptors can potentially be produced by each individual. The β-chains of these receptors are composed of one of about 25 (mouse) or 75 (man) V_β (variable) regions, $1/12$ J_β (junctional) regions and $1/2$ D_β (diversity) regions. The α chain is composed of about $1/75$ V_α elements. Deletion and addition of random nucleotide sequences at the V_α–J_α, V_β–D_β and the D_β–J_β junctions allows formation of this nearly unlimited repertoire. About $1/10^5$–$1/10^6$ T cells are specific for one particular immunogenic peptide (for a review see Acha-Orbea *et al.*, 1989).

Using monoclonal antibodies (MoAb) to CD4, MHC class II molecules or to non-variable parts of the TCR, several model autoimmune diseases could be blocked efficiently (Acha-Orbea *et al.*, 1989, also see chapters 8, 9 and 13 of this book). All of these forms of treatment are rather unspecific in that they eliminate mostly cells which are not involved in the autoimmune response.

Finding that T cells expressing a limited repertoire of the TCR molecules are responsible for an autoimmune disease would allow the specific destruction of the cells which are causing autoimmunity, leaving the rest of the immune system unaffected.

Diseases with limited heterogeneity of T-cell receptors

The classical model autoimmune disease with a limited repertoire of autoimmune T cells is experimental allergic encephalomyelitis (EAE) (Acha-Orbea *et al.*, 1988, 1989; Owashi & Heber-Katz, 1988; Padula *et al.*, 1988, 1991; Urban *et al.*, 1988; Zamvil *et al.*, 1988; Burns *et al.*, 1989; Chluba *et al.*, 1989; Heber-Katz & Acha-Orbea, 1989). This autoimmune disease can be induced by injecting biochemical extracts of brain in different species including man, rat and mouse. It was later shown that in mouse both myelin basic protein (MBP) and proteolipid protein (PLP) are able to induce the disease (for reviews see Acha-Orbea *et al.*, 1989). Furthermore the encephalitogenic peptides have been defined for a variety of mouse and rat strains. Depending on the MHC class II genes expressed, different peptides of a length of about nine amino acids are encephalitogenic.

The disease can also be transferred with such MBP- or PLP-specific cloned CD4$^+$ T cells. In this model of disease therefore both the MHC restriction elements as well as the encephalitogenic autologous peptides are well defined in a variety of rat and mouse strains.

Analysis of encephalitogenic T-cell clones revealed a highly restricted usage of TCR molecules by the disease causing T-cell clones in mouse and rat (see Table 10.1 for summary). In the PL/J mouse, for example, all the encephalitogenic T-cell clones share $V_\alpha 4.3$ and at least 80% $V_\beta 8.2$ expression (Acha-Orbea et al., 1988). In the congenic mice B10.PL, which share the MHC region and the encephalitogenic MPB peptides but differ in many other loci, the same types of receptors can be found, but in addition $V_\alpha 2$-bearing receptors are expressed by about 60% of these T-cell clones (Urban et al., 1988). Treatment of mice with anti-$V_\beta 8$ specific monoclonal antibodies before induction of the disease prevented induction of EAE with encephalitogenic T-cell clones, with encephalitogenic peptides and with whole MBP. Even reversal of established chronic relapsing disease induced with T-cell clones expressing $V_\beta 8$ or in disease induced with whole MBP was achieved with a single dose of anti-$V_\beta 8$ monoclonal antibodies (Acha-Orbea et al., 1988).

The c. 20% of T cells expressing receptors other than $V_\beta 8$ do not seem capable of continuing the autoimmune reaction. In addition, at least in the

Table 10.1. TCR usage of MBP-reactive T cells in rat and mice

Rat/ mouse strain	MBP peptide specific- ity	Restric- tion ele- ment	V_α	J_α	V_δ	J_β	Clones %
PL/J and (PL/J × SJL)F1 mouse	1–9	I-A^u	4.3	TA31	8.2	2.7	50.0
			4.3	TA31	8.2	2.3	25.0
			4.3	TT11	8.2	2.5	12.5
			4.3	F1-12	4	2.5	12.5
B10.PL mouse	1–9	I-A^u	2.3	39	8.2	2.7	51.0
			2.3	39	13	2.2	9.3
			4.2	39	8.2	2.7	32.6
			4.2	39	13	2.2	7.0
Lewis rat	68–88	RT1^1	2		8.2		72% V_α 100% V_β
Fischer rat	68–88	RT1^1	2		8.2		Majority
ACI rat	NK	RT1^a	2		8.2		Majority
Buffalo rat	NK	RT1^b	2		8.2		Majority

NK, not known.

early stages of the disease (see below), other encephalitogenic peptides which have been shown to be capable of inducing EAE in this mouse strain, are not perpetuating the disease process. This means that T cells expressing $V_\beta 8$ are actively involved in the induction and the continuation of the autoimmune disease and not just responsible for the triggering of a general inflammation in the brain. This form of treatment eliminates 10–20% of the peripheral T cells and it seems that this semispecific form of treatment leaves the rest of the immune system fully functional. There are no indications so far for a reduction of the immune response (Acha-Orbea et al., 1988).

Similar results were obtained in the Lewis rat. Since in this animal model the disease is not chronic only prevention of the disease with an antiidiotypic monoclonal antibody was shown (Owhashi & Heber-Katz, 1988). This monoclonal antibody is highly specific for the autoimmune T cells and recognizes practically no other cells of the peripheral immune repertoire.

In classical peptide-specific T cells limited heterogeneity was observed in numerous experimental systems (Acha-Orbea et al., 1989). However, different receptors were used for recognition of different peptides of the same protein in association with different MHC class II gene products. In EAE, however, both in PL/J and B10.PL mice as well as four strains of rats, which differ in MHC class II molecules expressed and MBP-peptides recognized, very similar receptor molecules were utilized by the encephalitogenic T cells (Owhashi & Heber-Katz, 1988; Burns et al., 1989; Chluba et al., 1989; Heber-Katz & Acha-Orbea, 1989). The rat strains utilize the closest homologues of the mouse TCR $V_\beta 8.2$ and $V_\alpha 2$ and 4. In the rat models both MHC class II I-A as well as I-E restricted encephalitogenic T-cell clones express these TCR structures.

In uveitis in rat again the same types of receptors were detected in the autoimmune T-cell clones (Gregerson et al., 1991; Merryman et al., 1991). For unknown reasons, T cells bearing these receptor combinations are highly over-represented in the autoimmune populations (Heber-Katz & Acha-Orbea, 1989). The same finding was made in experimental allergic neuritis (EAN) in rats (Heber-Katz, 1990). A common feature of these induced diseases is that the antigen is injected together with complete Freund's adjuvant (CFA). We tried to see whether CFA treatment alone would trigger a T-cell response bearing these receptor structures. However, the only striking feature of the local lymph nodes after injection of CFA was an increase of $\gamma\delta^+$ T cells, the $V_\beta 8$ population did not increase (H. Acha-Orbea, unpublished observations). We therefore reasoned that this finding does not represent an obvious artefact.

We formulated the V-region disease hypothesis to explain these findings (Heber-Katz & Acha-Orbea 1989). This hypothesis states that T cells bearing these receptor combinations fulfil another function in vivo.

For unknown reasons T cells bearing $V_\beta 8$ are the most abundant in most strains of mice and rats. These T cells are not pathogenic unless activated in the periphery. Under normal conditions these encephalitogenic autoantigens most likely never reach sufficient levels in the periphery to trigger an autoimmune reaction. One possibility is that these TCR molecules interact with other receptors or fulfil other functions such as regulation of the immune response. These functions would not lead to activation of the 'autoimmune' T cells.

The SJL mouse strain, however, represents an exception to the rule. In this mouse strain, EAE can be induced easily but $V_\beta 8$ together with several other V_β elements are deleted from the germline repertoire. Several overlapping epitopes at the C-terminus of the MBP molecule are recognized by the encephalitogenic T-cell clones (Kono et al., 1988; Sakai et al., 1988). One of these peptides specifically elicits $V_\beta 17$ bearing T cells but the disease cannot be blocked with anti-$V_\beta 17$ monoclonal antibodies. Both the $V_\beta 17$ expressing and non-expressing T-cell lines were able to transfer the disease. The transfer of $V_\beta 17$ expressing T cells could be blocked with the monoclonal antibody (Sakai et al., 1988). In another study it was indicated that the majority of SJL encephalitogenic T cells express $V_\beta 4$. Transfer of a line expressing 57% $V_\beta 4$ T cells was effectively blocked with anti-$V_\beta 4$-specific monoclonal antibodies (Padula et al., 1991). So far nothing has been reported on the usage of TCR V_α in these encephalitogenic T-cell lines.

Other diseases

Insulin-dependent diabetes mellitus

Non-obese diabetic (NOD) mice represent an excellent model for insulin-dependent diabetes mellitus (IDDM) in man. The disease occurs spontaneously in the majority of female mice and it has been shown that both $CD4^+$ and $CD8^+$ T cells are required to transfer the disease into healthy animals. In addition macrophages are required for transfer of the disease. Despite the preliminary results that T cells expressing $V_\beta 5$ are responsible for the disease, these findings could not be reproduced and have since been corrected (Reich et al., 1989). Several groups have found a large heterogeneity of the autoimmune response in both the $CD4^+$ as well as the $CD8^+$ autoimmune T-cell populations at the onset of clinical disease (Haskins et al., 1989; Nakano et al., 1991). Preliminary results of the early infiltrating T cells in the lesions revealed a more restricted heterogeneity of TCR usage, but so far no agreement has been achieved (Livingstone et al., 1991; U. Hurtenbach, personal communication).

In human IDDM, analysis of peripheral blood lymphocytes with the three available monoclonal antibodies anti-$V_\beta 5$, 8 and 12 revealed a slight

increase of all of them in the CD25[+] (high affinity IL-2 receptor expressing, activated) T-cell population shortly after onset of clinical disease. The
interpretation of these results was that in this disease no oligoclonality of
the autoimmune T cells is present (Posnett et al., 1988; Kontiainen et al.,
1990).

Multiple sclerosis

The autoantigen(s) responsible for multiple sclerosis (MS) is not known.
Analysis of peripheral T cells from MS patients indicate that MBP as in
EAE could be the relevant autoantigen. Since T cells going through
activation and proliferation have a higher chance of acquiring mutations
at any locus, peripheral T cells from MS patients and controls were
selected for drug resistance and these T-cell clones were analysed for fine
specificity. Several of the patients' T-cell clones were reactive with MBP
(Allegretta et al., 1990).

    Several recent studies addressed the oligoclonality of TCR molecules
in MS in man. Using restriction fragment length polymorphism (RFLP)
analysis of T-cell clones isolated from the spinal fluid of MS patients,
oligoclonal TCR rearrangements were detected which varied from individual to individual by one (Hafler et al., 1988) but not by another group
(Rotteveel et al., 1987).

    Analysis of MBP-reactive T-cell clones isolated from the blood of
healthy controls and MS patients, recognizing different epitopes of MBP,
revealed a restricted usage of TCR V_β elements. Particularly T cells
expressing TCR $V_\beta 12$ and 17 were found in the majority of MBP-reactive
T cells (Hafler et al., 1988). In another study oligoclonality was found
which differed from patient to patient (Ben-Nun et al., 1991). In addition,
preliminary results of TCR expression in the brain of MS patients using
the polymerase chain reaction (PCR) with TCR V-region specific oligo-
nucleotides, revealed a highly restricted usage of TCR V_α elements in the
lesions (Oksenberg et al., 1990). Analysis of a larger patient sample,
however, revealed that different patients express on the average four
different V_α as well as V_β gene elements in the lesions with patient to
patient variation (L. Steinman, personal communication).

Arthritis

Conflicting results have been obtained in rheumatoid arthritis in man
(Savill et al., 1987; Brennan et al., 1988; Stamenkovic et al., 1988; Duby et
al., 1989; Hakoda et al., 1990; Miltenburg et al., 1990; Sioud et al., 1991;
Sottini et al., 1991; Van Laar et al., 1991). After amplification of lymphocytes isolated from the synovial membrane of affected joints with IL-2 and
later expansion in phytohaemaglutinin (PHA), clear oligoclonality was

observed in most of the patients (13/14) by one group (Stamenkovic *et al.*, 1988) but not by another, which found oligoclonality only in a minority of patients (Savill *et al.*, 1987). Amplification of synovial fluid T cells without selection for IL-2 responsiveness prior to non-specific stimulation or Southern blot analysis of freshly isolated synovial fluid T cells did (Miltenburg *et al.*, 1990) or did not indicate oligoclonality (Duby *et al.*, 1989). In another study two out of 25 CD$^+$ T cells shared the same TCR V_β rearrangements and the same rearrangement was found in one peripheral T-cell clone (Hakoda *et al.*, 1990). With monoclonal antibodies specific for $V_\beta 5$ or 8, an increase of these populations was detected in the synovium and the synovial fluid of most patients analysed compared to peripheral blood lymphocytes (Brennan *et al.*, 1988). There was however an increase of different populations in individual patients. Two groups found oligoclonality only in a minority of patients by Southern blot analysis of synovial fluid T cells expanded in IL-2 or in IL-2 and anti-CD3 monoclonal antibodies (Savill *et al.*, 1987; Van Laar *et al.*, 1991). Amplification of predominant V regions in the lesions by PCR of fresh spinal fluid T cells indicated an increase in cells expressing $V_\beta 7$, V_α usage however was highly heterogenous (Sottini *et al.*, 1991). This group also showed that this population is not over-represented in peripheral blood lymphocytes. A recent result on frequencies of TCR V_β expression by PCR analysis indicated that in arthritis joints an increase of T cells expressing TCR $V_\beta 14$ is present whereas cells expressing this TCR element were strongly reduced in the peripheral blood (see below about superantigens) (Paliard *et al.*, 1991).

In mouse collagen-induced arthritis, conflicting results have been obtained by a number of groups (Banerjee *et al.*, 1988; Andersson *et al.*, 1991; Spinella *et al.*, 1991). David's group presented genetic evidence for an involvement of T cells expressing $V_\beta 6$. They showed that mice expressing the susceptible MHC haplotype but having a germline deletion of 10/18 TCR V_β elements were not susceptible to the disease (Banerjee *et al.*, 1988). In addition, they showed that crosses of susceptible mice with mice which induce clonal deletion of T cells bearing $V_\beta 6$, 7, 8.1 and 9, due to expression of the minor lymphocyte-stimulating antigen Mls-1[a], produce less arthritis than crosses with congenic mice not inducing this clonal deletion (Anderson *et al.*, 1991). The other two groups generated F2 mice between susceptible mice expressing the full TCR repertoire and the non-susceptible mice expressing the partially deleted repertoire. They could clearly separate disease susceptibility from TCR genotype (Andersson *et al.*, 1991; Spinella *et al.*, 1991). In addition they presented clear evidence against predominant usage of $V_\beta 6$ and 8 by the autoimmune T cells in both *in vivo* and *in vitro* experiments (Goldschmidt *et al.*, 1990). Similar crosses as described above, with Mls-1[a] expressing mouse strains, did not protect from arthritis development (Goldschmitt *et al.*, 1990). The choice of mouse strains in these crosses seems to be important for conferring protection since David's group found only partial protection in the strain combination used by Holmdahl's group (Goldschmitt *et al.*, 1990).

In rat arthritis, an arthritogenic and a non-arthritogenic T-cell line yielded at least three different rearrangements each in collagen specific T-cell hybridomas (Ku *et al.*, 1990).

T cells expressing $TCR_{\gamma\delta}$ expressing T cells are frequently found in the synovial fluid in both mice and humans. The possibility of responses against heat shock proteins of these $\gamma\delta$ T cells has been put forward but in humans the mycobacterium antigen specific T cells frequently recovered from the synovium were not reactive with heat shock proteins but with several other antigens (Holoshitz *et al.*, 1989a,b; Plater-Zuyberk *et al.*, 1989; Correale *et al.*, 1991; Mor, 1991; Sioud *et al.*, 1991). Contrary to peripheral blood T cells, which express mostly $V_\delta 2^+$ cells, the synovial cells preferentially express $V_\delta 1$ in humans (Sioud *et al.*, 1991). Analysis of the T cells indicated polyclonal expansion.

Several different antigens are recognized by T cells isolated from synovial fluid of lyme arthritis patients. The T cells reactive with these antigens reveal heterogeneity of their TCR repertoire (Yssel *et al.*, 1990).

Crohn's disease

Crohn's disease is an inflammatory bowel disease. Increase in $V_\beta 8$ but not three other TCR V_β families in CD4$^+$ as well as CD8$^+$ T cells was observed in the local lymph nodes (Posnett *et al.*, 1990). An increase in the periphery could be observed as well. In one patient a tenfold decrease of TCR $V_\beta 8^+$ cells was detected after surgery. The range of TCR $V_\beta 8$ expression in 15 patients was between 7.3–39.1% (average 16%) in mesenteric lymph nodes and a slighter increase in peripheral blood. This increase can be observed in about 20% of patients. Control patients suffering from a non-autoimmune condition, ulcerative colitis, did not show this increase and expressed on average about 5% TCR $V_\beta 8^+$ cells. No genetic linkage to germline $V_\beta 8$ polymorphisms was found. When mesenteric lymph nodes were analysed, 62% of patients had an increase of $V_\beta 8$, two of which had normal levels in the periphery. This increase of $V_\beta 8$ cells was not found in the gut mucosa. The interpretation of these results is that an afferent but not efferent limb gut-associated immune response takes place and thus this increase most likely represents a response to antigen.

Primary biliary cirrhosis

In primary biliary cirrhosis, an autoimmune liver disease, the same TCR rearrangements were found in 5/10 and 2/10 independently cloned liver infiltrating T cells from one patient and in 3/10 and 2.10 from another patient. T-cell clones isolated from blood did not show such oligoclonality and T-cell clones isolated from liver biopsies of hepatitis-related liver diseases no oligoclonality was found (Moebius *et al.*, 1990).

Pulmonary sarcoides

Pulmonary sarcoides is a chronic granulomatous disorder. Infiltration with activated $CD4^+$ T cells is generally observed. $V_\beta 8^+$ T cells are over-represented but this population is most likely polyclonal (Moller *et al.*, 1988).

Allografts

RFLP analysis of T-cell lines established from kidney graft infiltrating T cells during rejection have revealed oligoclonal TCR V_β bands in most of the lines. Samples taken 10 weeks apart showed the same V_β rearrangements (Miceli & Finn, 1989).

Tumour infiltrating lymphocytes

Using the PCR, an over-representation of $V_\alpha 7$ has been reported in several different tumours (Nitta *et al.*, 1990).

Germline polymorphisms of T-cell receptors in autoimmunity

As mentioned in the introduction, the peripheral repertoire of T cells is shaped during the development of tolerance towards self antigens. Therefore the peripheral repertoire of T cells expresses fewer TCR molecules than theoretically possible from rearrangements of the germline components. Nevertheless differences in the germline repertoire may play an important role in the induction of autoimmune diseases. Several groups have analysed the influences of the germline repertoire of TCR on the susceptibility of developing autoimmunity and several found genetic association between disease susceptibility and germline TCR repertoire. Several conflicting studies on this subject were reported most of them, however, indicate genetic linkage (Kotzin & Palmer, 1987; Banerjee *et al.*, 1988; Ito *et al.*, 1989; Katzin *et al.*, 1989; Oksenberg *et al.*, 1989; Tesch *et al.*, 1989; Concannon *et al.*, 1990; Fugger *et al.*, 1990; Hirose *et al.*, 1990; McMillan *et al.*, 1990; Noonan *et al.*, 1990; Reijonen *et al.*, 1990; Andersson *et al.*, 1991; Spinella *et al.*, 1991).

Superantigens

The recent discovery that bacterial as well as retroviral superantigens can stimulate T cells independently of their antigen specificity has led to new models for the initiation of an autoimmune response. (Fleischer & Schrezenmeier, 1988; White *et al.*, 1989; Woodland *et al.*, 1990, 1991; Acha-Orbea *et al.*, 1991; Acha-Orbea & Palmer, 1991; Choi *et al.*, 1991; Dyson *et al.*, 1991; Frankel *et al.*, 1991; Marrack *et al.*, 1991).

Superantigens are bacterial or retroviral gene products which are presented by MHC class II molecules and interact with T cells expressing particular TCR V_β chains. The other variable parts of the TCR seem not to be important. Therefore the frequencies of T cells interacting with a particular superantigen are in the order of 1–30% of the total T-cell repertoire. In classical specific T-cell responses, in the order of 1 in 10^5 T cells are specific for a particular peptide antigen. Therefore superantigens are capable of stimulating T cells with a wide variety of antigen-fine specificities, the only requirement being the expression of a particular TCR V_β region. When encounter with these superantigens occurs at birth, when the immune system is trained for self–non-self discrimination, T cells expressing these TCR V_β regions are clonally deleted during maturation in the thymus (Kappler *et al.*, 1988; MacDonald *et al.*, 1988). Encounter at later stages can result in expansion of these reactive T cells, secretion of lymphokines and polyclonal activation of B cells. This initial T-cell activation is followed by peripheral deletion or induction of unresponsiveness (anergy) (Rammensee *et al.*, 1989; Jones *et al.*, 1990; Webb *et al.*, 1990). So far over 16 different bacterial and over 15 endogenous, retrovirally encoded superantigens have been documented and the list is far from complete (Marrack & Kappler, 1990; Acha-Orbea & Palmer 1991; Herman *et al.*, 1991). Most likely, bacteria and retroviruses have adopted a strategy of exploiting the immune system allowing a more efficient infection.

Possible scenarios for superantigens involvement in the induction phase of autoimmunity are shown in Fig. 10.1.

Autoreactive T cells can easily be derived from healthy individuals. In experimental animals activation of such cells with the relevant autoantigen injected systemically, leads to autoimmunity in susceptible strains. It can be argued that presentation of autoantigens by professional antigen-presenting cells can lead to pathology, whereas presentation by other cells can lead to unresponsiveness. Another interpretation would be that the immune system is not even tolerant to such autoantigens because they are never encountered at high enough quantities to induce activation of an autoimmune response.

Figure 10.1a shows a model for peripheral activation of autoreactive T cells (along with many other T cells with other specificities). These activated autoreactive T cells then migrate to the target organ expressing these autoantigens and start the autoimmune reaction. In this model the predictions are not clear. These autoreactive cells can either be found in the lesions at later stages of the autoimmune disease or they just initiate an autoimmune reaction which then, due to an increase of tissue debris, is

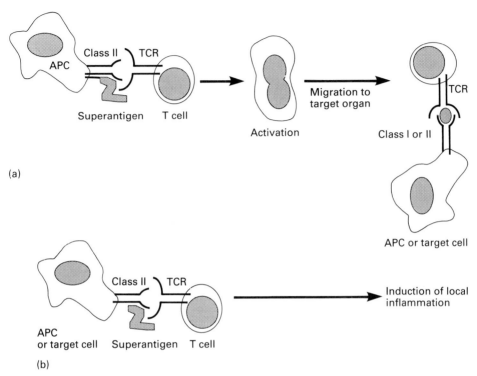

(a)

(b)

Fig. 10.1. Scenarios for an involvement of superantigens in the induction phase of autoimmunity. (a) Encounter in periphery: a model of peripheral activation of autoreactive T cells. (b) Encounter in target organ the site of autoimmune reaction showing the first encounter with the superantigen.

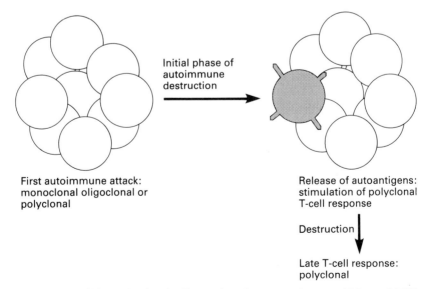

Fig. 10.2. Possible mechanism leading to broader autoantigen specificity and TCR heterogeneity in chronic autoimmune disease.

taken over by other, peptide-responsive, autoreactive T cells. In the first case oligoclonality of the infiltrating T cells might ensue. In the second case the response would be polyclonal at the onset of clinical symptoms.

Similar to the picture shown in Fig. 10.1a the first encounter with the superantigen could take place at the site of autoimmune reaction Fig. 10.1b. It could be expressed there from endogenous genes or after infection with a virus with specific tissue trophicity. Again the outcome of the local activation is not clear. Classical superantigen reactions lead to induction of anergy after an initial activation of the T cells. If the same is true for local activation in autoimmunity due to superantigen interaction, it is most likely that potential oligoclonality would not be detectable anymore at the onset of the clinical symptoms.

In an elegant model it has recently been shown that mice which express a target antigen for cytotoxic T cells in the β cells of the pancreas do not suffer from autoimmunity unless the antigen is encountered in the periphery. Then autoimmune destruction of the pancreatic β cells results within a short time and the mice become diabetic (Ohashi *et al.*, 1991; Oldstone *et al.*, 1991).

In rheumatoid arthritis in humans a recent report on the expression of T cells expressing TCR $V_\beta 14$ in the joints of patients and the periphery gave results which could be easily explained with superantigen activation in the periphery. Peripheral T cells showed a much lower percentage of TCR $V_\beta 14$ T cells in patients than in controls whereas this population was enriched in the joints (Bisno, 1991; Paliard *et al.*, 1991). This observation is similar to the classical superantigen peripheral deletion models. In other models of autoimmunity, roles for retroviruses have been indicated (Crawford *et al.*, 1980; Krieg & Steinberg, 1990). Expression of HTLV-1 genes in transgenic mice resulted in arthritis symptoms. Further studies are required to see whether superantigens are indeed involved in the induction of autoimmune diseases.

Interpretation of results

Induced autoimmune diseases represent model autoimmune diseases where the kinetics of disease induction can easily be manipulated. Autoimmune T-cell clones can be derived shortly after immunization from the local lymph nodes and the autoantigens are easily characterized. Injection of these autoreactive T-cell clones gives valuable information about their involvement in the disease process. These T-cell clones therefore represent the first response to these autoantigens.

In spontaneous autoimmune diseases it has been more difficult to derive an unbiased panel of autoimmune T-cell clones and practically always from subjects which were in a late phase of autoimmunity, already showing clinical symptoms. In these diseases the T-cell clones were either derived from the peripheral repertoire or less frequently from the local infiltrating lymphocytes in the target of autoimmune destruction. Due to the lack of monoclonal antibodies directed against the majority of TCR V_β regions, PCR analysis remains the best tool for an analysis of the TCR repertoire in the lesions.

For spontaneous autoimmunity the time between first histological signs of autoimmunity to onset of clinical disease is very long. For human IDDM, for example, this takes an average of 5 years (Eisenbarth, 1985). This slow progression of the disease is a puzzle for researchers in the field. Little is known about the phases of activation or the state of anergy of the cells in the lesions.

So far EAE, EAN and uveitis stand alone with the strikingly limited repertoire of TCR expression in the autoimmune T-cell clones. Other models of induced autoimmunity such as collagen-induced arthritis have so far not given such simple patterns. In spontaneous autoimmune diseases, at the onset of clinical disease, either wide heterogeneity is found as in NOD autoimmune-diabetes mellitus of conflicting result have been reported as in human rheumatoid arthritis and MS. In human arthritis most (but not all) groups have found a more profound oligoclonality after expansion of the activated T cells from the lesions in IL-2 containing medium. Whether this is due to outgrowth of rare clones or represents a limited repertoire of autoimmune T cells is not clear at this point. A large patient to patient variation was observed. Local inflammations in autoimmunity are usually as heterogenous as delayed type hypersensitivity reactions. Even in models such as EAE, where practically all the autoimmune T cells express $V_\beta 8$, the lesions do not show predominant expression of the TCR molecules found in encephalitogenic T-cell clones.

The results obtained with PCR, although highly interesting, have to be taken with caution. It is generally not easy to quantitate accurately with PCR. So far indications for limited heterogeneity of TCR molecules, using the PCR approach, have been reported in MS, rheumatoid arthritis and tumour-infiltrating lymphocytes. On the other hand, analysis of the peripheral T-cell repertoire directed at MBP shows clear oligoclonality.

A major problem in studies in humans is that there are no experimental systems to differentiate pathogenic from non-pathogenic T-cell clones. However, the lack of monoclonal antibodies reactive with the different V regions makes PCR the method of choice for analysis of TCR repertoires. Using this approach the oligoclonality in EAE would most likely not have been detected. Three studies using the three available anti-TCR V_β antibodies have given indications for and against a limited heterogeneity of TCR but, with the exception of Crohn's disease, a large patient to patient variation was observed. The studies with Crohn's disease are encouraging and need confirmation by independent groups.

Initial destruction of target cells leads to cellular debris. These debris antigens can be presented by local antigen-presenting cells (APCs) to T cells. Even if the triggering event for autoimmunity would be driven by an immunodominant peptide and the responsive T cells would be oligoclonal, one can easily imagine that the autoimmune T cells present at later stages of the disease could be much more polyclonal (see Fig. 10.2).

A possible scenario for the increase in autoantigen specificity during the course of an autoimmune disease is depicted in Fig. 10.2. Should this mechanism be true then in the majority of chronic autoimmune diseases potential oligoclonality at the initiation of the autoimmune disease would be hidden by the larger heterogeneity at the outbreak or after chronic disease. The problem then would be that treatment with anti-TCR monoclonal antibodies would have to start very early, long before clinical symptoms are apparent.

A recent study in EAE showed that the heterogeneity of autoantigens and in parallel the heterogeneity of T cells recognizing them, augments with chronicity of the disease (McCarron et al., 1990). Most likely chronic tissue damage exposes more and more different autoantigens to the immune system. For induction of EAE, activation of autoimmune T cells has to occur in the periphery to induce the inflammation within the brain. Normally T cells are excluded from the brain by the blood–brain barrier. There are indications that activated T cells can pass this barrier better.

The results presented in this review show that, especially in human autoimmune diseases, more analyses are required before a clear picture emerges about possible oligoclonality of TCR in autoimmune diseases. There are indications for, as well as against, such oligoclonality and this within the same diseases. These conflicts have to be resolved and it has to be clarified whether these results represent experimental problems or whether there are subgroups of patients which can be identified. To obtain a clearer picture it is definitively very important to develop more reagents for analysis of autoimmune T cells such as TCR-V_β-specific monoclonal antibodies. Characterization of immunodominant autoantigens in spontaneous autoimmune diseases is required for a better picture of the T-cell response towards these antigens. An additional requirement is to define strategies for the distinction of T cells which cause autoimmunity from the other infiltrating T cells.

Treatment results in EAE clearly showed that anti-TCR V_β treatment can be effective also when only about 80% of the encephalitogenic T cells share the TCR V_β region. The future will tell whether anti-TCR V_β treatment is effective in the treatment of human autoimmune diseases or whether combinations of different forms of treatments are synergistic.

The results obtained thus far are both encouraging and frustrating. Hopefully the near future will show whether this highly specific form of treatment is applicable to human autoimmune diseases.

References

Acha-Orbea, H., Mitchell, D. J., Timmerman, L., Wraith, D. C., Tausch, G. S., Waldor, M. K., Zamvil, S. S., McDevitt, H. O. & Steinman, L. (1988). Limited heterogeneity of T cell receptors in experimental allergic encephalomyelitis. *Cell* **54**, 263–273.

Acha-Orbea, H. & Palmer, E. (1991). Mls — a retrovirus exploits the immune system. *Immunology Today* **12**, 356–361.

Acha-Orbea, H., Shakhov, A. N., Scarpellino, L., Kolb, E. Müller, V., Vessaz-Shaw, A., Fuchs, R., Blöchlinger, K., Rollini, P., Billote, J., Sarafidou, M., MacDonald, H. R. & Diggelmann, H. (1991). Clonal deletion of $V_{\beta}14$ positive T cells in mammary tumor virus transgenic mice. *Nature* **350**, 207–211.

Acha-Orbea, H., Steinman, L. & McDevitt, H. O. (1989). T cell receptors in murine autoimmune diseases. *Annual Review of Immunology* **7**, 371–405.

Allegretta, M., Nicklas, J. A., Sriram, S. & Albertini, R. J. (1990). T cells responsive to myelin basic protein in patients with multiple sclerosis. *Science* **247**, 718–721.

Anderson, G. D., Banerjee, S., Luthra, H. S. & David, C. S. (1991). Role of Mls-1 locus and clonal deletion of T cells in susceptibility to collagen-induced arthritis in mice. *Journal of Immunology* **147**, 1189–1193.

Andersson, M., Goldschmidt, T. J., Michaelsson, E., Larsson, A. & Holmdahl, R. (1991). T cell receptor V_{β} haplotype and complement component C5 play no significant role for the resistance to collagen induced arthritis in the SWR mouse. *Immunology* **73**, 191–196.

Banerjee, S., Haqqi, T. M., Luthra, H. S., Stuart, J. M. & David, C. S. (1988). Possible role of V_{β} T cell receptor genes in susceptibility to collagen-induced arthritis in mice. *Journal of Experimental Medicine* **167**, 832–839.

Ben-Nun, A., Liblau, R. S., Cohen, L., Lehmann, D., Tourneir-Lasserve, E., Rosenzweig, A., Jingwu, Z., Raus, J. C. F. & Bach, M.-A. (1991). Restricted T-cell receptor V_{β} gene usage by myelin basic protein-specific T-cell clones in multiple sclerosis: Predominant genes vary in individuals. *Proceedings of the National Academy of Sciences USA* **88**, 2466–2470.

Bisno, A. L. (1991). Group A streptococcal infections and acute rheumatic fever. *New England Journal of Medicine* **325**, 783–793.

Brennan, F. M., Allard, S. Londai, M., Savill, C., Boylston, A., Carrel, S., Maini, R. N. & Feldman, M. (1988). Heterogeneity of T cell receptor idiotypes in rheumatoid arthritis. *Clinical Experimental Immunology* **73**, 417–423.

Burns, F. R., Li, X., Shen, N., Offner, H., Chou, Y. C., Vandenbark, A. A. & Heber-Katz, E. (1989). Both rat and mouse T cell receptors specific for the encephalitogenic determinant of myelin basic protein use similar V_{α} and V_{β} chain genes even though the major histocompatibility complex and encephalitogenic determinants are different. *Journal of Experimental Medicine* **169**, 27–39.

Chluba, J., Steeg, C., Becker, A., Wekerle, H. & Epplen, J. T. (1989). T cell receptor β chain usage in myelin basic protein-specific rat T lymphocytes. *European Journal of Immunology* **19**, 279–284.

Choi, Y., Kappler, J. W. & Marrack, P. (1991). A superantigen encoded in the open reading frame of the 3′ long terminal repeat of mouse mammary tumor virus. *Nature* **350**, 203–207.

Concannon, P., Wright, J. A., Wright, L. G., Sylvester, D. R. & Spielman, R. S. (1990). T-cell receptor genes and insulin-dependent diabetes mellitus (IDDM): no evidence for linkage from affected sib pairs. *American Journal of Human Genetics* **47**, 45–52.

Correale, J., Mix, E., Olsson, T., Kastulas, V., Fredrikson, S., Hojeberg, B. & Link, H. (1991). CD5^{+} B cells and CD4^{-}8^{-} T cells in neuroimmunological diseases. *Journal of Neuroimmunology* **32**, 123–132.

Crawford, R. B., Adams, D. S., Cheevers, W. P. & Cork, L. C. (1980). Chronic arthritis in goats caused by a retrovirus. *Science* **207**, 997.

Duby, A. D., Sinclair, A. K., Osborne-Lawrence, S. L., Zeldes, W., Kan L. & Fox, D. A. (1989). Clonal heterogeneity of synovial fluid T lymphocytes from patients with rheumatoid arthritis. *Proceedings of the National Academy of Sciences USA* **86**, 6206–6210.

Dyson, P. J., Knight, A. M., Fairchild, S., Simpson, E. & Tomonari, K. (1991). Genes encoding ligands for deletion of $V_\beta 11$ T cells cosegregate with mammary tumor virus genomes. *Nature* **349**, 531–532.

Eisenbarth, G. S. (1985). Type 1 diabetes. A chronic autoimmune disease. *New England Journal of Medicine* **314**, 1360–1368.

Fleischer, B. & Schrezenmeier, H. (1988). T cell stimulation by staphylococcal entero-toxins. Clonally variable response and requirements for major histocompatibility complex class II molecules on accessory or target cells. *Journal of Experimental Medicine* **167**, 1697–1707.

Frankel, W. N., Rudy, C., Coffin, J. M. & Huber, B. T. (1991). Linkage of MIs genes to endogenous mammary tumor viruses of inbred mice. *Nature* **349**, 526–528.

Fugger, L., Sandberg-Wollheim, M., Morling, N., Ryder, L. P. & Svejgaard, A. (1990). The germline repertoire of T-cell receptor β chain genes in patients with relapsing/remitting multiple sclerosis or optic neuritis. *Immunogenetics* **31**, 278–280.

Goldschmidt, T. J., Jansson, L. & Holmdahl, R. (1990) *In vivo* elimination of T cells expressing specific T-cell receptor V_β chains in mice susceptible to collagen-induced arthritis. *Immunology* **69**, 508–514.

Gregerson, D. S., Fling, S. P., Merryman, C.F., Zhang, X. Li, X. & Heber-Katz, E. (1991). Conserved T cell receptor V gene usage by uveitogenic T cells. *Clinical Immunology and Immunopathology* **58**, 154–161.

Hafler, D. A., Duby, A. D., Lee, S. J., Benjamin, D., Seidman, J. G. & Weiner, H. L. (1988). Oligoclonal T lymphocytes in the cerebrospinal fluid of patients with multiple sclerosis. *Journal of Experimental Medicine* **167**, 1313–1322.

Hakoda, M., Ishimoto, T., Yamamotoko, K., Inoue, K., Kamatani, N. & Nishioka, K. (1990). Clonal analysis of T cell infiltrates in synovial tissue of patients with rheumatoid arthritis. *Clinical Immunology and Immunopathology* **57**, 387–398.

Haskins, K., Portas, M., Bergman, B., Lafferty, K. & Brasley, B. (1989). Pancreatic islet-specific T-cells clones from nonobese diabetic mice. *Proceedings of the National Academy of Sciences USA* **86**, 8000–8004.

Heber-Katz, E. & Acha-Orbea, H. (1989). The V-region disease hypothesis: evidence from autoimmune encephalomyelitis. *Immunology Today* **10**, 164–169.

Heber-Katz, E. (1990). The autoimmune T cell receptor: Epitopes, Idiotopes and Malatopes. *Clinical Immunology and Immunopathology* **55**, 1–80.

Herman, A., Kappler, J. W., Marrack, P. & Pullen, A. M. (1991). Superantigens: mechanisms of T-cell stimulation and role in immune responses. *Annual Review of Immunology* **9**, 745–772.

Hirose, S., Tokushige, K., Kinoshita, K., Nozawa, S., Saito, J., Nishimura, H. & Shirai, T. (1990). Contribution of the gene linked to the T cell receptor β chain gene complex of NZW mice to autoimmunity of (NZB × NZW)F1 mice. *European Journal of Immunology* **21**, 823–826.

Hohlfeld, R., Toyka, K. V., Heininger, K., Gross-Wilde, H. & Kalies, I. (1984). Autoimmune T lymphocytes specific for acetylcholine receptor. *Nature* **310**, 244–246.

Holoshitz, J., Koning, F., Coligan, J. E., De Bruyn, J. & Strober, S. (1989). Isolation of $CD4^-$ $CD8^-$ mycobacteria-reactive T lymphocytes clones from rheumatoid arthritis synovial fluid. *Nature* **339**, 226–229.

Ito, M., Tanimoto, M., Kamura, H., Yoneda, M., Morishima, Y., Yamauchi, K., Itasu, T., Takatsuki, K. & Saito, H. (1989). Association of HLA antigen and restriction fragment length polymorphism of T cell receptor β-chain gene with Grave's disease and Hashimoto's thyroiditis. *Journal of Clinical Endocrinology and Metabolism* **69**, 100–104.

Jones, L. A., Chin, L. T., Longo, D. L. & Kruisbeek, A. M. (1990). Peripheral clonal elimination of functional T cells. *Science* **250**, 1726–1729.

Kappler, J. W., Roehm, N. & Marrack, P. (1987). T cell tolerance by clonal elimination in the thymus. *Cell* **49**, 273–280.

Kappler, J. W., Staerz, U. D., White, J. & Marrack, P. C. (1988). Self-tolerance eliminates T cells specific for Mls-modified products of the major histocompatibility complex. *Nature* **332**, 35–40.

Katzin, W. E., Fishleder, A. J. & Tubs, R. R. (1989). Investigation of the clonality of lymphocytes in Hashimoto's thyroid is using immunoglobulin and T-cell receptor gene probes. *Clinical Immunology and Immunopathology* **51**, 264–274.

Kisielow, P., Blüthmann, H., Staerz, U. D., Steinmetz, M. & von Boehmer, H. (1988). Tolerance in T-cell-receptor transgenic mice involves deletion of nonmature CD4$^+$8$^+$ thymocytes. *Nature* **333**, 742–746.

Konon, D. H., Urban, J. L., Horvath, S., Ando, D. G., Saavedra, R. A. & Hood, L. (1988). Two minor determinants of myelin basic protein induce experimental allergic encephalomyelitis in SJL/J mice. *Journal of Experimental Medicine* **168**, 213–227.

Kontiainen, S., Toomath, R., Lowder, J. & Feldman, M. (1990). Selective activation of T cells in newly diagnosed insulin-dependent diabetic patients: evidence for heterogeneity of T cell receptor usage. *Clinical and Experimental Immunology* **83**, 347–351.

Kotzin, B. L. & Palmer, E. (1987). The contribution of NZW genes to lupus-like disease in (NZB × NZW)F1 mice. *Journal of Experimental Medicine* **165**, 1237–1251.

Krieg, A. M. & Steinberg, A. D. (1990). Analysis of thymic endogenous retroviral expression in murine lupus. Genetic and immune studies. *Journal of Clinical Investigation* **86**, 809.

Ku, G., Brahn, E. & Kronenberg, M. (1990). Characterization of collagen-specific T cells from pathogenic and nonpathogenic rat T cell lines. *Cellular Immunology* **30**, 472–489.

Liblau, R., Tournier-Lasserve, E., Maciazek, J., Duams, G., Siffert, O., Hashim, G. & Bach, M.-A. (1991). T cell response to myelin basic protein epitopes in multiple sclerosis patients and healthy subjects. *European Journal of Immunology* **21**, 1391–1395.

Livingstone, A., Edwards, C. T., Shizuru, J. A. & Fathman, C. G. (1991). Genetic analysis of diabetes in the nonobese diabetic mouse. I. MHC and T cell receptor β gene expression. *Journal of Immunology* **146**, 529–.

MacDonald, H. R., Schneider, R., Lees, R. L., Howe, R. K., Acha-Orbea, H., Festenstein, H., Zinkernagel, R. M. & Hengartner, H. (1988). T-cell receptor V$_\beta$ use predicts reactivity and tolerance to Mls^a-encoded antigens. *Nature* **332**, 40–45.

Marrack, P. & Kappler, J. (1990). The staphylococcal enterotoxins and their relatives. *Science* **248**, 705–711.

Marrack, P., Kushnir, E. & Kappler, J. (1991). A maternally inherited superantigen encoded by a mammary tumor virus. *Nature* **349**, 524.

Martin, R., Jaraquemada, D., Flerlage, M., Richert, J., Whitacker, J., Long, E. O., McFarlin, D. E. & McFarland, H. F. (1990). Fine specificity and HLA restriction of myelin basic protein-specific cytotoxic T cell lines from multiple sclerosis patients and healthy individuals. *Journal of Immunology* **145**, 540–548.

McCarron, R. M., Fallis, R. J. & McFarlin, D. E. (1990). Alterations in T cell antigen specificity and class II restriction during the course of chronic relapsing experimental allergic encephalomyelitis. *Journal of Neurology* **29**, 73–79.

McMillan, S. A., Graham, C. A., Hart, P. J., Hadden, D. R. & McNeil, T. A. (1990). A T cell receptor beta chain polymorphism is associated with patients developing insulin-dependent diabetes after the age of 20 years. *Clinical and Experimental Immunology* **82**, 538–541.

Merryman, C. F., Donoso, L. A., Zhang, X., Heber-Katz, E. & Gregerson, D. (1991). Characterization of a new potent immunopathogenic epitope in S-antigen that elicits T cells expressing $V_\beta 8$ and $V_\alpha 2$-like genes. *Journal of Immunology* **146**, 75–80.

Miceli, M. C. & Finn, O. J. (1989). T cell receptor β-chain selection in human allograft rejection. *Journal of Immunology* **142**, 81–86.

Miltenburg, A. M. M., Van Laar, J. M., Daha, M. R., De Bries, R. R. P., Van den Elsen, P. J. & Breedveld, F. C. (1990). Dominant T-cell receptor β-chain gene rearrangements indicate clonal expansion in the rheumatoid joint. *Scandinavian Journal of Immunology* **31**, 121–125.

Moebius, U., Manns, M., Hess, G., Kober, G., Meyer zum Büschenfelde, K.-H. & Meuer, S. C. (1990). T cell receptor gene rearrangements of T lymphocytes infiltrating the liver in chronic active hepatitis B and primary biliary cirrhosis (PBC): oligoclonality of PBC-derived T cell clones. *European Journal of Immunology* **20**, 889–896.

Moller, D. R., Konishi, K., Kirby, M., Balbi, B. & Crystal, R. G. (1988). Bias towards use of a specific T cell receptor β-chain variable region in a subgroup of individuals with sarcoides. *Journal of Clinical Investigation* **82**, 1183–1191.

Mor, F. (1991). Polymyositis mediated by T lymphocytes expressing the gamma/delta receptor. *New England Journal of Medicine* **325**, 587–588.

Nakano, N., Kikutani, H., Nishimoto, H. & Kishimoto, T. (1991). T cell receptor V gene usage of islet β cell-reactive T cells is not restricted in non-obese diabetic mice. *Journal of Experimental Medicine* **173**, 1091–1097.

Nitta, T., Oksenberg, J. R., Rao, N. A. & Steinman, L. (1990). Predominant expression of T cell receptor $V_\alpha 7$ in tumor-infiltrating lymphocytes of uveal melanoma. *Science* **249**, 672–674.

Noonan, D. J., McConahey, P. J. & Cardenas, G. J. (1990). Correlations of autoimmunity with H-2 and T cell receptor β chain genotypes in (NZB × NZW)F2 mice. *European Journal of Immunology* **20**, 1105–1110.

Ohashi, P. S., Oehen, S., Bürki, K., Pricher, H., Ohashi, C. T., Odermatt, B., Malissen, B., Zinkernagel, R. M. & Hengartner, H. (1991). Ablation of 'tolerance' and induction of diabetes by virus infection in viral antigen transgenic mice. *Cell* **65**, 305–317.

Oksenberg, J. R., Sherritt, M., Begovich, A. B., Erlich, H. A., Bernard, C. C. Cavalli-Sforza, L. L. & Steinman, L. (1989). T-cell receptor V_α and C_α alleles associated with multiple sclerosis and myasthenia gravis. *Proceedings of the National Academy of Sciences USA* **86**, 988–992.

Oksenberg, J. R., Stuart, S., Begovich, A. B., Bell, R. B., Erlich, H. A., Steinman, L. & Bernard, C. C. A. (1990). Limited heterogeneity of rearranged T cell receptor V_α transcripts in brains of multiple sclerosis patients. *Nature* **345**, 344–346.

Oldstone, M. B. A., Nerenberg, M. & Lewicki, H. (1991). Virus infection triggers insulin-dependent diabetes mellitus in a transgenic model: role of anti-self (virus) immune responses. *Cell* **65**, 319–331.

Owhashi, M. & Heber-Katz, E. (1988). Protection from experimental allergic encephalomyelitis conferred by a monoclonal antibody directed against a shared idiotype on rat T cell receptors specific for myelin basic protein. *Journal of Experimental Medicine* **168**, 2153–2164.

Padula, S. J., Lingenheld, E. G., Stabach, P. R., Chou, C.-H. J., Kono, D. H. & Clark, R.

B. (1991). Identification of encephalitogenic $V_\beta4$-bearing T cells in SJL mice. Further evidence for the V region disease hypothesis? *Journal of Immunology* **146**, 879–883.

Padula, S. J., Sgroi, D. C., Lingenheld, E. G., Love, J. T., Chaou, C.-H. J. & Clark, R. B. (1988). T cell receptor beta chain gene rearrangement shared by murine T cell lines derived from a site of autoimmune inflammation. *Journal of Clinical Investigation* **81**, 1810–1818.

Paliard, X., West, S. G., Lafferty, J. A., Clements, J. R., Kappler, J. W., Marrack, P. & Kotzin, B. L. (1991). Evidence for the effects of a superantigen in rheumatoid arthritis. *Science* **253**, 325–329.

Pette, M., Fujita, K., Wilkinson, D., Altman, D. M., Trowsdale, J., Giegerich, G., Hinkkanen, A., Epplen, J. T., Kappos, L. & Wekerle, H. (1990). Myelin autoreactivity in multiple sclerosis: recognition of myelin basic protein in the context of HLA-DR2 products by T lymphocytes of multiple sclerosis patients and healthy donors. *Proceedings of the National Academy of Sciences USA* **87**, 7968–7972.

Plater-Zyber, C., Brennan, F. M.k, Feldmann, M. & Maini, R. N. (1989). 'Fetal-type' B and T lymphocytes in rheumatoid arthritis and primary Sjörgen's syndrome. *Journal of autoimmunity* **2**, 233–241.

Posnett, D. N., Gottlieb, A., Bussel, J. B., Friedman, S. M., Chiorazzi, N., Li, Y., Szabo, P., Farid, N. R. & Robinson, M. A. (1988). T cell antigen receptors in autoimmunity. *Journal of Immunology* **141**, 1963–1969.

Posnett, D. N., Schmelkin, I., Burton, D. A., August, A., McGrath, H. & Mayer, L. F. (1990). T cell antigen receptor V gene usage. Increases in $V_\beta8^+$ T cells in Crohn's disease. *Journal of Clinical Investigation* **85**, 1770–1776.

Rammensee, H.-G., Kroschewsky, R. & Frangoulis, B. (1989). Clonal anergy induced in mature $V_\beta6$ T lymphocytes on immunizing Mls-1^b mice with Mls-1^a expressing cells. *Nature* **339**, 541–544.

Reich, E. P., Sherwin, R. S., Kanagawa, O. & Janeway, C. A. Jr. (1989). An explanation for the protective effect of the MHC class II I-E molecule in murine diabetes. *Nature* **341**, 326–328.

Reijonen, H., Silvenoinen-Kassinen, S., Ilonen, J. & Knip, M. (1990). Lack of association of T cell receptor beta-chain constant region polymorphisms with insulin-dependent mellitus in Finland. *Clinical and Experimental Immunology* **181**, 396–399.

Rotteveel, F. T. M., Kokkelink, H. K., Polman, C. H., Van Dongen, J. J. M. & Lucas, C. J. (1987). Analysis of T cell receptor-gene rearrangement in T cells from the cerebrospinal fluid of patients with multiple sclerosis. *Journal of Neurology* **15**, 243–249.

Sakai, K., Sinha, A. A., Mitchell, D. J., Zamvil, S. S., Rothbard, J. B., McDevitt, H. O. & Steinman, L. (1988). Involvement of distinct murine T-cell receptors in the autoimmune encephalitogenic response to nested epitopes of myelin basic protein. *Proceedings of the National Academy of Sciences USA* **85**, 8608–8612.

Savill, C. M., Delves, P. J., Kioussis, D., Walker, P., Lydyard, P. M., Colaco, B., Shipley, M. & Roitt, I. M. (1987). A minority of patients with rheumatoid arthritis show a dominant rearrangement of T-cell receptor β chain genes in synovial lymphocytes. *Scandinavian Journal of Immunology* **25**, 629–635.

Sioud, M., Forre, O. & Natvig, J. B. (1991). T cell receptor diversity of freshly isolated T lymphocytes in rheumatoid synovitis. *European Journal of Immunology* **21**, 239–241.

Sottini, A., Imberti, L., Gorla, R., Cattaneo, R. & Primi, D. (1991). Restricted expression of T cell receptor V_β but not V_α genes in rheumatoid arthritis. *European Journal of Immunology* **21**, 461–466.

Spinella, D. G., Jeffers, J. R., Reife, R. A. & Stuart, J. M. (1991). The role of C5 and T-cell receptor V_β genes in susceptibility to collagen-induced arthritis. *Immunogenetics* **34**, 23–27.

Stamenkovic, I., Stegagno, M., Wright, K. A., Krane, S. M., Amento, E. P., Colvin, R. B.,

Duquesnoy, R. J. & Kurnick, J. T. (1988). Clonal dominance among T-lymphocyte infiltrates in arthritis. *Proceedings of the National Academy of Sciences USA* **85**, 1179–1183.

Sun, J.-B., Olsson, T., Wang, W.-Z., Xiao, B.-G., Kostulas, V., Fredrikson, S., Ekre, H.-P. & Link, H. (1991). Autoreactive T and B cells responding to myelin proteolipid protein in multiple sclerosis and controls. *European Journal of Immunology* **21**, 1461–1468.

Tesch, H., Hohlfeld, R. & Toyka, K. V. (1989). Analysis of immunoglobulin and T cell receptor gene rearrangements in the thymus of myasthenia gravis patients. *Journal of Neuroimmunology* **21**, 169–176.

Urban, J. L., Kumar, V., Kono, D. H., Gomez, C., Horvath, S. J., Clayton, J., Ando, D. G., Sercarz, E. E. & Hood, L. (1988). Restricted use of T cell receptor genes in murine autoimmune encephalomyelitis raises possibilities for antibody therapy. *Cell* **54**, 577–592.

Van Laar, J. M., Miltenburg, A. M. M., Verdonk, M. J. A., Daha, M. R., De Vries, R. R. P., Van den Elsen, P. J. & Breedveld, F. C. (1991). Lack of T cell oligoclonality in enzyme-digested synovial tissue and in synovial fluid in most patients with rheumatoid arthritis. *Clinical Experimental Immunology* **83**, 352–358.

Webb, S., Morris, C. & Sprent, J. (1990). Extrathymic tolerance of mature T cells: clonal elimination as a consequence of immunity. *Cell* **63**, 1249–1256.

White, J., Herman, A., Pullen, A. M., Kubo, R., Kappler, J. W. & Marrack, P. (1989). The V_β-specific superantigen staphylococcal enterotoxin B: stimulation of mature T cells and clonal deletion in neonatal mice. *Cell* **56**, 27–35.

Woodland, D., Happ, M. P., Bill, J. & Palmer, E. (1990). Requirement for cotolerogenic gene products in the clonal deletion of I-E reactive T cells. *Science* **247**, 964–967.

Woodland, D. L., Happ, M. P., Gollub, K. J. & Palmer, E. (1991). An endogenous retrovirus mediating deletion of $\alpha\beta$ T cells? *Nature* **349**, 529–530.

Wucherpfenning, K. W., Ota, K., Endo, N., Seidman, J. G., Rosenzweig, A., Weiner, H. L. & Hafler, D. A. (1990). Shared human T cell receptor V_β usage to immunodominant regions of myelin basic protein. *Science* **248**, 1016–1019.

Yssel, H., Nakamoto, T., Schneider, P., Freitas, V., Collins, C., Webb, D., Mensi, N., Soderberg, C. & Peltz, G. (1990). Analysis of T lymphocytes cloned from synovial fluid and blood of a patient with lyme arthritis. *International Immunology* **2**, 1081–1089.

Zamvil, S. S., Mitchell, D. J., Lee, N. E., Moore, a. C., Waldor, M. K., Sakai, K., Rothbard, J. B., McDevitt, H. O., Steinman, L. & Acha-Orbea, H. (1988). Predominant expression of a T cell receptor V_β-subfamily in autoimmune encephalomyelitis. *Journal of Experimental Medicine* **167**, 1586–1596.

Chapter 11

Interleukin-2 receptor-directed immunosuppressive therapies: antibody- or cytokine-based targeting molecules

Terry B. Strom, Vicki Rubin Kelley,
Thasia G. Woodworth and John R. Murphy

Introduction

The ideal immunosuppressive therapy can be realized by breaking the lock and key arrangement leading to T-cell activation that intimately engages cellularly bound antigens with those T cells bearing receptors that stereospecifically recognize the stimulating antigen. This approach would leave the overwhelming majority of immune cells involved in protective host defence mechanisms untouched, thereby avoiding the undesirable consequences of generalized immunosuppression. This solution would be obtained by developing antibodies or tolerogenic peptides that react with the antigen-combining site of T-cell-antigen receptors for disease stimulating antigens. This strategy has been deterred, at least temporarily, by the vast genetic diversity of the T-cell receptor for antigen. Many reagents would be required to execute clone-specific immunosuppressive therapy. This approach will not provide a practical therapeutic solution unless autoreactive T-cell clones are oligoclonal and similar in each patient with a given disease.

    We have developed the simpler approach of targeting the high affinity interleukin-2 receptor (IL-2R). In essence, only recently activated lymphocytes, especially T cells, bear this structure. This structure is absent from the surface of resting T cells and non-lymphoid tissues (Smith, 1987). The *de novo* acquisition of high affinity IL-2Rs is a critical event in the course of T-cell activation (Leonard *et al.*, 1982; Cantrell & Smith, 1984; Maddock *et al.*, 1985; Smith, 1987). Interaction of IL-2 with its receptor is required for the clonal expansion and continued viability of activated T cells (Maddock *et al.*, 1985). The IL-2R is present on the cell surface as high-, intermediate- and low-affinity binding sites. The high-affinity site is a complex of a 55 kD α chain (CD25) and a 70 kD β chain. The isolated 70 kD chain possesses intermediate binding affinity, while the isolated 55 kD chain is a low-affinity binding site (Tsudo *et al.*, 1986). The β-chain is sparsely expressed on some resting T cells while the α chain is not expressed upon resting T cells. With T-cell activation, marked amplification of expression of the β-chain and *de novo* expression of the α chain ensue.

As the IL-2Rα chain is only transiently expressed during the brief proliferative burst of lymphocytes triggered in response to antigen, we first wondered whether administration of anti-IL-2R monoclonal antibody (MoAb) in the early post-transplant period or to autoimmune hosts would provide a utilitarian approach to achieving selective immunosuppression directed solely at activated lymphocytes. In theory, an MoAb directed against the IL-2R chain — a protein expressed in the common pathway of T-cell activation — can be used in every situation of unwanted T-cell dependent immunity to achieve selective immunosuppression.

Antibody-based therapeutic ligands

Conventional monoclonal antibodies

First generation anti-IL-2Rα, but not anti-IL-2Rβ, MoAbs have been tested for immunosuppressive efficacy in mice, rats, monkeys and man. Rat-anti-mouse and mouse-anti-rat pan-T cell, anti-CD4 and anti-CD25, i.e. IL-2R α-chain, MoAbs exert remarkable immunosuppressive effects in rodent transplant and autoimmune models whereas only select first generation rodent anti-human IL-2R MoAbs exert meaningful immuno-suppression in clinical practice. While graft tolerance can be achieved with anti-IL-2R MoAbs in rodents, immunosuppression, but not tolerance, occurs with clinical application of first generation anti-CD25 MoAbs. One of the reasons for the failure of anti-IL-2R or anti-T cell MoAb treatment to live up to expectations in clinical practice must be due to the failure of the constant, e.g. Fc, region of most murine MoAbs to facilitate lysis of human target cells in the treated human host. These antibodies do not fix human complement or activate human Fc receptor positive phagocytic/cytolytic cells. As a consequence, clinical application of the first generation rodent anti-human MoAbs do not effect destruction of the targeted human cells while *in vivo* treatment with mouse anti-rat or rat anti-mouse, i.e. rodent anti-rodent, MoAbs can destroy the target cell population. It is not surprising that the most immunosuppressive first generation MoAbs in clinical practice target functionally important domains of vitally important T-cell-surface proteins, e.g. the T-cell antigen/CD3 complex or the IL-2R. These MoAbs probably function as receptor site blockers. In addition to the failure of the first generation MoAbs to destroy the target-cell population, these rodent MoAbs are 'foreign proteins' for humans. Thus, the potential for repetitive therapy is limited by the formation of anti-MoAbs, especially anti-idiotypic, antibodies. Hence, efforts now are proceeding in many quarters to use genetic engineering strategies to replace the constant and framework regions of murine antibodies with human sequences in order to produce MoAbs that will lyse the targeted human cell *in vivo* and eliminate immunogenicity.

Humanized anti-CD25 monoclonal antibodies

Morrison *et al.* (1984) developed a strategy for transforming a murine MoAb into a chimeric murine–human antibody. Using genetic engineering, the mouse variable (V) antigen binding domain is fused to a human constant (C), i.e. Fc, domain. These MoAbs cause target cell lysis *in vivo* because they fix human complement and activate human FcR⁺ cells. This tactic does not, however, obviate antibody responses against the murine V region. Winter *et al.* (1988) addressed this shortcoming of chimeric MoAbs by 'humanizing' framework residues within the murine (V) region of a chimeric rat/human MoAb. The V region consists of discrete complementarily determining regions (CDRs) that are woven into the fabric of the scaffolding, i.e. framework regions. The Winter laboratory (Reichmann *et al.*, 1988) genetically altered the murine framework sequences to human framework sequences. This strategy permits retention of murine CDRs while replacing the more numerous mouse framework sequences with human sequences. CAMPATH-1H which binds to an antigen expressed upon all lymphocytes was the first 'humanized' MoAb to be developed (Reichmann *et al.*, 1988).

A mouse anti-human IL-2Rα chain MoAb, anti-Tac MoAb, has recently been humanized (Queen *et al.*, 1989). In constructing the humanized anti-Tac MoAb, Queen *et al.* learned that it was not possible to retain antigen binding if all the mouse framework residues were converted to human sequences. Using a computer model of anti-Tac MoAb structure as a guide, certain key contact points between the murine CDRs and the murine framework regions were retained. The affinity of antigen binding of the humanized MoAb was restored to near but not to equivalency of the murine anti-human MoAb. The binding affinity of anti-Tac or humanized anti-Tac for the IL-2R is at least 100-fold less efficient than IL-2.

IL-2/Ig fusion proteins

More recently, MoAbs have also been genetically engineered so that IL-2 replaces the V_H region of the Ig molecule (Landolfi, 1991). Since IL-2 binds to its receptor with a much higher affinity than an MoAb, this fusion protein binds to the IL-2R with a very high affinity. In the absence of complement or FcR$^+$ phagocytes, this human IL-2/IgG chimer powerfully stimulated the growth of IL-2-dependent cells. In the presence of complement, the IL-2/IgG chimer triggers target cell lysis of IL-2R$^+$ cells. Our laboratory has now expressed murine IL-2/IgG chimer and will soon test this molecule for therapeutic efficacy in various pre-clinical models. Souilliou's laboratory has prepared a human IL-2/IgM chimer (personal communication). Since pentameric IgM is not readily internalized, this fusion protein does not produce IL-2 like agonist activities.

Cytokine-toxin fusion proteins

The great German scientist Paul Erhlich first suggested that Zauberkugeln, i.e. 'magic bullet' hybrid molecules, consisting of cell-specific antibodies linked to a toxin (immunotoxin) be constructed for therapeutic purposes. He envisioned that immunotoxins could be used as magic bullets to destroy a highly selective population of target cells. This vision has been realized.

Functional domains of diphtheria toxin and *Pseudomonas* exotoxin

Each mature holotoxin used in the construction of hybrid molecules possesses at least three functionally specialized domains that: (i) bind to specific target cell surface receptors; (ii) translocate the toxin into the appropriate subcellular compartment; and (iii) enzymatically intoxicate the target cell (Pastan *et al.*, 1986; Olsnes *et al.*, 1989). An enzymatically active domain, the toxophore, is responsible for catalysing the chemical reaction that intoxicates the target cell. In the case of both diphtheria toxin (DT) and *Pseudomonas* exotoxin A (PEA) (Fig. 11.1), the enzymatically active core is an ADP-ribosyltransferase which targets elongation factor-2 (EF-2). EF-2 is an essential element in the translational apparatus of the cell. Following ADP-ribosylation, EF-2 is inactivated and the cell dies as a consequence of a failure to manufacture new cellular proteins. The extreme carboxy terminus of DT and the amino terminus of PEA function as a receptor-binding element and are responsible for the binding of the toxin to specific eukaryotic cell surface receptors (Fig. 11.1). The third centrally located domain of both toxins serves as a translocating element and enables the intact toxin to traverse the target cell membrane. This activity

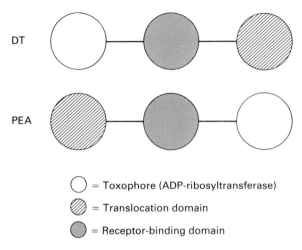

Fig. 11.1. Function/structure relationships of diphtheria toxin (DT) and *Pseudomonas* exotoxin A (PEA).

gains access of the toxin to the endosome and subsequent delivery of the toxophore to the cytosol (Pastan *et al.*, 1986; Olsnes *et al.*, 1989).

As outlined previously, biochemical and genetic analyses of DT has clearly shown that the toxin molecule is composed of at least three functional domains: (i) the enzymatically active fragment A; (ii) the membrane-associating domains; and (iii) receptor-binding domain of fragment B (Fig. 11.2). Moreover, each domain of DT has been shown to play an essential role in the intoxication of eukaryotic cells (Pappenheimer, 1977). In mature form, DT is a single polypeptide chain of 585 amino acids in length (Fig. 11.2), and contains four cysteine residues which form two disulphide bridges: Cys^{186}–Cys^{201} and Cys^{461}–Cys^{471} (Greenfield *et al.*, 1983; Kaczorek *et al.*, 1983; Ratti *et al.*, 1983). The 14 amino acid loop subtended by the first disulphide bridge contains three arginine residues (Arg^{190}, Arg^{192} and Arg^{193}) and this loop is extremely sensitive to proteolytic attack by serine proteases. Upon trypsin 'nicking' and reduction of the first disulphide bridge, DT can be separated under denaturing conditions into two polypeptide fragments (Collier *et al.*, 1971; Gill & Pappernheimer, 1971). Fragment A, the N-terminal 21.2 kDa polypeptide, carries the catalytic centres for the nicotinamide adenine dinucleotide (NAD^+) dependent adenosine diphosphoribosylation (ADPR) of eukaryotic EF-2 (Uchida *et al.*, 1971). The B fragment of DT, carries at least two functional domains: the hydrophobic membrane-associating domains which are responsible for the translocation of fragment A through the cell membrane and into the cytosol (Boquet *et al.*, 1976), and the native DT receptor-binding domain (Uchida *et al.*, 1971). The toxin receptor-binding domain has been recently tracked to the

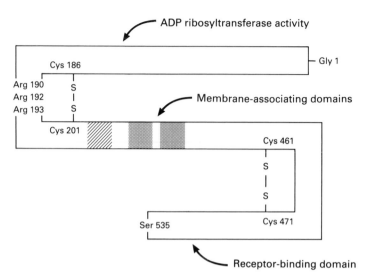

Fig. 11.2. Diphtheria toxin. DT possesses three functional domains: the enzymatically-active (ADP-ribosyltransferase active) toxophore, a translocating domain and a receptor-binding domain. An additional feature of note is a protease-sensitive region within the stretch of amino acids that subtend the first disulphide loop. Proteolytic nicking of the toxin at this site results in separation of fragment A from fragment B.

extreme C-terminal end of the toxin molecule (Greenfield *et al.*, 1987; Rolf *et al.*, 1990).

Interactions between DT and toxin-sensitive eukaryotic cells involve: (i) the binding of intact toxin to the cell-surface receptor (Middlebrook *et al.*, 1978); (ii) internalization of bound toxin by receptor-mediated endocytosis into acidification competent vesicles (Moya *et al.*, 1985) and upon 'nicking' of the toxin in this acidic environment (pH 5.3–5.1) (Middlebrook *et al.*, 1978; Sandvig *et al.*, 1986); (iii) insertion of the hydrophobic domain(s) into the vesicle membrane (Donovan *et al.*, 1981; Kagan *et al.*, 1981); thereby facilitating (iv) the delivery of fragment A to the cytosol. Once delivered to the cytosol, fragment A catalysed ADP-ribosylation of EF-2 abolishes cellular protein synthesis and as a result leads to the death of the cell. Yamaizumi *et al.* (1978) have determined that a *single* molecule of fragment A delivered to the cytosol of a cell is sufficient to be lethal for that cell.

Pseudomonas exotoxin A

A detailed analysis of the structure/function relationships of PEA have revealed that; (i) amino acids 1–252 function as the receptor-binding domain; (ii) amino acids 253–364 constitute the translocation domain;

and (iii) amino acids 400–613 bear the enzymatically active ADP-ribosyl-transferase (Hwang *et al.*, 1987). Amino acids 365–399 do not possess any functional activities (Siegall *et al.*, 1989). The steps leading to intoxication of the target cell are quite similar to those described for DT (Pastan & FitzGerald, 1991).

Recombinant cytokine-toxin fusion proteins

Within the last 3 years, the design and genetic construction of eukaryotic cell surface-receptor specific toxins has become a reality. A detailed understanding of the structure/function relationships of both DT and PEA, the nucleic acid sequence of their respective structural genes as well as the technical ability to precisely construct recombinant toxin-related peptide fusion proteins has allowed the development of a number of unique receptor-specific cytokines.

Since structure/function analysis of DT has shown that the toxin's receptor-binding domain of DT is positioned at the C-terminal end of the molecule, and that the first step in the intoxication process involves the binding of DT to its receptor, we reasoned several years ago that the replacement of the receptor-binding domain with either a cytokine, polypeptide hormone or cell-specific growth factor should result in the formation of *new* toxins. Moreover, the cellular target of these new toxins should be determined by the polypeptide hormone or growth factor used in its construction (Murphy *et al.*, 1986; Chaudhary *et al.*, 1987, 1988; Williams *et al.*, 1987; Lorberboum-Galski *et al.*, 1988a; Siegall *et al.*, 1988).

The genetic replacement of the receptor-binding domain native to DT or PEA with eukaryotic cell receptor-specific cytokine, polypeptide hormones or growth factors has resulted in the development of a new class of biological response modifiers — the fusion toxin (Murphy *et al.*, 1986; Chaudhary *et al.*, 1987, 1988; Williams *et al.*, 1987, 1988, 1990a,b; Bacha *et al.* 1988; Lorberboum-Galski *et al.*, 1988a,b; Siegall *et al.*, 1988). The first of these fusion toxins, DAB_{486}-Il-2 (Williams *et al.*, 1987), is currently in human phase I clinical trials.

Unlike the immunotoxins (i.e. fragments of microbial or plant toxins cross-linked to MoAbs), we chose to assemble these chimeric toxins at the level of the gene rather than by chemically coupling the toxophore with the ligand. Rather than chemically cross-linking the toxophore and ligand components through a disulphide bond, we have employed protein and genetic engineering methods to create gene fusion whose chimeric products are joined by a peptide bond at a defined site. The precision of the genetic fusion strategy enables the assembly of isomeric fusion proteins, while chemical cross-linking yields racemic mixtures. Moreover, following interaction with cell-surface receptors, the genetically engineered fusion toxins would be expected to be internalized by receptor-mediated endocytosis which would deliver the toxin to the acidic environment of the endosome and facilitate the delivery of the ADP-ribosyltransferase to the cytosol. Monoclonal antibodies can insure the delivery of immunotoxins to the cell surface; however, they do not provide assured delivery of the toxophore to either the endosome or the cytosol. Moreover, cytokines, polypeptide hormones and growth factors bind to their target receptor proteins with a higher binding affinity than MoAbs. Hence, it is likely that cytokine toxin hybrids will possess a greater therapeutic 'window' than conventional immunotoxins. Therefore, rather than to employ MoAbs as the cellular targeting component, we have used cytokines and growth factors whose receptors are known to undergo receptor-mediated endocytosis. Since cytokines and growth factors are known to be internalized into vesicles that become acidified, we reasoned that the internalization of a given toxin-related fusion protein should follow the same route of entry into the cell as DT itself.

First generation IL-2 toxin (DAB$_{486}$-IL-2)

DAB$_{486}$-IL-2 is a bipartite fusion protein composed of DT fragment A and truncated fragment B sequences to Ala^{486} linked to Pro^2 through Thr^{133} of human IL-2 (Williams et al., 1987) (Fig. 11.3). This chimeric protein is the product of a genetic fusion between a truncated DT gene (Fig. 11.3) encoding fragment A and the membrane-associating domains of fragment B of DT and a synthetic gene encoding human IL-2 (Williams et al., 1988). In this construct, the 3'-end of the tox structural gene encoding the C-terminal receptor-binding domain of DT was removed and replaced by a synthetic gene encoding amino acids 2 through 133 of human IL-2 (Fig. 11.3). Since the native DT receptor-binding domain was replaced with IL-2 sequences, the resulting fusion toxin is directed towards IL-2R$^+$ cells. DAB$_{486}$-IL-2 has been shown to selectively bind to the high affinity IL-2R, be internalized by receptor-mediated endocytosis, and facilitate the delivery of DT fragment A to the cytosol of target cells bearing high affinity IL-2Rs (Bacha et al., 1988). Recent studies have defined the minimal size of fragment B that is required to deliver fragment A across the endocytic vesicle membrane in target cells, and defined the site of proteolytic processing involved in the release of fragment A from the intact fusion toxin molecule (Williams et al., 1990a,b).

Importantly, IL-2R$^-$ cells were found to be resistant to the inhibitory action of DAB$_{486}$-IL-2. Bacha et al. (1988) have confirmed that the cytotoxic action of this fusion toxin is mediated through the IL-2R. Moreover, since lysozomatrophic agents (e.g. chloroquine) also block the cytotoxic action of DAB$_{486}$-IL-2, the fusion toxin must pass through an acidic compartment in order to deliver its ADP-ribosyltransferase to the cytosol of target cells. Bacha et al. (1988) also demonstrated that inhibition

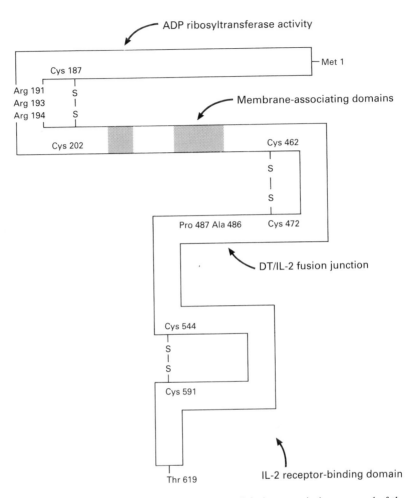

Fig. 11.3. DAB_{486}-IL-2 toxin. The DAB_{486}-IL-2 fusion protein is composed of the entire DT toxophore (fragment A), a truncated fragment B component, lacking the receptor-binding domain and human IL-2.

of protein synthesis in target cells was, in fact, due to the specific ADP-ribosylation of EF-2 in the target cell cytosol. Thus, the cytotoxic action of DAB_{486}-IL-2: (i) is directed through the IL-2R; (ii) requires passage through an acidic compartment in a manner analogous to native DT; and (iii) catalyses the ADP-ribosylation of EF-2 in a manner indistinguishable from that of native DT fragment A.

Walz et al. (1989) reported that the sequential events following the binding of DAB_{486}-IL-2 to the IL-2R on phytohaemaglutinin (PHA) activated T cells reflects both the IL-2 and the ADP-ribosyltransferase components of the fusion toxin. In a manner identical to native IL-2, DAB_{486}-IL-2 stimulated the expression of c-*myc*, interferon (IFN)γ, IL-2R and IL-2 mRNAs for the first 7 h of exposure. However, after the 7h exposure the action of the fusion toxin is analogous to that of cyclohexi-mide — an inhibitor of protein synthesis. By this time, the effects of protein synthesis inhibition by the ADP-ribosylation of EF-2 predominate, and the steady-state levels of c-*myc* and IL—2R mRNA are decreased. This study establishes that the functional activity of each of DAB_{486}-IL-2 component parts is retained: (i) interaction of the fusion toxin with the IL-2R results in signal transduction; and (ii) the delivery of the ADP-ribosyltransferase to the cytosol results in an inhibition of protein synthe-sis and elicits a series of effects which are similar to those imposed by cycloheximide.

It is well known that the high-affinity form of the IL-2R is composed of at least two subunits: a low affinity 55 kDa glycoprotein (p55, α chain) and an intermediate affinity 75 kDa glycoprotein (p75, β chain) (Tsudo *et al.*, 1986, 1987; Sharon *et al.*, 1986; Weissman *et al.*, 1986; Dukovich *et al.*, 1987; Robb *et al.*, 1987; Teshigawara *et al.*, 1987; Tanaka *et al.*, 1988). Moreover, it is known that both the high-affinity (p55 + p75) and p75 intermediate-affinity receptor, but not the p55 low-affinity IL-2R, undergo accelerated internalization after binding native IL-2 (Fujii *et al.*, 1986; Weissman *et al.*, 1986; Robb *et al.*, 1987; Tanaka *et al.*, 1988). Based on these observations, Waters *et al.* (1990) have examined the receptor-binding requirements of DAB_{486}-IL-2 for the efficient intoxication of target cells. Dose–response analysis of high-, intermediate- and low-affinity IL-2R bearing cells demonstrates that only cell lines which bear the high-affinity form of the IL-2R are sensitive to the cytotoxic action of DAB_{486}-IL-2 ($IC_{50} \le 10^{-10}$ M). In marked contrast, cell lines which bear either isolated p55 or p75 chains are resistant to the action of the fusion toxin and require exposure to *c*. 1000-fold higher concentrations ($IC_{50} \ge 1 \times 10^{-7}$ M) of DAB_{486}-IL-2.

Since peripheral blood mononuclear cells (PBMC) with natural killer (NK) activity have been reported to bear only the p75 subunit of the IL-2R on the cell surface and these cells are responsive to IL-2 and appear to be precursors of lymphokine activated killer (LAK) cell activity, Waters *et al.* (1990) examined the effect of DAB_{486}-IL-2 on human NK cell activity. Human NK cells proved to be as resistant to the action of DAB_{486}-IL-2 as continuous cell lines which bear only the p75 subunit of the IL-2R.

Weissman *et al.* (1986) have shown that the p55 subunit of the IL-2R does not internalize IL-2. By comparison, native IL-2 bound to the p75 subunit of the receptor is known to be internalized as rapidly as the high-affinity receptor ($t_{1/2} = 15$ min) (Robb & Greene, 1987). Since interme-diate affinity $p75^+$, $p55^-$ bearing cell lines were resistant to the action of DAB_{486}-IL-2, we reasoned that this resistance was due to altered binding of the fusion toxin to this subunit of the receptor. Waters *et al.* (1990) have also determined the receptor-binding properties of DAB_{486}-IL-2 by competitive displacement experiments using $[^{125}I]$-labelled IL-2. Approximately 200-fold higher concentrations of DAB_{486}-IL-2 are required to displace radiolabelled IL-2 from the high-affinity (p55 + p75) receptor. It is of interest to note that only 18-fold higher concentrations of DAB_{486}-IL-2 than native IL-2 are required to displace radiolabelled IL-2 from the p55 subunit; whereas, 120-fold higher concentrations are required for the p75 subunit.

These receptor-binding experiments indicate that the relative resistance of intermediate affinity IL-2R$^+$ cells to intoxication by DAB_{486}-IL-2 is due to altered binding to the p75 subunit of the receptor. Although both the p75 and the high-affinity heterodimer share the common property of rapidly internalizing bound ligand, the intermediate-affinity receptor site is characterized by slow kinetics of IL-2 association/dissociation. In contrast, the high-affinity receptor displays the fast 'on' rate of p55 and the slow 'off' rate of p75 (Lowenthal & Greene, 1987; Wang & Smith, 1987). Thus, an alteration in DAB_{486}-IL-2 binding to the p75 subunit may influence more dramatically the kinetics of this fusion toxin's binding to the intermediate vis-à-vis high-affinity receptor. As determined by the concentration of fusion toxin required to inhibit radiolabelled IL-2 binding, it is evident that DAB_{486}-IL-2 displays altered binding to *both* subunits of the IL-2R; however, binding to the p75 subunit appears to be more greatly affected than binding to the p55 subunit.

Since Collins *et al.* (1988) have reported that the N-terminal sequences of native IL-2, particularly Asp^{20}, are essential for binding to the p75 subunit of the IL-2R, it is likely that the altered binding of DAB_{486}-IL-2 to this subunit results from stearic constraints imposed on the fusion toxin: p75 IL-2R interaction. In the case of DAB_{486}-IL-2, human IL-2 sequences are fused to the C-terminal end of a truncated form of the toxin. Therefore, the fusion junction between DT-related and IL-2 sequences are likely to place Asp^{20} (Asp^{505} in DAB_{486}-IL-2) in an internal or less favourable position to bind to the p75 subunit.

Second generation IL-2 toxin (DAB_{389}-IL-2)

Williams *et al.* (1990) have demonstrated that the in-frame deletion of 97 amino acids from Thr^{387} to His^{485} of DAB_{486}-IL-2 increases both the potency ($IC_{50} \approx 2 - 5 \times 10^{-11}$ M) and the apparent dissociation constant (K_d) of the resulting DAB_{389}-IL-2 for high-affinity IL-2R bearing T cells (Fig. 11.4). In marked contrast, the deletion of an additional 94 amino acids (Asp^{291} to Gly^{483}) results in a greater than 1000-fold loss of cytotoxic potency in the fusion toxic DAB_{295}-IL-2. It is important to note that the structural regions between Asp^{291} and Gly^{483} include the hydrophobic putative membrane spanning helical regions of fragment B that have been postulated to facilitate the delivery of fragment A across the

Fragment A

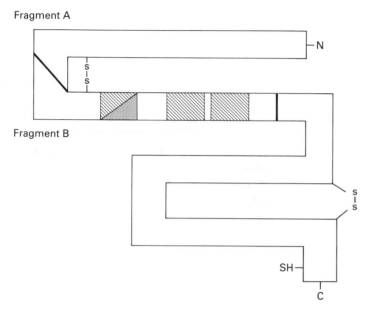

Fig. 11.4. DAB$_{389}$-IL-2 toxin. The DAB$_{389}$-IL-2 fusion protein was created by deleting the codons for the second disulphide loop of DT from the DAB$_{486}$ construct. This streamlined molecule is a more efficient toxin than DAB$_{386}$-IL-2.

endocytic vesicle membrane (Boquet *et al.*, 1976). The results of experiments described by Williams *et al.* (1990a,b) strongly suggest that the putative membrane spanning helices of fragment B are essential in the intoxication process.

In addition, Williams *et al.* (1990a,b) have shown that the amphipathic membrane surface binding region of fragment B contained between Asn^{204} and Ile^{290} is also essential to the cytotoxicity of the DAB-IL-2 fusion toxins. It is important to note that the genetic deletion of this region of fragment B in both DAB (205-289)$_{486}$-IL-2 and DAB(205-289)$_{389}$-IL-2 also decreases biological activity of the fusion toxin by *c.* 1000-fold. Most interestingly, these in-frame internal deletion mutations also effect the apparent K_d of the fusion toxin for the high-affinity IL-2R. Since the region that has been deleted carries an amphipathic domain(s) (Lambotte, *et al.*, 1986), it is reasonable to postulate that this region of fragment B associates with the T-cell membrane surface forming a non-specific secondary binding event and appears to stabilize the interaction of the fusion toxin with the target cell surface.

It is of particular interest to note that analysis of the DAB-IL-2 toxins has revealed a common predicted 'most' flexible region — amino acids 1 through 10 of human IL-2. Since this region was also found to be unordered in the crystal structure of IL-2 (Brandhuber *et al.*, 1987), we postulated that the apparent flexibility of the fusion toxin might allow for some degree of mobility of the IL-2 component with respect to the DT-related sequences. Were this the case, duplication of the flexible region might result in a fusion toxin with increased receptor-binding affinity and potency. In order to test this hypothesis, Kiyokawa *et al.* (1991) have genetically constructed mutants of DAB_{486}-IL-2 and DAB_{389}-IL-2 in which amino acids 2 through 8 of IL-2 were duplicated at the fusion junction (Fig. 10.4). This was done to provide a flexible 'spacer' between the toxin and IL-2 components of the fusion protein.

The dose–response curve of the duplication mutant DAB_{389}-(1-10)IL-2 on high-affinity IL-2R bearing HUT 102 cells reveals that the IC_{50} for DAB_{389}-(1-10)IL-2 (6×10^{-12} M) is 40- to 60-fold higher than that of DAB_{486}-IL-2 and approximately tenfold higher than DAB_{389}-IL-2. These studies establish that the application of protein engineering methodologies towards the development of second and third generation DAB-IL-2 fusion toxins will result in variants with increased biological potency.

Tripartite IL-2 fusion toxin, Shiga-A-DT 'B'-IL-2

Recently Murphy *et al.* (in preparation) have selected the A chain of Shiga-like toxin to replace DT fragment A in the construction of the first tripartite toxin for the following reasons: (i) both Shiga-like A and diphtheria fragment A are similar in molecular mass; (ii) the introduction of a single molecule of Shiga-like A chain to the cytosol of a target cell will result in an irreversible inhibition of protein synthesis, and, as a result, the measurement of biological activity of the tripartite fusion would be both convenient and sensitive; and (iii) the modification of the gene for Shiga-like A chain required to construct the tripartite fusion toxin gene is straightforward and could be readily accomplished.

The A subunit of Shiga-like toxin contains a single disulphide bridge that subtends a protease sensitive loop. Upon trypsin nicking an A1 and A2 fragment are released. The A1 fragment of Shiga-like toxin has been shown to be an enzyme which specifically cleaves the N-glycosidic bond at an adenine in the 28S ribosomal RNA (Calderwood *et al.*, 1987). Thus, Shiga-like toxin inhibits protein synthesis in a manner that is identical to that of the plant toxin ricin (Endo & Tsurugi, 1987).

A tripartite toxin, the Shiga-like A-DT 'B' (the protease sensitive site and the translocating domain of DT-IL-2 fusion toxin was purified to apparent homogeneity. The tripartite toxin is biologically active against high-affinity IL-2R bearing T lymphocytes. Intoxication by the tripartite toxin can be specifically blocked with either excess IL-2 or MoAb to the IL-2 binding domain of the IL-2Rα chain. It is notable that both DT and Shiga toxin intoxicate target cells by poisoning the translational apparatus of the target cell. However, these toxins target different molecules. DT inactivates EF-2 while Shiga toxin directly targets the ribosome. Although as yet unproved, we believe it likely that combined treatment with diphtheria toxin based and Shiga toxin based IL-2 fusion proteins will provide synergistic effects.

First generation IL-2 PE40

A variety of recombinant cytokine PE-related fusion proteins have been created using the same strategy that had been established for DT-related fusion proteins. The codons for the receptor-binding domain (amino acids 1–252 were deleted and replaced with various targeting molecules including human IL-2) (Lorberboum et al., 1988b; Pastan et al., 1991). Thus, the orientation of the functional domains of DAB_{486}-IL-2 and IL-2 PEA are reversed. In the DT-based molecule the N-terminus of IL-2 is joined to the COOH-terminus of the truncated DT molecule while the COOH-terminus of IL-2 is joined to the N-terminus of a truncated PEA. Probably owing to the α helix at the COOH-terminus of IL-2, the IL-2 PEA molecules binds poorly to activated human T cells. Nonetheless, IL-2 PE40 readily intoxicates activated murine T cells and has been tested in several immunological models.

Second generation IL-2 PEA, IL-2 PE664 Glu

Because human IL-2 PEA readily intoxicates activated murine, but not human T cells, an improved IL-2 PE-based fusion protein, was developed. In this construct, codons for the receptor-binding domain were not deleted. Instead, the codons for four amino acids were altered to eliminate the function of the receptor-binding domain. The resultant fusion protein IL-2 PE664Glu is far superior to IL-2 PE40 in binding to and intoxicating activated human T cells (Lorberboum-Galski et al., 1989).

In short, a variety of fusion proteins in which the native receptor-binding domain of either DT or PE has been genetically replaced with IL-2. The chimeric toxins selectively intoxicate IL-2 receptor bearing target cells in vitro. The IL-2 DT and IL-2 PE fusion proteins are immunosuppressive in vivo.

Pre-clinical therapeutic trials

Anti-IL-2R MoAb (M7/20) reduces delayed-type hypersensitivity: the role of complement and epitope

The delayed-type hypersensitivity (DTH) reaction is blocked by the anti-IL-2R MoAb, M7/20, (Kelley et al., 1987). While it is often assumed that anti-T cell antibodies mediate immunosuppression by targeting T cells for destruction, other activities warrant consideration. Antibodies reacting with vital surface proteins may mediate immunosuppression by blocking the function of the targeted protein. In order to dissect the mechanisms by which anti-IL-2R MoAbs mediate immunosuppression, the activity of two IgM, κ complement-fixing rat anti-mouse IL-2R MoAbs, but defining functionally distinct epitopes, were probed in a DTH model using BALB/c as well as two C5-deficient mouse strains. Low doses of M7/20 anti-IL-2R MoAb, which competitively blocks IL-2 binding, inhibits DTH in BALB/c mice, while another anti-IL-2R MoAb which does not block the IL-2 binding site did not abrogate DTH (Kelley et al., 1987). Interestingly, an anti-L3T4 MoAb, but not M7/20 anti-IL-2R MoAb blocked DTH in the C5-deficient strains (Kelley et al., 1987). Thus, M7/20 did not cause immunosuppression solely by blocking the IL-2-binding domain of IL-2Rs, as M7/20 binding to T blasts is equivalent in BALB/c and C5-deficient strains. Consequently, immunosuppression mediated by this IgM anti-IL-2R MoAb is dependent on both IL-2R site blockade and the presence of C5. This dual requirement was, frankly, contrary to our expectations. Ideally, anti-IL-2R MoAbs used in the clinic should lyse target cells and block IL-2 binding.

DAB_{486}-IL-2 blocks delayed-type hypersensitivity

As described above, the appearance of the high-affinity receptor for IL-2 marks a critical and pivotal point in the maturation of an immune response. As noted herein, targeting of the low-affinity p55 subunit of the IL-2 receptor with the MoAb M7/20 has been shown to effectively suppress a variety of T-cell-mediated reactions, including acute transplant rejection, autoimmunity and DTH. In the case of suppression of DTH with M7/20, it is clear that successful therapy requires complement activation and the use of an antibody that defines the IL-2-binding domain of p55 (Kelley et al., 1987). Given these results, Kelley et al. (1988a) have examined the action of DAB_{486}-IL-2 as an immunosuppressive agent in a murine model of DTH. In these experiments, mice were immunized trinitrobenzensesulphonate, rested for 7 days, and then challenged by footpad injection (Fig. 11.5). In this hypersensitivity model, the vigor of the immune response is determined by the degree of induration and swelling of the footpad 24 h after challenge. Daily treatment with DAB_{486}-IL-2 in doses as low as 50 μg/day for 6 days induced profound immunosuppression (Table 11.1). Indeed, the fusion protein proved more potent than M7/20 MoAbs (Table 11.1). Moreover, flow cytometric characterization of $CD4^+$ and $CD8^+$ T cells in single-cell suspensions from draining lymph nodes established that DAB_{486}-IL-2 prevented the expansion of IL-2 receptor-positive lymph node T cells (Table 11.2).

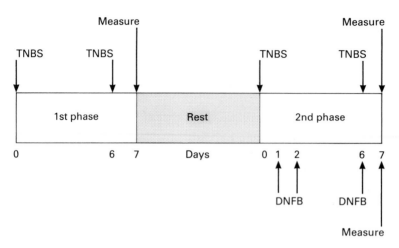

Fig. 11.5. Schema for DTH experiments. On day 0 mice received an i.p. injection of TNBS (a hapten). On day 6, they were challenged with TNBS by footpad injection. Following a rest period lasting 7–28 days, the mice were administered and rechallenged with either TNBS (original hapten) or DNFB (new hapten).

Table 11.1. IL-2-toxin (DAB_{486}-IL-2) is a more potent suppressor of DTH than anti-IL-2R MoAb and is not dependent on complement

Strain	Treatment	n	DTH units
BALB/c			
	Untreated	5	42.5 ± 2.0
	IL-2-toxin	5	20.6 ± 1.3[1]
	CRM 45	5	34.4 ± 0.7[1]
BALB/c			
	Untreated	9	51.6 ± 0.5[1]
	IL-2-toxin	5	18.6 ± 0.9
	Anti-IL-2R MoAb	5	35.6 ± 0.8[2]
DAB/2 (C5 deficient)			
	Untreated	5	20.0 ± 1.7[1]
	IL-2-toxin	5	20.0 ± 1.7[1]
	CRM 45	5	47.0 ± 4.1

Dose of IL-2 toxin, CRM 45, and anti-IL-2 MoAb (M7/20) is 5 µg/day/mouse.
[1] $P = 0.001$.
[2] $P = 0.005$.

Table 11.2. IL-2 toxin (DAB_{486}-IL-2) destroys activated IL-2R$^+$ cells during a DTH response

Lymph node	IL-2R$^+$%	
	CD4$^+$	CD8$^+$
Non-immunized	3	2
Immunized	14	18
Immunized, treated IL-2 toxin	5	3

Analysis of 0.5×10^4 cells/sample.

Importantly, Kelley *et al.* (1988a) also examined if diphtheria toxoid pre-immunization neutralized the subsequent immunosuppressive effect of IL-2-toxin. Pre-immunization with toxoid had little effect on the development of an immune response against trinitrobenzenesulphonate. Most interestingly, prior immunization with diphtheria toxoid had only a modest neutralizing effect on the ability of IL-2-toxin to induce antigen-specific immunosuppression. These results are consistent with the observations of Zucker and Murphy (1984), who demonstrated that only those monoclonal anti-diphtheria toxoid antibodies that prevented native toxin from binding to its receptor were neutralizing. In the case of DAB_{486}-IL-2, the receptor-binding domain of the native toxin was deleted and replaced with human IL-2 sequences.

IL-2 targeted therapy mouse organ allograft models

The utility of IL-2R targeted immunosuppressive therapy was first established in a murine model of heterotopic cardiac transplantation using the rat anti-mouse M7/20 MoAb (IgM) (Kirkham *et al.*, 1985). Gaulton *et al.* (1985) previously reported that this MoAb defined the IL-2 binding domain of the IL2Rα chain and inhibited IL-2 driven proliferation. Treatment with M7/20 (5 ug/mouse i.p.) for 10 days after grafting at least doubled graft survival in two inbred mice strain combinations. It is remarkable that many H-2 mismatched mouse cardiac transplant recipients are permanently engrafted following a single 10-day course of rat antimouse anti-IL-2Rα chain MoAb (Kirkman *et al.*, 1985). Delayed therapeutic application of M7/20 MoAb can totally reverse ongoing cardiac graft rejection (Kirkman *et al.*, 1985). The notion that targeting a small population of IL-2R$^+$ cells with an MoAb could block cardiac allograft rejection was soon confirmed using AMT-13, a rat anti-mouse IL-2Rα chain (IgG2a), which also defined the IL-2R-binding site (Kirkman *et al.*, 1987).

Skin allograft survival could also be prolonged using M7/20 (Kirkman *et al.*, 1987). Although a 10-day course of MoAb treatment resulted in a modest graft prolongation (*c.* 15 days versus 8 days in untreated mice), none of the skin grafts survived indefinitely. A low dose of X-irradiation (350 R) as an adjunct to M7/20 therapy extended graft survival further to *c.* 1 month (Granstein *et al.*, 1986).

IL-2 toxin fusion proteins suppress transplant rejection

Courses of treatment with either *Pseudomonas* exotoxin (IL-2 PE40) or DT related IL-2 (DAB_{486}-IL-2) fusion proteins routinely produce tolerance in a heterotopic mouse heart transplant model employing H-2 incompatible donors (Kirkman *et al.*, 1989; Lorberboum-Galski, *et al.*, 1989; Table 11.3).

In a series of cardiac allografts using the strain combination of B10.BR donor to C57BL/10 recipient, Kirkman *et al.* (1989) and Lorberboum-Galski *et al.*, (1989) have shown that a single 10-day course of DAB_{486}-IL-2 PE40 therapy greatly prolongs allograft survival. In the IL-2DT experiments, allografts in the untreated control, as well as allografts in animals treated with CRM-45 (a non-toxic 45 000 D fragment of native diphtheria toxin) or A197-IL-2 toxin (a non-toxic ADP-ribosyl-transferase mutant of IL-2-toxin) were rejected between days 10 and 20. In marked contrast, allograft survival was prolonged in animals that received 1 μg of DAB_{486}-IL-2/day.

IL-2 toxin fusion protein (DAB_{486}-IL-2) also prolonged engraftment in a murine model of pancreatic islet transplantation (Pankewycz *et al.*, 1989). Pancreatic islets were transplanted from DBA/2 donors into diabetic $B6AF_1$ recipients, a strain combination disparate in both class I and II histocompatibility antigens. This strain combination evokes a strong rejection response, and both skin and islet grafts are rapidly rejected. During treatment with DAB_{486}-IL-2 rejection was never noted; however, the kinetics of islet graft rejection in recipients receiving

Table 11.3. DAB_{486} IL-2 prolongs cardiac allograft survival

Treatment	Graft survival days
DAB_{486}-IL-2 1.0 μg	20, > 50, > 50, > 50, > 50, > 50
CRM45 0.66 mg	11, 12, 12, 13, 19
None	10, 14, 15, 18, 20

i.p. qd for 10 days $P < 0.01$; mice = B10.BR into C57Bl/10; CRM45 (DT lacking the receptor binding domain).

DAB_{486}-IL-2 once daily for 20 days demonstrated a prolonged allograft survival but not tolerance.

As the IL-2 toxin molecule has a short serum half-life, subsequent experiments were designed to prolong the bioavailability of the chimeric molecule in the treated host. $B6AF_1$ recipients of islet grafts were given an identical dose of DAB_{486}-IL-2 (5 µg/day) for 10 days divided in two daily injections. Half of the animals in this group had long-term graft survival of > 100 days. Thus, a shorter course of intensive IL-2 toxin immunosuppression leads to more frequent induction of graft 'tolerance'.

IL-2R targeted therapy in rat recipients of organ allografts cardiac allograft survival in anti-IL-2Rα MoAb treated rats

ART-18 a mouse IgG1 antibody that like M7/20 defines the IL-2-binding domain of the rat IL-2Rα chain and inhibits *in vitro* IL-2 driven T-cell proliferation (Osawa & Diamantstein, 1983). This MoAb was used to test the efficacy of IL-2R targeted therapy in acute rejection of heterotopic cardiac allografts in a Lew × BN) F_1 to LEW inbred rat strain combination (Kupiec-Weglinski *et al.*, 1986). Monotherapy with ART-18 administered i.v. for 10 consecutive post-transplant days increased allograft survival in a dose-dependent fashion to *c.* 21 days (acute rejection in untreated hosts occurred within 8 days). When treatment was delayed until 5 days after grafting, the time of major rejection activity, and continued for a total of 4 days, graft survival improved to *c.* 18 days, whereas treatment of two consecutive rejection episodes (5–9 and 15–19 days) with ART-18 extended survival to *c.* 1 month. The outcome of IL-2R targeted therapy was not unique to one strain combination; comparable cardiac graft prolongation was observed in several strongly histoincompatible recipients (Kupiec-Weglinski *et al.*, 1986). To confirm that these results were related to the specificity of ART-18 for IL-2R, a group of animals was treated with ART-62 (IgG1), an antibody which recognizes rat class 1 MHC antigens and inhibits IL-2 driven T-cell growth but does not bind to rat IL-2R (Osawa *et al.*, 1985). ART-62 treatment did not inhibit rejection. Thus, therapy with ART-18 targeted selectively at IL-2R$^+$ cells can be successfully utilized to delay or treat acute rejection of cardiac allografts in rats.

IL-2 targeted therapy: the role of antibody isotype

ART-18 switch variants apparently possessing the same (V) region residues but distinct isotype specificities (IgG2a and IgG2b) were compared to the parental IgG1 clone, and their immunosuppressive efficacy was probed in rat cardiac allograft recipients (Kupiec-Weglinski *et al.*, 1988).

Indeed, acute rejection could be prevented in a dose-dependent fashion following a 10-day treatment with all three ART-18 isotypes. In contrast, long-term engraftment is dependent on the isotype of antibody; the IgG2b preparation facilitated the longest graft survival (c. 28 days), followed by IgG1 (c. 21 days) and IgG2a, which was the least beneficial (17 days). The survival rate was not additively increased when MoAbs of distinct isotypes were administered concomitantly or alternately (DiStefano et al., 1988). Preliminary studies suggest that differences in phagocytosis and in the ability to induce antibody dependant cell-mediated cytotoxicity (ADCC) are primarily responsible for the divergent in vivo efficacy of ART-18 switch variants. Alternatively, as already described, treatment of mice with M7/20, an anti-IL-2R MoAb of IgM isotype, obviated DTH responses in normal but not in complement (C5) deficient mice (Kelley et al., 1988), suggesting that IgM MoAbs ideally should both fix terminal complement components and inhibit T-cell function.

The role of epitope IL-2R targeted therapy

In contrast to ART-18, ART-65 does not inhibit IL-2 binding or IL-2-driven proliferation. Interestingly, ART-54 given to cardiac allograft recipients in a dose and time course similar to ART-18, did abrogate acute rejection and extended graft survival to c. 16 days (DiStefano et al., 1988).

A revealing observation has come from the studies in which rat recipients of cardiac allografts were treated with ART-18 and ART-65 in combination to target distinct IL-2R epitopes. Concomitant administration of these MoAbs to recipient animals in relatively low doses proved highly successful, with 30% of transplants surviving indefinitely and 50% undergoing late rejection at c. 40 days. These results provide evidence that anti-IL-2R MoAbs should simultaneously target functionally different epitopes of the IL-2R molecule to obviate rejection effectively. In ART-65-treated hosts, $CD4^+$ cells conferred profound specific suppression to naive rats following adoptive transfer and prolonged test graft survival to an unprecedented length (c. 45 days). Whether the long lasting benefit of a cocktail of MoAbs is achieved by preventing association of p55 β and p75 α chains so that no high-affinity receptors can be formed, remains to be determined.

ART-18 treatment suppresses host alloreactivity

Following a 10-day course of ART-18 therapy, T cells harvested from treated but not control donors, were able to transfer donor-specific suppression of rejection of the grafts' original donor (Kupiec-Weglinski et al., 1986, 1987). Rejection of third-party grafts were not influenced. $CD8^+$ T cells, but not $CD4^+$ T cells, were active in this system. In addition,

ART-18 caused a quantitative defect in host $CD4^+$ T cells that hastened donor-specific rejection in a passive transfer model (Kupiec-Weglinski *et al.*, 1987).

In vivo *synergy between anti-IL-2R MoAbs and cyclosporine A*

In so far as cyclosporin A (CsA) inhibits expression of IL-2 and anti-IL-2R MoAbs must compete with IL-2 for occupation of the IL-2R, one might predict an additive or synergistic effect would be produced by combined therapy. Indeed, a combination of ART-18 treatment (which prolongs cardiac allograft survival to *c.* 21 days on its own) with subtherapeutic dose of CsA (one-tenth of the effective dose, which is ineffectual by itself) was strikingly synergistic in preventing rejection; one-third of the transplants survived indefinitely with the remainder rejecting at *c.* 50 days following a 10-day post-operative course of therapy (Diamantstein *et al.*, 1986). This combination therapy also reversed well-established rejection, with 20% of hearts surviving 100 days.

Transient benefit of anti-IL-2R MoAbs in primate kidney allografts

The prolonged engraftment achieved using anti-IL-2R MoAbs in murine and rat transplantation models provided the incentive for pre-clinical trials in primates. Two IgG_{2a} mouse anti-human IL-2R MoAb, 1-HT4-4H3 and anti-Tac, react with concanavalin A (Con A)-activated *Macaca fascicularis* monkey lymphocytes (Shapiro *et al.*, 1987; Reed *et al.*, 1989). These antibodies were tested in an *M. fascicularis* renal transplantation model (Shapiro *et al.*, 1987; Reed *et al.*, 1989). It is noteworthy that mouse IgG2a antibodies do not fix human or monkey complement nor activate FcR^+ phagocytes. Administration of 1-HT4-4H3 did not prolong graft survival despite clearly demonstrable serum mouse antibody titres. In contrast, anti-Tac MoAb infused as an i.v. bolus of 2 mg/kg into nephrectomized hosts pre-operatively and every other day post-transplant until rejection occurred, was modestly effective, i.e. mean recipient survival in anti-Tac MoAb treated group was 19 days versus 12 days in untreated recipients. Although addition of low-dose CsA therapy resulted in a modest prolongation of graft survival beyond that achieved with anti-Tac MoAb alone, all grafts were still eventually rejected.

In treated hosts, the appearance of circulating $IL-2R^+$ T cells was delayed from day 4–5 to day 12–13 and coincided with an initial rise in serum creatinine. The number of circulating $IL-2R^+$ cells in the treated group IL-2R expression peaked on day 12–13, i.e. preceded the creatinine rise and subsequent allograft rejection. Given the relative success of anti-IL-2R MoAb in rodent transplantation models, the ability of anti-Tac MoAb to prolong the renal graft in *M. fascicularis* is not surprising. Thus, the major question arising is why is the anti-Tac MoAb effect so transient? Nearly all monkeys treated with anti-Tac MoAb develop anti-mouse antibodies. Therefore, it is highly probable that the loss of anti-Tac efficacy is associated with the development of anti-murine antibodies by the host. Indeed, nearly all monkeys treated with anti-Tac MoAb formed anti-mouse antibodies 7–10 days following initiation of therapy, i.e. the time anti-Tac MoAb has lost its ability to bind to IL-2R. The development of monkey antibodies against anti-Tac MoAb exactly heralded the initiation of rejection.

M7/20 IL-2MoAb suppresses insulitis in murine autoimmune diabetes mellitus

In order to assess the importance of IL-2R$^+$ lymphocytes and macro-phages in the pathogenesis of autoimmunity, we tested the therapeutic efficacy of M7/20 MoAb in several distinct autoimmune models. For example, we hypothesized that anti-IL-2R MoAb treatment would reduce the autoimmune insulitis in the non-obese diabetic (NOD) mouse. Hence, we treated NOD mice with 5 μg of M7/20 daily beginning at 5 weeks of age for 5 weeks (Kelley et al., 1988; Table 11.4). Control mice were given a rat anti-mouse Forrsman IgM MoAb. Treatment with anti-IL-2R MoAb suppressed insulitis in this strain. However, the therapeutic benefit of M7/20 was compromised by the formation of anti-idiotypic antibodies to this anti-IL-2R MoAb (Pankewycz et al., 1988). These anti-idiotypic antibodies neutralize the biological activity of M7/20 after several weeks and thereby limit the therapeutic period.

DAB$_{486}$ IL-2 suppresses murine autoimmune diabetes mellitus

We put DAB$_{486}$-IL-2 to the challenging task of preventing an accelerated form of autoimmune insulin-dependent diabetes mellitus induced by transferring spleen cells from diabetic NOD mice into younger pre-diabetic NOD mice. Doses of 5–10 μg/day, DAB$_{486}$-IL-2 given on the

Table 11.4. Therapeutic efficacy of M7/20 MoAb in murine autoimmune diabetes mellitus

MoAb	Insulitis[1,2]	Number with insulitis
Anti-IL-2	0.7 ± 0.4	3/7
Control	2.1 ± 0.4	6/6

[1], $P < 0.05$; [2], 0–4 scale.

same day of adoptive transfer protected pre-diabetic NOD mice from becoming diabetic (Pacheco-Silva *et al.*, 1992). Even after the termination of DAB_{486}-IL-2 these mice only developed a milder form of diabetes.

M7/20 anti-IL-2R MoAb retards development of murine lupus nephritis

Using the extensively studied mouse hybrid, NZB × NZW F1 female which dies from autoimmune lupus nephritis, we investigated the therapeutic benefit of IL-2R targeted strategies. NZB × NZW F1 female mice were treated with M7/20 MoAb from 2 months, monitored for urinary proteins and sacrificed at 8 months of age. Treatment with M7/20 decreased proteinuria, reduced the amount of IgG and gp70 deposition in glomeruli, and diminished renal pathological changes characteristic of this strain (Table 11.5; Kelley *et al.*, 1988b). These studies indicate that highly selective therapeutic targeting to activated IL-2R$^+$ lymphocytes and macrophages provides a discrete method of dampening of autoimmunity. Obviously, IL-2R$^+$ cells are of vital importance in the expression of this form of autoimmunity.

DAB_{486}-IL-2 suppresses expression of murine systemic lupus erythematosus

A preliminary analysis indicates that DAB_{486}-IL-2 treatment prolongs survival of mice with systemic lupus erythematosus (SLE). Treatment of NZB × NZW F1 female hybrids for 28 days beginning at 4 months of age decreased the time at which 50% mortality occurred from 7.5 to 9.5 months (Kelley *et al.*, unpublished data). Since this study was terminated when the mice were 9.5 months of age, we are evaluating the possibility of permanent protection in additional experiments. Because of the promising therapeutic result in the NZB × NZW F1 hybrid we investigated another lupus prone strain, the MRL-lpr mouse. DAB_{486}-IL-2 was injected into MRL-lpr mice for 28 days beginning at 2.5 months of age. In treated mice, there was a delay in lymphadenopathy ($P < 0.02$) and the incidence of renal disease was reduced (proteinuria, $p < 0.05$) (data unpublished).

Table 11.5. Therapeutic efficacy of M7/20 MoAb in murine SLE

	Proteinuria (%)	Histology[1]	IgG (%)	gp70 (%)
Anti-IL-2R	38	1.1[2]	37[2]	12[2]
Control	75	2.5	85	50

[1] 0–4 scale; [2] $P < 0.05$.

Prophylactic treatment of SLE prone mice with DAB_{486}-IL-2 provides a method for reducing the severity of this autoimmune disease.

ART-18 + CsA dampens autoimmune diabetes mellitus in a rat model

Short-term treatment with ART-18 in combination with low dose CsA cured the majority of diabetic BB rats while ART-18 alone temporarily halted the destruction of β cells by autoreactive lymphocytes and delayed the onset of fatal hyperglycaemia but failed to cure BB rats (Hahn *et al.*, 1987).

ART-18 + CsA in a local graft-versus-host model

In local graft-versus-host (GVH) reaction, as determined by a popliteal lymph node assay, ART-18 or ART-65 treatment reduced the GVH index; addition of subtherapeutic doses of CsA completely abolished this classic experimental immune disorder (Volk *et al.*, 1986).

ART-18 + CsA increase on pancreatic islet allograft survival

When pancreatic islets from LEW.1A Ma × K rats are grafted into streptozotocin-diabetic LEW.1W Ma × K rats, the recipients become hyperglycaemic again within 8 days because of a rejection of the islets. Treatment with ART-18 (1mg/kg/day for 10 days following transplantation) doubled islet survival and produced permanent (> 120 days) graft acceptance in 30% of animals (Hahn *et al.*, 1987). Combined therapy with ART-18 and CsA in subtherapeutic doses (1.5 mg/kg) resulted in a further prolongation of graft survival to about 3 weeks.

IL-2 PE40 and DAB_{486}-IL-2 fusion toxins inhibit rodent autoimmunity

IL-2 PE treatment has been shown to inhibit experimental autoimmune uveoretinitis (Roberge *et al.*, 1989) and relapsing experimental allergic encephalomyelitis in Lewis rats (Rose *et al.*, 1991). DAB_{486}-IL-2 also inhibits experimental allergic encephalomyelitis in a mouse model (manuscript in preparation).

IL-2 PE40 and DAB_{486}-IL-2 fusion toxin reduce rat adjuvant arthritis

Given the short half-life of the IL-2 toxins, it is interesting to note that IL-2 PE40 treatment in the adjuvant arthritis model is far more effective when administered by osmotic pumps than by bolus injection (Case *et al.*, 1989;

Lorberboum-Galski *et al.*, 1989). DAB$_{486}$-IL-2 is also effective in this model (manuscript in preparation).

Clinical therapeutic trials

Monoclonal antibodies

Anti-IL-2R MoAb prolongs engraftment of human renal transplants

Clinical trials targeting the IL-2R with MoAb have only been directed against the 55 kDa chain of the human IL-2 receptor. Two different MoAbs, 33B3.1 and anti-Tac, sharing the same isotype, IgG$_{2a}$ and function, i.e. the ability to block the binding of IL-2 to its receptor and the inhibition of IL-2 driven T-cell proliferation, have successfully suppressed early renal allograft rejection episodes. When 33B3.1 treatment was compared with antithymocyte globlulin (ATG), 33B3.1 was not only as effective as ATG when used in a quadruple agent sequential immunosuppressive protocol in first kidney transplants, but was remarkably better tolerated (Soulillou *et al.*, 1990). Recently, a similar randomized study comparing ATG and 33B3.1 MoAb has been started in second kidney transplants.

Trials with the second antibody, anti-Tac, were conducted in kidney transplant recipients at the Beth Israel and Brigham and Women's Hospital in collaboration with Dr T. Waldmann at the NIH (Kirkman *et al.*, 1991). Because the antibody treatment was more beneficial when administered with CsA, a randomized trial administered anti-Tac in combination with standard dose CsA based triple therapy. There was a marked reduction in the incidence of early rejection episodes but no long-term differences in graft or patient survival. Of interest, patients receiving anti-Tac were successfully treated with anti-human CD3 (OKT3) (also mouse IgG$_{2a}$ MoAb) for acute rejection. This suggests that sequential therapy with multiple mouse MoAbs is possible providing there is no idiotype cross-reactivity. Taken together, targeting the IL-2R with MoAb is immunosuppressive in recipients of first cadaveric kidney grafts.

Anti-IL-2R MoAb prevents acute rejection
episodes in liver transplant recipients

Clinical trials directed by Stephan Meuer in Heidelberg report that the murine anti-IL-2R MoAb, BT563, has the capacity to prevent acute graft rejection in liver transplantation. The original pilot study has been extended to 19 consecutive liver transplants using three regimens (Otto *et al.*, 1989, 1991). Even when conventional immunosuppression was much reduced the rate of rejection remained remarkably low among patients who received BT563.

Prevention of acute graft-versus-host disease by anti-IL-2R MoAb

Improved treatment of graft-versus-host disease (GVHD) has made bone marrow transplantation a safer procedure. The benefit of targeting IL-2R in established GVHD was first reported by Herve *et al.* (1988). This study prompted the investigation of a combination therapy of an anti-IL-2R MoAb with CsA using the 33B3.1 MoAb which prevents early kidney graft rejection. Patients were treated daily after established marrow engraftment (day 15–30), before evidence of engraftment (day 10–30) and from the time of transplant (day 0–30). GVDH did not occur during anti-IL-2R MoAb therapy. GVHD was observed after day 35 in 3/8 patients treated for 30 days. In a follow-up of 3–16 months, 12/18 patients are in remission (Blaise *et al.*, 1989).

Clinical studies at the Hutchinson Cancer Research Center reported that treatment with the murine IgG_1 MoAb, 2A3, which is specific for the α chain of IL-2R caused no toxicity and improved acute GVHD in patients treated with the highest dose of antibody early after transplantation (Anasetti *et al.*, 1990). These studies were extended to examine the efficacy of the 2A3 MoAb used in conjunction with CsA and methotrexate for prophylaxis of acute GVHD in 11 patients with advanced leukaemia transplanted with unmodified marrow from related haploidentical donors incompatible for 2–3 HLA loci (Anasetti *et al.*, 1991). The control group of 36 patients received standard CsA + methotrexate and were compared to 11 patients receiving these drugs plus 2A3 on days 1–19. During treatment with 2A3, IL-2Rs on circulating cells were saturated with antibody. Patients receiving 2A3 MoAb tolerated more CsA than controls with lower serum creatinine during the first month. Acute GVHD in patients given 2A3 was documented in 70% with an onset median of 20 days compared to 87% with an onset median of 13 days in controls. The incidence of survival was not improved with 2A3 MoAb treatment. Two patients treated with 2A3 MoAb and two controls survived more than 1 year. These studies suggest that the 2A3 MoAb suppresses and delays the activation of alloantigen-specific T cells but does not permanently eliminate them.

DAB_{486}-IL-2 fusion toxin treatment in man

Because the malignant cells of some leukaemis and lymphomas express IL-2R, initial safety, pharmacokinetic and biological effect studies were performed in patients with refractory IL-2R expressing haematopoietic malignancies. More than 100 patients have been evaluated. Doses of 0.007–0.4 mg/kg/day administered intravenously by 5–90 min infusion daily for 5–7 days/month have shown acceptable tolerability. At the highest doses the side-effects include transient hepatic transaminase elevations and mild hypoalbuminaemia, occasional transient elevation of serum creatinine with urinalysis abnormalities suggesting tubular cell dysfunction and an occasional transient decrease in platelet count. A more curious observation has been the occurrence in patients (2/10) receiving the highest dose (0.3–0.4 mg/kg) of transient haemolysis, thrombocytopenia, and renal insufficiency, all of which were reversible over 7–10 days, responding to intravenous fluids and blood replacement. Thirty per cent of patients had anti-diphtheria toxoid (DT)-antibody pre-study and about 60% had antibody post-study. Occasional patients had anti-IL-2 activity pre-study and a few had low titre activity post-study. Occasional patients experienced reversible bronchospasm at the beginning of a repeat course of agent administration, but in most patients, including those with anti-DT antibodies, repeat courses were well tolerated.

Pharmacokinetic analysis for single and multiple doses has indicated that DAB_{486}-IL-2 has a monophasic half-life of 5–7 min and a volume of distribution which approximates the plasma volume. Importantly, *in vitro* studies have consistently shown that the minimum cell contact time to induce irreversible cytoxicity is 5–15 min at concentrations of 7–700 ng/ml (10^{-10} to 10^{-8} M) DAB_{486}IL-2.

While these studies have been designed primarily to assess safety, tolerability and pharmacokinetics/pharmocodynamics, DAB_{486}IL-2 reduced tumour burden in 30% of patients for at least 4 weeks. The responses in some patients occurred despite the presence of anti-DT antibody, and two patients, one with large cell B-cell lymphoma, one with cutaneous T-cell lymphoma (CTCL), are in complete remission while off therapy for 30, 20 and 12 months, respectively (LeMaistre *et al.*, 1991; Schwartz *et al.*, 1991).

DAB_{486}IL-2 may benefit patients with severe methotrexate refractory rheumatoid arthritis

A pilot evaluation of DAB_{486}-IL-2 safety, tolerability, pharmacokinetic and biological effects in patients with active severe refractory rheumatoid arthritis was recently completed at Beth Israel Hospital, Boston under the direction of Drs David Trentham and K. Lea Sewell (Sewell & Trentham, 1991). Nineteen patients with methotrexate refractory, prednisone-requiring ($\leq$ 10 mg/day) rheumatoid arthritis were evaluated in a dose-response, safety and pharmacokinetic pilot study. Duration of disease varied from 3 to 25 years. Patients underwent a 3-week washout period from methotrexate (or another experimental therapy) and also discontinued non-steroidal anti-inflammatory drugs (NSAIDs) for the week before, week of, and 2 weeks after DAB_{486}IL-2 administration. Six patients received 0.04 mg/kg/day for five daily doses. Six patients received 0.07 mg/kg/day as a 60-min infusion for seven daily doses and seven patients received 0.10 mg/kg/day as a 60-min infusion for seven daily doses. All patients in the two higher dose groups showed significant improvement in one or more clinical parameters.

At the end of the 4-week observation period, 3/6 patients treated at the 0.07 mg/kg/day dose level, and 1/7 patients treated at the 0.10 mg/kg/day level improved by American Rheumatic Association (ARA) criteria (> 50% improvement in painful and swollen counts sustained for > 4 weeks). Further, the group of 12 evaluable patients in the two higher dose groups as a whole showed improvement in four important measures of disease activity as shown in Table 11.6. The therapeutic action of a single course of $DAB_{486}IL$-2 begins during the treatment period, is maximal at 2–3 weeks after treatment is initiated, and the duration varies from 5–16 weeks. Seven patients improved with retreatment despite the presence of anti-DT antibodies. Side-effects were transient, and consisted of superficial phlebitis at the intravenous sites, nausea/malaise and sporadic fevers. Minimal to moderate elevations of hepatic transaminases were transient, returning to baseline within 2–3 weeks, and unassociated with other abnormalities of liver function. Renal function remained normal in all patients. Although total peripheral blood CD4 numbers were normal, the number of activated CD25-expressing cells appeared to increase during the washout period and decrease in association with $DAB_{486}IL$-2 administration. A small number of patients have received second and third courses of $DAB_{486}IL$-2. In this group, the therapeutic effect is 50% improvement. These data provide initial indirect evidence that activated lymphocytes are important in the pathogenesis of rheumatoid arthritis.

In December 1991, a two-centre, 60 patient, randomized, double-blind placebo-controlled study was initiated to further characterize the anti-rheumatic action of $DAB_{486}IL$-2 in this type of patient. Patients with no effect during the placebo treatment will be allowed to enter the treatment arm following completion of the placebo arm, and arthritis status is being evaluated by a third party blinded observer.

Table 11.6. DAB_{486}-IL-2 improves rheumatoid arthritis

Parameter	Entry/baseline	Day 21	Day 8	Improvement[1] d21/d28
Painful joints (number)	17/20	9	11	54/45%
Swollen joints (number)	12/12	6	8	50/35%
Morning stiffness (min)	123/156	53	61	66/61%
Grip strenth (mmHg)	61/41	68	62	67/52%

[1]Compared to baseline.

Potential clinical benefit of DAB$_{486}$IL-2 patients with recent onset insulin-dependent diabetes

A phase I/II study of safety, tolerability, pharmacokinetic and biological response of DAB$_{486}$IL-2 in patients with recent onset insulin-dependent diabetes mellitus (IDDM) is being conducted by Professors Jean-Francois Bach and Christian Boitard at Hopital Necker, Paris, France.

This pilot study was designed to evaluate the safety and tolerability of DAB$_{486}$IL-2 in IDDM patients and to assess pharmacokinetic and immune function effects, together with changes in diabetic status as determined by insulin requirement, C-peptide levels and control of hyperglycaemia. Based on experience in similar studies, such preliminary effects can be assessed over a 4–6-week period following administration of immunosuppressive drugs. Thus, recent onset IDDM provides a clinical model for the evaluation of a new immunosuppressive agent like DAB$_{486}$IL-2.

DAB$_{486}$IL-2 has been administered to individuals over 15 years of age with symptoms $\leq$ 4 months duration, HLA DR3 or 4 and/or anti-islet cell antibody formation. Patients received a 60-min intravenous infusion daily for 7 days in a cohort dose-escalation protocol, evaluating dose levels of 0.025, 0.05 and 0.075 mg/kg. This pilot study has evaluated 18 patients, each receiving a single course.

To date, 18 patients are being evaluated for safety and seven for response. DAB$_{486}$IL-2 has been well tolerated in this group of patients; there has been mild transient hepatic transaminase elevations in 15–20% of patients, one transient episode of oedema and two instances of mild rash suggestive of hypersenstivity-like effects. Four of these patients (two in the 0.025 mg/kg and two in the 0.05 mg/kg dose groups) have had a substantial decrease in insulin requirement, together with a sustained increase in C-peptide and a normalization of glycosylated haemoglobin. Data analysis for the other 11 patients is underway.

In conclusion, clinical trials in autoimmune disease and transplantation provide evidence that strategies that target the IL-2R can prevent destructive immunological events.

References

Anasetti, C., Martin, P. J., Hansen, J. A., Appelbaum, F. R., Beatty, P. G., Doney, K., Harkonen, S., Jackson, A., Reichert, T., Stewart, P., *et al.* (1990). A phase I-II study evaluating the murine anti-IL-2 receptor antibody 2A3 for treatment of acute graft-versus-host disease. *Transplantation* **50**, 49–54.

Anasetti, C., Martin, P. J., Storb, R., Appelbaum, F. R., Beatty, P. G., Calori, E., Davis, J., Doney, K., Reichert, T., Stewart, P., Sullivan, K. M., Thomas, E. D., Witherspoon, R. P. & Hansen, J. A. (1991). Prophylaxis of graft-versus-host disease by administration of the murine anti-IL-2 receptor antibody 2A3. *Bone Marrow Transplantation* **7**, 375–381.

Bacha, P., Williams, D. P., Waters, C., Williams, J. M., Murphy, J. R. & Strom, T. B. (1988). Interleukin-2 receptor targeted cytotoxicity: interleukin-2 receptor mediated action of a diphtheria toxin-related interleukin-2 fusion protein. *Journal of Experimental Medicine* **167**, 612–22.

Boquet, P., Silverman, M. S., Pappenheimer, A. M., Jr & Vernon, W. B. (1976). Binding of triton X-100 to diphtheria toxin, cross-reacting material 45, and their fragments. *Proceedings of the National Academy of Sciences USA* **73**, 4449–4453.

Brandhuber, B. J., Boone, T., Kenney, W. C. & McKay, D. B. (1987). Three-dimensional structure of interleukin-2. *Science* **238**, 1707–1709.

Calderwood, S. B., Auclair, F., Donohue-Rolfe, A., Keusch, G. T. & Mekalanos, J. J. (1987). Nucleotide sequence of the Shiga-like toxin genes of *Escherichia coli*. *Proceedings of the National Academy of Sciences USA* **84**, 4364–4368.

Cantrell, P. A. & Smith, K. A. (1984). The interleukin-2 T-cell system: a new cell growth model. *Science* **224**, 1312–1316.

Case, J. P., Lorberboum-Galski, H., Lafyatis, R., FitzGerald, D., Wilder, R. L. & Pastan, I. (1989). Chimeric cytotoxin IL-2-PE40 delays and mitigates adjuvant-induced arthritis in rats. *Proceedings of the National Academy of Sciences USA* **86**, 287–91.

Chaudhary, V. K., FitzGerald, D. J., Adhya, S. & Pastan, I. (1987). Selective killing of HIV infected cells by recombinant human CD4-*Pseudomonas* exotoxin hybrid protein. *Proceedings of the National Academy of Sciences USA* **84**, 4538–4542.

Chaudhary, V. K., Mizukami, T., Fuerst, T. R., FitzGerald, D. J., Moss, B., Pastan, I. & Berger, E. A. (1988). Activity of a recombinant fusion protein between transforming growth factor type alpha and *Pseudomonas* toxin. *Nature* **335**, 369–372.

Collier, R. J. & Kandel, J. (1971). Structure and activity of diphtheria toxin. I. Thiol-dependent dissociation of a fraction of toxin into enzymically active and inactive fragments. *Journal of Biological Chemistry* **246**, 1496–1503.

Collins, L., Tsien, W. H., Seals, C., Hakami, J., Weber, D., Bailon, P., Hoskings, J., Greene, W. C., Toome, V. & Ju, G. (1988). Identification of specific residues of human interleukin-2 that affect binding to the 7-kDa subunit (p 70) of the interleukin-2 receptor. *Proceedings of the National Academy of Sciences USA* **85**, 7709–7713.

Diamantstein, T., Volk, H. D., Tilney, N. L. & Kupiec-Weglinski, J. W. (1986). Specific immunosuppressive therapy by monoclonal anti-IL-2 receptor monoclonal antibody and its synergistic action with cyclosporine. *Immunobiology* **172**, 391–399.

DiStefano, R., Mouzaki, A., Araneda, D., Diamantstein, T., Tilney, N. L. & Kupic-Weglinski, J. W. (1988). Anti-interleukin-2 receptor monoclonal antibodies spare phenotypically distinct T suppressor cells *in vivo* and exert synergistic biological effects. *Journal of Experimental Medicine* **167**, 1981–1986.

Donovan, J. J., Simon, M. I., Draper, R. K. & Montal, M. (1981). Diphtheria toxin forms transmembrane channels in planar lipid layers. *Proceedings of the National Academy of Sciences USA* **78**, 172–176.

Dukovich, M., Wanos Y., Bich-Thuy, L. T., Katz, P., Cullen, D., Kehrl, J. H. & Greene, W. C. (1987). A second human IL-2 binding protein that may be a component of high-affinity IL-2 receptors. *Nature* **327**, 518–522.

Endo, Y. & Tsurugi, K. (1987). RNA *N*-glucosidase activity of ricin A-chain. Mechanism of action of the toxic lectin ricin on eukaryotic ribosomes. *Journal of Biological Chemistry* **262**, 8128–8130.

Fujii, M., Sugamura, K., Sano, K., Nakai, M., Sagita, K. & Hinuma, Y. (1986). High affinity receptor mediated internalization and degradation of IL-2 in human T-cells. *Journal of Experimental Medicine* **163**, 550–562.

Gaulton, G. N., Bangs, J., Maddock, S., Springer, T., Eardley, D. D. & Strom, T. B. (1985). Characterization of a monoclonal rat anti-mouse interleukin-2 (IL2) receptor antibody and its use in the biochemical characterization of the murine IL-2 receptor. *Clinical Immunology and Immunopathology* **36**, 18–29.

Gill, D. M. & Papenheimer, A. M., Jr. (1971). Structure activity relationships in diphtheria toxin. *Journal of Biological Chemistry* **246**, 1492–1495.

Granstein, R. D., Goulston, C. & Gaulton, G. N. (1986). Prolongation of murine skin allograft survival by immunologic manipulation with anti-IL-2 receptor antibody. *Journal of Immunology* **136**, 898–902.

Greenfield, L., Bjorn, M., Horn, G., Fong, D., Buck, G. A., Collier R. J. & Kaplan, D. A. (1983). Nucleotide sequence of the structural gene for diphtheria toxin carried by corynbacteriophage beta. *Proceedings of the National Academy of Sciences USA* **80**, 6853–6857.

Greenfield, L., Johnson, V. & Youle, R. J. (1987). Mutations in diphtheria toxin separate binding from entry and amplify immunotoxin selectivity. *Science* **238**, 536–539.

Hahn, H. J., Kuttler, B., Dunger, A., Kloting, I., Lucke, S., Volk, H. D., vonBaehr, R. & Diamantstein, T. (1987). Prolongation of rat pancreatic islet allografts by a temporary recipient rats with monoclonal anti-interleukin-2 receptor antibody and cyclosporine. *Diabetologia* **30**, 44–46.

Hahn, H. J., Lucke, S., Kloting, I., Volk, H. D., Baehr, R. & Diamantstein, T. (1987). Curing BB rats of freshly manifested diabetes by short-term treatment with a combination of monoclonal anti-interleukin-2 receptor antibody and a subtherapeutic dose of cyclosporine. *European Journal of Immunology* **17**, 1075–1078.

Hwang, J., Fitzgerald, D. J., Adhya, S. & Pastan, I. (1987). Functional domains of *Pseudomonas* exotoxin identified by deletion analysis of the gene expressed in *E. coli*. *Cell* **48**, 129.

Kaczorek, M., Delpeyroux, F., Chenciner, N., Streeck, R. E., Murphy, J. R., Boquet, P. & Tiollais, P. (1983). Nucleotide sequence and expression of the diphtheria tox228 gene in *Escherichia coli*. *Science* **221**, 855–858.

Kagan, B. L., Finkelstein, A. & Colombini, M. (1981). Diphtheria toxin fragment forms large pores in phospholipid bilayer membranes. *Proceedings of the National Academy of Sciences USA* **78**, 4950–4954.

Kelley, V. E., Bacha, P., Pankewycz, O. G., Nichols, J. C., Murphy, J. R. & Strom, T. B. (1988a). Interleukin-2 diphtheria toxin fusion protein can abolish cell-mediated immunity *in vivo*. *Proceedings of the National Academy of Sciences USA* **85**, 3980–3984.

Kelley, V. E., Gaulton, G. N., Hattori, M., Ikegami, H., Eisenbarth, G. & Strom, T. B. (1988b). Anti-interleukin-2 receptor antibody suppresses murine diabetic insulitis and lupus nephritis. *Journal of Immunology* **140**, 59–61.

Kelley, V. E., Gaulton, G. N. & Strom, T. B. (1987). Inhibitory effects of anti-interleukin-2 receptor and anti-L3T4 antibodies on delayed type hypersensitivity: the role of complement and epitope. *Journal of Immunology* **138**, 2771–2775.

Kirkman, R. L., Bacha, P., Barrett, L. V., Forte, S., Murphy, J. R. & Strom, T. B. (1989). Prolongation of cardiac allograft survival in murine recipients treated with a diphtheria toxin-related interleukin-2 fusion protein. *Transplantation* **47**, 327–330.

Kirkman, R. L., Barrett, L. V., Gaulton, G. N., Kelley, V. E., Koltun, W. A., Schoen, F. J., Ythier, A. A. & Strom, T. B. (1985a). The effect of anti-interleukin-2 receptor monoclonal allograft rejection. *Transplantation* **40**, 719–721.

Kirkman, R. L., Barrett, L. V., Gaulton, G. N., Kelley, V. E., Ythier, A. A. & Strom, T. B. (1985b). Administration of anti-interleukin-2 receptor-monoclonal antibody prolongs cardiac allograft survival in mice. *Journal of Experimental Medicine* **162**, 358–362.

Kirkman, R. L., Barrett, L. V., Koltun, W. A. & Diamantstein, T. (1987). Prolongation of murine cardiac allograft survival by the anti-interleukin-2 receptor monoclonal antibody AMT 13. *Transplant Proceedings* **19**, 618–619.

Kirkman, R. L., Shapiro, M. E., Carpenter, C. B., McKay, D. B., Milford, E. L., Ramos, E. L., Tilney, N. L., Waldmann, T. A., Zimmerman, C. E. & Strom, T. B. (1991). A randomized prospective trial of anti-Tac monoclonal antibody in human renal transplantation. *Transplantation* **51**, 107–113.

Kiyokawa, T., Williams, D. P., Snider, C. E., Strom, T. B. & Murphy, J. R. (1991). Protein engineering of diphtheria toxin-related interleukin-2 fusion toxins to increase cytotoxic potency for high-affinity IL-2-receptor-bearing target cells. *Protein Engineering* **4**, 463–468.

Kupiec-Weglinski, J. W., Diamantstein, T., Tilney, N. L. & Strom, T. B. (1986). Anti-interleukin-2 receptor monoclonal antibody spares T suppressor cells and prevents or reverses acute allograft rejection. *Proceedings of the National Academy of Sciences USA* **83**, 2624–26278.

Kupiec-Weglinski, J. W., DiStefano, R., Stunkel, K. G., Grutzmann, R., Theisen, P., Araneda, D., Tilney, N. L. & Diamantstein, T. (1988). Anti-interleukin-2 receptor monoclonal antibody (IL-2R mAb) therapy in rat recipients of cardiac allografts: the role of antibody isotype. *Transplant Proceedings* **20**, 272–275.

Kupiec-Weglinski, J. W., Padberg, W., Uhteg, L. C., Ma, L., Lord, R. H., Araneda, D., Strom, T. B., Diamantstein, T. & Tilney, N. L. (1987). Selective immunosuppression with anti-interleukin-2 receptor targeted therapy: helper and suppressor cell activity in rat recipients of cardiac allografts. *European Journal of Immunology* **17**, 313–319.

Lambotte, P., Falnagne, P., Capiau, C., Zanen, J., Ruysschaert, J. M. & Dirk, J. (1980). Primary structure of diphtheria toxin fragment B: structural similarities with lipid-binding domains. *Journal of Cellular Biology* **87**, 837–840.

Lambotte, P., Kalmagne, P., Capiau, C. *et al.* (1986)

Landolfi, N. F. (1991). A chimeric IL-2/Ig molecule possesses the functional activity of both proteins. *Journal of Immunology* **146**, 915–919.

LeMaistre, C. F., Craig, F., Meneghetti, C., McMullin, B., Banks, P., Reuben, L., Rosenblum, M., Parker, K., Woodworth, T. & VonHoff, D. (1991). Phase I-II trial of an IL-2 fusion toxin (DAB486-IL-2) in IL-2 receptor positive and negative malignancies. *Blood* **78**, 126a.

Leonard, W. J., Depper, J. M., Uchiyama, T., *et al.* (1982). A mAb that appears to recognize receptor for human T-cell growth factor; partial characterization of the receptor. *Nature* **300**, 267.

Lorberboum-Galski, H., Barrett, L. V., Kirkman, R. L., Ogata, M., Willingham, M. C., FitzGerald, D. J. & Pastan, I. (1989). Cardiac allograft survival in mice treated with IL-2 PE40. *Proceedings of the National Academy of Sciences USA* **86**, 1008–12.

Lorberboum-Galski, H., FitzGerald, D., Chaudhary, V., Adhya, S., Pastan, I. (1988a). Cytotoxic activity of an interleukin-2 — *Pseudomonas* exotoxin chimeric protein produced in *Escherichia coli*. *Proceedings of the National Academy of Sciences USA* **85**, 1922–1926.

Lorberboum-Galski, H., Garsia, R. J., Gately, M., Brown, P. S., Clark, R. E., Waldmann, T. A., Chaudhary, V. K., FitzGerald, D. J. & Pastan, I. (1990). IL-2-PE664Glu, a new chimeric protein cytotoxic to human activated T lymphocytes. *Journal of Biological Chemistry* **25**, 16311–1637.

Lorberboum-Galski, H., Kozak, R. W., Waldmann, T. A., Bailon, P., FitzGerald, D. J., & Pastan, I. (1988b). Interleukin-2 (IL-2) PE40 is cytotoxic to cells displaying either the p55 or p70 subunit of the IL-2 receptor. *Journal of Biological Chemistry* **263**, 18650–18656.

Lowenthal, J. L. & Greene, W. C. (1987). Contrasting interleukin-2-binding properties of the alpha (p55) and beta (p70) protein subunits of the human high-affinity interleukin-2 receptor. *Journal of Experimental Medicine* **166**, 1156–1161.

Maddock, E. O., Maddock, S. W., Kelley, V. E. & Strom, T. B. (1985). Rapid stereospecific stimulation of lymphocytic metabolism by interleukin-2. *Journal of Immunology* **135**, 4004.

Middlebrook, J. L., Dorland, R. B. & Leppla, S. (1978). Association of diphtheria toxin with Vero cells. Demonstration of a receptor. *Journal of Biological Chemistry* **253**, 7325–7330.

Morrison, S. L., Johnson, M. J., Herzenberg, L. A. & Oi, V. T. (1984). Chimeric human antibody molecules: mouse antigen-binding domains with human constant region domains. *Proceedings of the National Academy of Sciences USA* **81**, 6851–6855.

Moya, M., Dautry-Versat, A., Goud, B., Louvard, D., & Boquet, P. (1985). Inhibition of coated pit formation in Hep2 cells blocks the cytotoxicity of diphtheria toxin but not that of ricin toxin. *Journal of Cellular Biology* **101**, 548–559.

Murphy, J. R., Bishai, W., Borowski, A., Miyanohara, A., Boyd, J. & Nagle, S. (1986). Genetic construction, expression, and melanoma-selective cytotoxicity of a diphtheria toxin-related alpha-melanocyte-stimulating hormone fusion protein. *Proceedings of the National Academy of Sciences USA* **83**, 8258–8262.

Olsnes, S., Sandrig, K., Petersen, O. W. & Van Deurs, B. (1989). Immunotoxins—entry into cells and mechanism of action. *Immunology Today* **10**, 291–295.

Osawa, H. & Diamantstein, T. (1983). The characteristics of a monoclonal antibody that binds specifically to rat T lymphoblasts and inhibits IL-2 receptor functions. *Journal of Immunology* **130**, 51–55.

Osawa, H., Herrmann, T. & Diamantstein, T. (1985). Inhibition of IL-2 dependent proliferation of rat T lymphoblasts by the monoclonal antibody ART-62 which reacts with MHC class I antigens. *Journal of Immunology* **134**, 3901–3906.

Otto, G., Thies, J., Kabelitz, D., Schlag, H., Hofman, W. J., Herfarth, C. H. & Meuer, S. (1989). Anti-CD25 monoclonal antibody prevents early rejection in liver transplantation — a pilot study. *Transplantation Proceedings* **23**, 1387–1389.

Otto, G., Thies, J., Kraus, T., Manner, M., Herfarth, C. H., Hoffmann, W. J. & Schlag, H. (1991). Monoclonal anti-CD25 for acute rejection after liver transplantation. *Lancet* **338**, 195.

Pacheco-Silva, A., Bastos, M. G., Muggia, R. A., Pankewycz, O., Nichols, J., Murphy, J. R., Strom, T. B. & Rubin-Kelley, V. E. (1992). Interleukin-2 receptor targeted fusion toxin (DAB$_{486}$ IL-2) Treatment blocks diabetogenic autoimmunity in mice. *European Journal of Immunology* **22**, 697–702.

Pankewycz, O. G., Hassarjian, R., Chang, C., Strom, T. B. & Kelley, V. E. (1988). Anti-interleukin-2 receptor monoclonal antibody therapy induces anti-idiotypic antibodies in mice that block both *in vitro* and *in vivo* activity. *Journal of Autoimmunity* **1**, 119–130.

Pankewycz, O., Mackie, J., Hassarjian, R., Murphy, J. R., Strom, T. B. & Kelley, V. E. (1989). Interleukin-2 diphtheria toxin fusion protein prolongs murine islet cell engraftment. *Transplantation* **47**, 318–322.

Pappenheimer, A. M., Jr. (1977). Diphtheria toxin. *Annual Review of Biochemistry* **46**, 69–94.

Pastan, I. & FitzGerald, D. (1991). Recombinant toxins for cancer treatment. *Science* **254**, 1173–1177.

Pastan, I., Willingham, M. C., FitzGerald, D. S. P. (1986). Immunotoxins. *Cell* **47**, 641–48.

Queen, C., Schneider, W. P., Selick, H. E., Payne, P. W., Landolfi, N. F., Duncan, J. F.,

Avdalovic, N. M., Levitt, M., Junghans, R. P. & Waldmann, T. A. (1989). A humanized antibody that binds to the interleukin-2 receptor. *Proceedings of the National Academy of Sciences USA* **86**, 10029–10033.

Ratti, G., Rappuoli, R. & Giannini, G. (1983). The complete nucleotide sequence of the gene coding for diphtheria toxin in the corynephage omega (tox +) genome. *Nucleic Acids Research* **11**, 6589–6595.

Reed, M. H., Shapiro, M. E., Strom, T. B., Carpenter, C. B., Letvin, N. L., Reimann, K., Weinberg, D. S., Waldmann, T. A. & Kirkman, R. L. (1989). Anti-Tac MoAb prolongs renal allografts in cynomolgus monkeys. *Transplant Proceedings* **21**, 1028–1030.

Reichmann, L., Clark, M., Waldmann, H. & Winter, G. (1988). Reshaping human antibodies for therapy. *Nature* **332**, 323–327.

Robb, R. J. & Greene, W. C. (1987). Internalization of interleukin-2 is mediated by the beta chain of the high-affinity interleukin-2 receptor. *Journal of Experimental Medicine* **165**, 1201–1206.

Robb, R. J., Rusk, C. M., Yodoi, J. & Greene, W. C. (1987). Interleukin-2 binding molecule distinct from the Tac protein: analysis of its role in formation of high-affinity receptors. *Proceedings of the National Academy of Sciences USA* **84**, 2001–2006.

Roberge, F. G., Lorberboum-Galski, H., LeHoang, P., deSmet, M., Chan, C. C., Fitzgerald, D. & Pastan, I. (1989). Selective immunosuppression of activated T-cells with the chimeric toxin IL-2-PE40. Inhibition of experimental autoimmune uveo-retinitis. *Journal of Immunology* **143**, 3498–3502.

Rolf, J. M., Gaudin, H. M. & Eidels, L. (1990). Localization of the diphtheria toxin receptor-binding domain to the carboxyl-terminal Mr approximately 6000 region of the toxin. *Journal of Biological Chemistry* **265**, 7331–7337.

Rose, J. W., Lorberboum-Galski, H., Fitzgerald, D., McCarron, R., Hill, K. E., Townsend, J. J. & Pastan, I. (1991). Chimeric cytotoxin IL-2-PE40 inhibits relapsing experimental allergic encephalomyelitis. *Journal of Neuroimmunology* **32**, 209–217.

Sandvig, K., Tonnessen, T. I., Sand, O. & Olsnes, S. (1986). Requirement of a transmembrane pH gradient for the entry of diphtheria toxin into cells at low pH. *Journal of Biological Chemistry* **261**, 11639–11645.

Schwartz, G., Tepler, L., Charcun, L., Kadin, M., Parker, K., Woodworth, T. & Schninner, L. (1991). Complete response Hodgkin's lymphoma in a phase I trial of DAB_{486}-IL-2, an IL-2-diphtheria fusion toxin. *Blood* **78**, 175a.

Sewell, K. L. & Trentham, D. E. (1991). Improvement in refractory rheumatoid arthritis by interleukin-2 receptor targeted therapy. *55th Annual Meeting of the American College of Rheumatology* p. 43. Program (A141) Boston, MA.

Siegall, C. B., Chaudhary, V. K., FitzGerald, D. J. & Pastan, I. (1988). Cytotoxic activity of an interleukin-6 *Pseudomonas* exotoxin fusion protein on human myeloma cells. *Proceedings of the National Academy of Sciences USA* **85**, 9738–9742.

Siegall, C. B., Chaudhary, V. K., FitzGerald, D. J. & Pastan, I. (1989). Functional analysis of domains II, Ib, and III of *Pseudomonas* exotoxin. *Journal of Biological Chemistry* **264**, 14256–14261.

Shapiro, M. E., Kirkman, R. L., Reed, M. H., Puskas, J. D., Mazoujian, G., Letvin, N. L., Carpenter, C. B., Milford, E. L., Waldmann, T. A., Strom, T. B. & Schlossman, S. H. (1987). Monoclonal anti-IL-2 receptor antibody in primate renal transplantation. *Transplantation Proceedings* **19**, 594–598.

Sharon, M., Klausner, R. D., Cullen, B. R., Chizzonite, R. & Leonard, W. L. (1986). Novel interleukin-2 receptor subunit detected by cross-linking under high-affinity conditions. *Science* **234**, 859–863.

Smith, K. A. (1987). The two chain structure of high-affinity IL-2 receptors. *Immunology Today* **8**, 11–13.

Soulillou, J. P., Cantarovich, D., Le Mauff, B., Giral, M., Hourmant, M., Hirn, M. & Jacques, Y. (1990). Randomized trial of an anti-interleukin 2 receptor monoclonal antibody (33B3.1) versus rabbit antithymocyte globulin (ATG) in prophylaxis of early rejection in human renal transplantation. *New England Journal of Medicine* **322**, 1175–1182.

Tanaka, T., Saiki, O., Doi, S., Fuji, M., Sugamura, K., Hara, H., Negoro, S. & Kishimoto, S. (1988). Novel receptor-mediated internalization of interleukin-2 in B cells. *Journal of Immunology* **140**, 866–870.

Teshigawara, K., Wang, H. M., Kato, K. & Smith, K. A. (1987). Interleukin-2 high-affinity receptor expression requires two distinct binding proteins. *Journal of Experimental Medicine* **165**, 223–238.

Tsudo, M., Kozak, R. W., Goldman, C. K. & Waldmann, T. A. (1987). Contribution of a p75 interleukin-2 binding peptide to a high-affinity interleukin-2 receptor complex. *Proceedings of the National Academy of Sciences USA* **84**, 4215–4218.

Tsudo, M., Kozak, R. W., Goldman, C. K. *et al.* (1986). Demonstration of a new peptide (non-Tac) binds IL-2: a potential participant in a multichain IL-2 receptor complex. *Proceedings of the National Academy of Sciences USA* **83**, 9694–9698.

Uchida, T., Gill, D. M. & Pappenheimer, A. M., Jr. (1971). Mutation of the structural gene for diphtheria toxin carried by temperate phage. *Nature* **233**, 8–11.

Volk, H. D., Brocke, S., Osawa, H. & Diamantstein, T. (1986). Suppression of local graft versus host reaction in rats by treatment with a monoclonal antibody specific for the interleukin-2 receptor. *European Journal of Immunology* **10**, 1309–1312.

Walz, G., Zanker, B., Brand, K., Waters, C., Genbauffe, F., Zeldis, J. B., Murphy, J. R. & Strom, T. B. (1989). Sequential effects of interleukin-2 diphtheria toxin fusion protein on T-cell activation. *Proceedings of the National Academy Sciences USA* **86**, 9485–9488.

Wang, H. M., & Smith, K. A. (1987). The interleukin-2 receptor. Functional consequences of its biomolecular structure. *Journal of Experimental Medicine* **166**, 1055–1069.

Waters, C. A., Schimke, P., Snider, C. E., Itoh, K., Smith, K. A., Nichols, J. C., Strom, T. B. & Murphy, J. R. (1990). Interleukin-2 binding requirements for entry of a diphtheria toxin related interleukin-2 fusion protein into cells. *European Journal of Immunology* **20**, 785–791.

Weissman, A. M., Harford, J. B., Svetlik, P. B., Leonard, W. L., Depper, J. M., Waldmann, T. A., Greene, W. C. & Kalusner, R. D. (1986). Only high-affinity receptors for interleukin-2 mediate internalization of ligand. *Proceedings of the National Academy of Sciences USA* **83**, 1463–1466.

Williams, D. P., Parker, K., Bacha, P., Bishai, W., Borowski, M., Genbauffe, F., Strom, T. B. & Murphy, J. R. (1987). Diphtheria toxin receptor binding domain substitution with interleukin-2: genetic construction and properties of a diphtheria toxin-related interleukin-2 fusion protein. *Protein Engineering* **1**, 493–498.

Williams, D. P., Regier, D., Akiyoshi, D., Genbauffe, F. & Murphy, J. R. (1988). Design, synthesis and expression of a human interleukin-2 gene incorporating the codon usage bias found in highly expressed *Escherichia coli* genes. *Nucleic Acids Research* **16**, 10453–10467.

Williams, D. P., Snider, C. E., Strom, T. B. & Murphy, J. R. (1990a). Structure/function analysis of interleukin-2 toxin (DAB_{486} IL-2). Fragment B sequences required for the delivery of fragment A to the cytosol of target cells. *Journal of Biological Chemistry* **265**, 11885–11889.

Williams, D. P., Wen, Z., Watson, R. S., Strom, T. B. & Murphy, J. R. (1990b). Cellular processing of the interleukin-2 fusion toxin DAB_{486} IL-2 and efficient delivery of diphtheria fragment A to the cytosol of target cells requires Arg194. *Journal of Biological Chemistry* **265**, 20673–20677.

Yamaizumi, M., Mekada, E., Uchida, T. & Okada, Y. (1978). One molecule of diphtheria toxin fragment A introduced into a cell can kill the cell. *Cell* **15**, 245–250.

Zucker, D. & Murphy, J. R. (1984). Monoclonal antibody analysis of diphtheria toxin. I. Localization of epitopes and neutralization of cytotoxicity. *Molecular Immunology* **21**, 785–793.

Part 4
Other approaches

Chapter 12
Towards idiotype specific therapy in autoimmune disease

Felix Mor and Irun R. Cohen

Introduction

Current therapeutic modalities in autoimmune disease have evolved empirically with the introduction of adrenal corticosteroid hormones more than 40 years ago (Hench *et al.*, 1949), later followed by cytotoxic drugs (Kaplan *et al.*, 1973), and more recently by antilymphocytic globulin, total lymphoid irradiation (Kotzin *et al.*, 1981), lymphoplasmapheresis (Wallace *et al.*, 1982) and cyclosporine (Assan *et al.*, 1985).

As a common denominator, these forms of therapy exert their effect by affecting either the number or the function of the lymphocytes involved in mediating the autoimmune disease. Since the pathways of activation and differentiation are similar for lymphocytes having a beneficial role (control of infection and surveillance against neoplasia) and for those having a detrimental role in perpetuating the autoimmune disease, an inherent problem with non-specific modalities of immunosuppression is an increased risk of infection and malignant disease. Moreover, in addition to immunosuppression, these drugs often have serious side-effects, e.g. the hormonal and metabolic effects of steroids, the haemorrhagic cystitis of cyclophosphamide (Plotz *et al.*, 1979) or the nephrotoxicity of cyclosporine (Kahan, 1989).

An ideal treatment for autoimmune disease, should fulfil several requirements:

1 It should selectively affect the function of the autoimmune T cells mediating the disease without affecting the immune system in general.
2 It should lack toxicity.
3 It could be used to abort the disease at an early stage.
4 It should retain its effectiveness in future exacerbations of the disease.

The most important characteristic of an ideal therapy would be its specificity, i.e. its ability to control the function of the one or few clones involved in mediating the disease process without adversely affecting the function or the repertoire of the entire immune system. In other words, its mechanism of action should involve amplification of the activity of cells engaged in regulation of the autoimmune effector cells.

In recent years we have gained new information about the basic mechanisms of antigen processing and presentation, T-cell recognition, T-cell activation and differentiation, and regulation of the immune response. This information could yield more specific forms of treatment for autoimmune disease. The purpose of this chapter is to review new developments in the treatment of autoimmune diseases. Although most of the work is in animal models, there are already clinical trials in human autoimmune diseases that are based on the results achieved in the animal models.

The autoimmune process

Figure 12.1 shows a scheme describing various cells and interactions involved in the generation and control of the autoimmune process. In a genetically susceptible individual having the appropriate major histocompatibility complex (MHC) genes, some stimulus (usually unknown) triggers the presentation of an autoantigen peptide in the MHC groove to autoreactive T cells together with the ancillary signals required for T-cell activation. Upon activation the T cells secrete various lymphokines that can influence other T cells, B cells and macrophages and can amplify the expression of MHC molecules on a variety of cells. Thus the activated T cells can cause damage by triggering inflammation, by exerting helper functions for the generation of pathogenic autoantibodies, or as cytotoxic cells that attack the cells expressing the self peptide MHC complex. In the past 10 years, considerable experience with T-cell lines and clones in autoimmune diseases such as adjuvant arthritis (AA), experimental autoimmune encephalomyelitis (EAE), experimental autoimmune thyroiditis (EAT), collagen arthritis, insulin-dependent diabetes mellitus (IDDM) in non-obese diabetic (NOD) mice, experimental autoimmune uveoretinitis (EAU) and others, has repeatedly shown that autoantigen specific T cells are pivotal in disease induction.

Many of these experimental diseases are transient and the autoaggressive T cells can be recovered from animals long after the disease has abated (Ben-Nun & Cohen, 1982); therefore there must be regulatory cells that can downregulate the activity of the pathogenic T cells. In characterizing these regulatory cells Lider et al. (1988) isolated CD4 and CD8 T cells that specifically recognized the autoimmune effector clone (see Fig. 12.1). Since the specific autoimmune T cells could be distinguished from other T cells, the regulatory T cells can be termed anti-idiotypic T cells (Lider et al., 1988). It is assumed that another set of regulatory T cell exists, T cells that are triggered by different epitopes on the autoantigen to amplify or

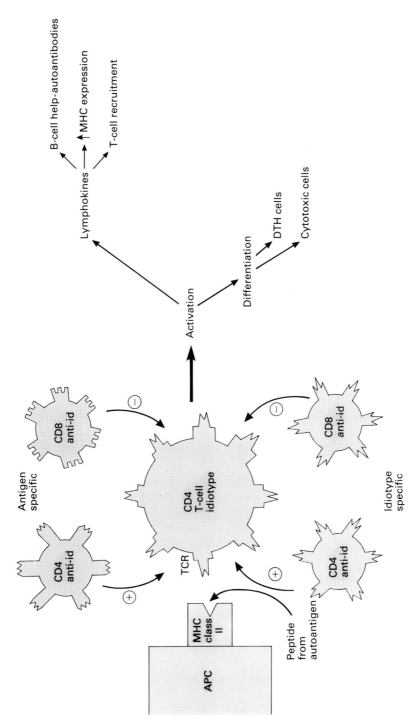

Fig. 12.1. Schematic representation of the cells and interactions involved in the generation and control of the autoimmune process.

attenuate the activity of the idiotype. These cells may be termed antigen-specific regulatory cells. The newer forms of immunotherapy are derived from these concepts of the pathogenetic mechanisms involved in the autoimmune process. This chapter will focus on some of these novel modalities of treatment.

The autoantigen

Detailed knowledge of the nature of the antigen involved in the autoimmune process and the specific epitopes recognized by effector cells and regulatory cells can be utilized to modify the disease. These experiments can be divided into two groups: those designed to induce tolerance to the antigen and those aimed at blocking MHC binding by the autoantigen.

Induction of tolerance to autoantigen

Classical experiments in immunology using ovalbumin as the antigen have shown that oral feeding of the experimental animal with the antigen (Mowat, 1987), or neonatal exposure to it (Billingham et al., 1953), can induce specific tolerance to subsequent immunization. The principle of oral tolerance has been exploited in EAE (Higgins & Weiner, 1988), experimental autoimmune uveitis (Nussenblatt et al., 1990) and collagen arthritis (Thompson & Staines, 1985) to demonstrate that feeding animals with the autoantigen (myelin basic protein, protein S and collagen type II, respectively), can prevent the subsequent attempts to induce these diseases using immunogenic protocols. Lider et al. (1989a) examined the mechanisms involved in oral tolerance to myelin basic protein. They found that feeding the autoantigen induces in the small intestine lymphatic tissue specific suppressor T cells that are capable of passively transferring the tolerance to naive recipients. The suppressor cells are thought to downregulate the immune response to the antigen upon subsequent immunization (Lider et al., 1989a). Using neonatal exposure to induce tolerance, Clayton et al. demonstrated the prevention of EAE (1989).

However, the target epitope can also be used to induce resistance to an autoimmune disease without the special procedures of oral administration or neonatal tolerance. Elias et al. (1991) defined a peptide of the mammalian 65 kDa heat shock protein (hsp65) recognized by diabetogenic T-cell clones in NOD mice; inoculation of adult, pre-diabetic mice with the peptide prevented the spontaneous development of IDDM. Moreover, administration of mycobacterial 65 kDa shock protein intraperitoneally rendered rats resistant to attempts to induce adjuvant arthritis with dead mycobacteria (van Eden et al., 1988) or streptococcal cell walls (van de Broek et al., 1989). Recently, Billingham et al. (1990) showed that the mycobacterial 65 kDa protein did not protect rats collagen or synthetic adjuvant arthritis.

Blocking peptides and antibodies

Knowledge of the specific encephalitogenic epitopes of myelin basic protein has enabled several groups of workers to synthesize short peptides that are able to bind to the MHC molecule, without having the ability to activate the encephalitogenic clone. These substituted peptides can protect animals from attempts to induce EAE (Sakai *et al.*, 1989, Wraith *et al.*, 1989). However, since blocking peptides are bound to the MHC, this form of therapy is not idiotype specific and it may stimulate T cells reactive to the synthetic blocking peptide. Moreover, blocking peptides will block MHC molecules to respond to other antigens. Thus, MHC blocking is not specific for the disease. The principle of MHC blocking was first demonstrated using monoclonal antibodies against class II molecules in EAE. Sriram & Steinmnan (1983) found that prior treatment with anti-class II antibodies protected mice against active induction of EAE.

The autoreactive T cell and T-cell vaccination

In the early 1980s it was established that T-cell lines and clones responsive to autoantigens could mediate autoimmune diseases. Repeated stimulation with the antigen *in vitro* led to the establishment of pathogenic T-cell lines had clones in a variety of autoimmune disease models: EAE (Ben-Nun *et al.*, 1981a), EAT (Maron *et al.*, 1983), adjuvant arthritis (Holoshitz *et al.*, 1983), EAU (Caspi *et al.*, 1988), collagen arthritis (Kakimoto *et al.*, 1988), streptococcal cell wall arthritis (van der Broek *et al.*, 1989) and others. Soon after the discovery that a T-cell line could mediate autoimmune disease, our group found that the same T-cell line rendered avirulent by irradiation or treatment with mitomycin C could induce protection against the disease (Ben-Nun *et al.*, 1981b). By analogy with a similar procedure used in preventing infectious diseases, this mode of therapy is termed T-cell vaccination (Cohen & Weiner, 1988). In experiments performed in the various animal models it was found that effective vaccination required that the T cells be activated prior to inoculation. We later found that the ability of some T cells to vaccinate could be enhanced by treatment of the T cells which chemical cross-linkers such as glutaraldehyde or formaldehyde, or by hydrostatic pressure (Lider *et al.*, 1987).

   In a disease model in which clinical signs could be followed for weeks, such as AA, it was possible to show that T-cell treatment could be therapeutic when administered shortly after the onset of clinical signs (Lider *et al.*, 1987). An additional form of T-cell vaccination can be achieved by administrating subencephalitogenic doses of activated T-cell clones (10^2–10^4/cells) without any additional modification (Beraud *et al.*, 1989). Investigation of the immunological consequences of T-cell vaccination has revealed that this form of intervention generates in the recipient anti-idiotypic responses composed of both T-helper and T-suppressor cells

(Lider *et al.*, 1988). Apart from EAE, T-cell vaccination was found to be effective in AA (Holoshitz *et al.*, 1983), EAT (Maron *et al.*, 1983), collagen arthritis (Kakimoto *et al.*, 1988), and IDDM in NOD mice (Cohen, 1989). Instead of using T-cell lines or clones that take many weeks to grow we have subsequently found that the procedure can be simplified and shortened by using a heterogenous population of lymphocytes, such as lymph node cells primed with the autoantigen in adjuvant. Inoculation of this mixed cell population enriched with the relevant idiotype has led to the creation of effective vaccines in EAE and AA (Lider *et al.*, 1987).

Our laboratory has investigated culture conditions for enriching a heterogenous population of lymphocytes with the relevant autoimmune T cells (Mor *et al.*, 1990). We found that upon incubation with medium containing IL-2, there was no enrichment in antigen activity in AA. However, stimulation of the cells with the mitogen concanavalin A (Con A) prior to culture in the IL-2-containing medium caused a significant increase (up to 40-fold) in the frequency of the antigen-specific T cells. Apparently, upon mitogen stimulation, the antigen-primed cells respond with accelerated kinetics relative to the naive T-cell population in their IL-2 receptor expression and cell division. Memory cells have been shown to respond more than naive cells to a variety of stimuli including anti-CD2, anti-CD3 antibodies (Sanders *et al.*, 1989) and Con A (Hedlund *et al.*, 1989).

In the last 2 years the therapeutic modality of T-cell vaccination has been explored in patients. In Boston, cells were cloned by non-specific activation from the celebrospinal fluid of patients with progressive multiple sclerosis (MS). When the cells reached adequate numbers, a vaccine was prepared by membrane modulation with glutaraldehyde and the vaccine was injected subcutaneously. It is still too early to draw conclusions from this limited experience with regard to efficacy, however, patients seem to tolerate the treatment and no significant side-effects have been reported. In two medical centres in Europe, synovial fluid T lymphocytes obtained from patients with rheumatoid arthritis (RA) are being used in T-cell vaccination. Since RA, MS and other autoimmune diseases are characterized by spontaneous exacerbations and remissions, it will take several years until this mode of treatment can be adequately explored in human autoimmunity.

Recently, two groups of workers have reported their results on the prevention of EAE by prior vaccination of rats with peptides of the T-cell receptor of encephalitogenic clones. One group used peptides from the V region of the T-cell receptor (TCR) (Vanderbark *et al.*, 1989) and the other used peptides from the hypervariable region (VDJ) that is involved in binding the autoantigen epitope (Howell *et al.*, 1989). However, experience with this modality is still limited and it remains to be established whether this form of molecular T-cell therapy will be effective in other animal models of autoimmune disease. The mechanism of protection is not known, but it has been proposed that the immune response mounted against the TCR downregulates the encephalitogenic clones generated during induction of the disease (Vandenbark *et al.*, 1989).

A similar approach was proved to be successful when monoclonal antibodies against the TCR were tested for their ability to block EAE. Several groups who characterized the sequence of TCR from encephalitogenic clones from various strains of rats and mice found that the pathogenic clones often used the same $V\beta$ and $V\alpha$ genes (Heber-Katz & Acha-Orbea, 1989). As monoclonal antibodies to the $V\beta8.2$ were available, it was possible to test their therapeutic potential. Acha-Orbea *et al.* (1988) found that pre-treatment of the animals with the antibody prevented the induction of EAE. This monoclonal antibody could also abort T-clone-induced EAE (Acha-Orbea *et al.*, 1988) and, recently, has been reported to prevent cyclophosphamide-induced diabetes in NOD/Wehi mice (Bacelj *et al.*, 1989). However, it should be emphasized that this form of therapy is not idiotype specific and has the potential of affecting some 15–30% of the T lymphocyte pool utilizing this TCR segment (Acha-Orbea *et al.*, 1988). With the cloning of TCR genes from encephalitogenic T-cell clones, it may be possible to isolate the hypervariable idiotype-specific autoantigen binding peptide and to create monoclonal antibodies to it that might specifically attack the autoimmune T cells without affecting other T cells.

Regulatory T cells

The availability of pathogenic autoimmune T cell clones has prompted researchers to try and culture *in vitro* anti-idiotypic T cells that may have a therapeutic effect. Although the idea is logical, it has been difficult to grow regulatory cells. By culturing in limiting dilution conditions Lider *et al.* (1988) showed that in rats protected against EAE it is possible to grow *in vitro* two populations of regulatory cells. Some clones were CD8[+] and were found to specifically suppress the response of an encephalitogenic clone to basic protein; some clones were CD4[+] and were found to stimulate the encephalitogenic clone and to enhance its response to the antigen (Lider *et al.*, 1988). Sun *et al.* (1988) have been able to culture *in vitro* CD8 cells that specifically lyse the encephalitogenic T-cell clone, and these cells are also capable of mediating protection against EAE. Using the same disease model, Ellerman *et al.* (1988) were able to isolate a CD4 suppressor-inducer T-cell line able to prevent the induction of EAE.

Over the last few years, additional modes of immunotherapy of autoimmune disease have been tried that are not idiotype specific, but are more restricted than the present therapies: monoclonal antibodies against the CD4 molecule (Brostoff & Mason, 1984; Wang *et al.*, 1987), the CD8 molecule (Sedgwick, 1988), the IL-2 receptor (Hayosh *et al.*, 1987) or ricin conjugated antibody to the IL-2 molecule (Case *et al.*, 1989). Our group discovered that autoimmune T-cell clones produce upon activation an enzyme that degrades heparan sulphate from the extracellular matrix, low doses of heparin caused inhibition of the activity of this enzyme (Naparstek *et al.*, 1984) and when tested in AA was found to attenuate severity of disease (Lider *et al.*, 1989a). However, monoclonal antibodies against common T-cell-surface molecules (Brostoff & Mason, 1984) or class II MHC molecules, as well as the heparin therapy, do not distinguish between the pathogenic autoimmune T cells and other T cells and hence are not idiotype specific. Therefore, we should expect that additional immunological functions will be affected when they are used to treat autoimmune disease.

Common autoimmune diseases such as IDDM, MS, RA, and systemic lupus erthymatosus (SLE) and others tend to develop in relatively young patients, and then have an enormous effect on the quality of life as well as on survival. So far the treatment of these diseases has been disappointing with many untoward side-effects. It is hoped that the impressive achievements gained in the treatment of animal models of these diseases will help to develop a more effective and less toxic therapy of this form of human disease.

References

Acha-Orbea, H., Mitchel, D. J., Timmermann, L., Wraith, D. C., Tausch, G. S., Waldor, M. K., Zamuil, S. S., McDevitt, H. O. & Steinman, L. (1988). Limited heterogeneity of T cell receptors from lymphocytes mediating autoimmune encephalomyelitis allows specific immune intervention. *Cell* **54**, 263–273.

Assan, R., Feutren, G., Debray-Sachs, M., Quiniou-Debrie, M. C., Laborie, C., Thomas, G., Chatenaud, L. & Bach, J.-F. (1985). Metabolic and immunological effects of cyclosporin in recently diagnosed type 1 diabetes mellitus. *Lancet* **i**, 67–71.

Bacelj, A., Charlton, B. & Mandel, T. E. (1989). Prevention of cyclophosphamide-induced diabetes by anti-Vβ 8 T-lymphocyte receptor monoclonal antibody therapy in NOD/Wehi mice. *Diabetes* **38**, 1492–1495.

Ben-Nun, A. & Cohen, I. R. (1982). Spontaneous remission and acquired resistance to autoimmune encephalomyelitis (EAE) are associated with suppression of T cell reactivity: suppressed EAE effector T cells recovered as T cell lines. *Journal of Immunology* **128**, 1450–1457.

Ben-Nun, A., Wekerle, H. & Cohen, I. R. (1981a). The rapid isolation of clonable antigen-specific T lymphocyte line capable of mediating autoimmune encephalomyelitis. *European Journal of Immunology* **11**, 195–199.

Ben-Nun, A., Wekerle, H. & Cohen, I. R. (1981b). Vaccination against autoimmune encephalomyelitis with T lymphocyte line cells reactive against myelin basic protein. *Nature* **292**, 60–61.

Beraud, E., Lider, O., Baharav, E., Reshef, T. & Cohen, I. R. (1989). Vaccination against experimental autoimmune encephalomyelitis using a subencephalitogenic dose of autoimmune effector cells. 1. Characteristics of vaccination. *Journal of Autoimmunity* **2**, 75–86.

Billingham, M. E. J., Carney, S., Butler, R. & Colston, M. J. (1990). A mycobacterial 65 kD heat shock protein induces antigen specific suppression of adjuvant arthritis, but is not itself arthritogenic. *Journal of Experimental Medicine* **171**, 339-344.

Billingham, R. E., Brent, L. & Medawar, P. B. (1953). Actively acquired tolerance of foreign cells. *Nature* **172**, 603-605.

Brostoff, S. W. & Mason, D. W. (1984). Experimental allergic encephalomyelitis: successful treatment in vivo with monoclonal antibody that recognizes T helper cells. *Journal of Immunology* **133**, 1938-1942.

Case, J. P., Lorberbaum-Galski, H., Lefyatis, R., FitzGerald, D., Wilder, R. L. & Pastan, I. (1989). Chemiric cytotoxin IL2-PE40 delays and mitigates adjuvant-induced arthritis in rats. *Proceedings of the National Academy of Sciences USA* **86**, 287-291.

Caspi, R. R., Kuwabara, T. & Nussenblatt, R. B. (1988). Characterization of a suppressor cell line which downgrades experimental autoimmune uveoretinits. *Journal of Immunology* **140**, 2579-2584.

Clayton, J. P., Gammon, G. M., Ando, D. G., Kono, D. H., Hood, L. & Sercarz, E. E. (1989). Peptide specific prevention of experimental allergic encephalomyelitis. Neonatal tolerance induced to the dominant T cell determinant of myelin basic protein. *Journal of Experimental Medicine* **169**, 1681-1691.

Cohen, I. R. & Weiner, H. L. (1988). T cell vaccination. *Immunology Today* **9**, 332-335.

Cohen, I. R. (1989). The physiological basis of T cell vaccination against autoimmune disease. In *Immunologic Recognition*, Vol. LIV, pp879-884. Symposium on Quantitative Biology, Cold Spring Harbor.

Elias, D., Reshef, T., Birk, O. S. van der Zee, R., Walker, M. D. & Cohen, I. R. (1991). Vaccination against autoimmune mouse diabetes with a T cell epitope of the human 65 kD heat shock protein. *Proceedings of the National Academy of Sciences USA* **88**, 3088-3091.

Ellerman, K. E., Powers, J. M. & Brostoff, S. W. (1988). A suppressor T lymphocyte line for autoimmune encephalomyelitis. *Nature* **331**, 265-267.

Hayosh, N. S. & Swanborg, R. H. (1987). Autoimmune effector cells. IX. Inhibition of adoptive transfer of autoimmune encephalomyelitis with a monoclonal antibody specific for interleukin 2 receptor. *Journal of Immunology* **138**, 3771-3775.

Heber-Katz, E. & Acha-Orbea, H. (1989). The V-region disease hypothesis: evidence from autoimmune encephalomyelitis. *Immunology Today* **10**, 164-169.

Hedlund, G. M. & Dohlsten, P. O., Ericsson O. & Sjorgren, H. O. (1989). Rapid response to Con A by $CD4^+$ $CD45R^-$ rat memory lymphocytes as compared to $CD4^+$ $CD45R^-$ lymphocytes. *Cellular Immunology* **119**, 317-326.

Hench, P. S., Kendall, E. C., Slocumb, C. H. & Polley, H. F. (1949). The effect of a hormone of the adrenal cortex 17-hydroxy-11-dehydrocorticosterone; compound E and of pituitary adrenocorticotropic hormone on rheumatoid arthritis. *Proceedings of the Staff Meeting Mayo Clinic* **24**, 181-197.

Higgins, P. J. & Weiner, H. L. (1988). Suppression of experimental autoimmune encephalomyelitis by oral administration of myelin basic protein and its fragments. *Journal of Immunology* **140**, 440-445.

Holoshitz, J., Naparstek, Y., Ben-Nun, A. & Cohen, I. R. (1983). Lines of T lymphocytes induce or vaccinate against autoimmune arthritis. *Science* **219**, 56-58.

Howell, M. D., Winters, S. T., Opee, T., Powell, H. C., Carlo, D. J. & Brostoff, S. W. (1989). Vaccination against experimental allergic encephalomyelitis with T cell receptor peptides. *Science* **246**, 668-670.

Kahan, B. D. (1989). Drug therapy: cyclosporine. *New England Journal of Medicine* **321**, 1725-1738.

Kakimoto, K., Katsuki, M., Hirofuji, T., Iwata, H. & Koga, T. (1988). Isolation of T cell line capable of protecting mice against collagen-induced arthritis. *Journal of Immunology* **140**, 78-83.

Kaplan, S. R. & Calbresi, P. (1983). Drug therapy: immunosuppressive agents. Part I. *New England Journal of Medicine* **289**, 952-954.

Kotzin, B. L., Strober, S., Engleman, E. G., Colis, A., Hoppe, R. T., Kansas, G. S., Terrell, C . P. & Kaplan, H. S. (1981). Treatment of intractable rheumatoid arthritis with total lymphoid irradiation. *New England Journal of Medicine* **305**, 969-976.

Lider, O., Baharav, E., Mekori, Y. A., Miller, T., Naparstek, Y., Vlodavsky, I. & Cohen, I. R. (1989a). Suppression of experimental autoimmune disases and prolongation of allograft survival by treatment of animals with low doses of heparins. *Journal of Clinical Investigation* **83**, 752-756.

Lider, O., Karin, N., Shinitzky, M. & Cohen, I. R. (1987). Therapeutic vaccination against adjuvant arthritis using autoimmune T cells treated with hydrostatic pressure. *Proceedings of the National Academy of Sciences USA* **84**, 4577-4580.

Lider, O., Reshef, T., Beraud, E., Ben-Nun, A. & Cohen, I. R. (1988). Anti-idiotypic network induced by T cell vaccination against experimental autoimmune encephalomyelitis. *Science* **239**, 181-183.

Lider, O., Santos, L. M. B., Lee, C. S. Y., Higgins, P. J. & Weiner, H. L. (1989b). Suppression of experimental autoimmune encephalomyelitis by oral administration of myelin basic protein. II. Suppression of disease and *in vitro* immune responses is mediated by antigen specific CD8 T lymphocytes. *Journal of Immunology* **142**, 748-752.

Maron, R., Zerubavel, R., Rriedman, R. & Cohen, I. R. (1983). T lymphocyte line specific for thyroglobulin produces or vaccinates against autoimmune throiditis in mice. *Journal of Immunology* **131**, 2316-2322.

Mor, F., Lohse, A. W., Karin, N. & Cohen, I. R. (1990). Clinical modelling of T cell vaccination against autoimmune disease in rats, selection of antigen specific T cells using a mitogen. *Journal of Clinical Investigation* **85**, 1594-1598.

Mowat, A. L. (1987). The regulation of immune responses to dietary protein antigens. *Immunology Today* **8**, 93-98.

Naparstek, Y., Cohen, I. R., Fuks, Z. & Vlodavsky, I. (1984). Activated T lymphocytes produce a matrix-degrading heparan sulfate endoglycosidase. *Nature* **310**, 241-243.

Nussenblatt, R. B., Caspi, R. R., Mahdi, R., Chan, C. C., Roberge, F., Lider, O. & Weiner, H. L. (1990). Inhibition of S-antigen induced experimental autoimmune uveoretinitis by oral induction of tolerance with S-antigen. *Journal of Immunology* **144**, 1689-1693.

Plotz, P. H., Klippel, J. H., Decker, J. L., Grauman, D., Wolff, B., Brown, B. C. & Rutt, G. (1979). Bladder complications in patients receiving cyclophosphamide for systemic lupus erythematosus or rheumatoid arthritis. *Annals of Internal Medicine* **91**, 221-223.

Sakai, K., Zamvil, S. S., Mitchell, D. J., Hodgkinson, S., Rothbard, J. B. & Steinman, L. (1989). Prevention of experimental encephalomyelitis with peptides that block interaction of T cells with major histocompatibility complex proteins. *Proceedings of the National Academy of Sciences USA* **86**, 9470-9474.

Sanders, M. E., Makoba, M. W., June, C. H., Young, H. A. & Shaw, S. (1989). Enhanced responsiveness of human memory T cells to CD2 and CD3 receptor mediated activation. *European Journal of Immunology* **19**, 803-808.

Sedgwick, J. D. (1988). Long-term depletion of CD8 positive T cells *in vivo* in the rat: no observed role for CD8 (cytotoxic/suppressor) cells in the immunoregulation of experimental allergic encephalomyelitis. *European Journal of Immunology* **18**, 495-502.

Sriram, S. & Steinman, L. (1983). Anti IA antibody suppresses active encephalomyelitis: treatment model for diseases linked to IR genes. *Journal of Experimental Medicine* **158**, 1362-1367.

Sun, D., Qin, F., Chluba, J., Epplen, J. T. & Wekerle, H. (1988). Suppression of experimentally induced autoimmune encephalomyelitis by cytolytic T-T cell interactions. *Nature* **332**, 843–845.

Thomspon, H. S. G. & Staines, N. A. (1985). Gastric administration of type II collagen delays the onset and severity of collagen-induced arthritis in rats. *Journal of Clinical Experimental Immunology* **64**, 581–586.

van der Broek, M. F., Hogervorst, E. J. M., van Bruggen, M. C. J., van Eden, W., van de Zee, R. & van den Berg, W. (1989). Protection against streptococcal cell wall-induced arthritis by pretreatment with the 65 kD mycobacterial heat shock protein. *Journal of Experimental Medicine* **170**, 449–556.

van Eden, W., Thole, J. E. R., van der Zee, R., Noordiz, A., Embden, J. D. A., Hensen, E. J. & Cohen, I. R. (1988). Cloning of the mycobacterial epitope recognized by T lymphocytes in adjuvant arthritis. *Nature* **331**, 171–173.

Vanderbark, A. A., Hashim, G. & Offner, H. (1989). Immunization with a synthetic T cell receptor V-region peptide protects against experimental autoimmune encephalomyelitis. *Nature* **341**, 541–544.

Wallace, D., Goldfinger, D., Lowe, C., Nichols, S., Weiner, J., Brachman, M. & Klinenberg, J. R. (1982). A double blind controlled study of lymphoplasmapheresis versus sham apheresis in rheumatoid arthritis. *New England Journal of Medicine* **306**, 1406–1410.

Wang, Y., Hao, L., Gill, R. G. & Laffergy, K. J. (1987). Autoimmune diabetes in NOD mouse is L3T4 T lymphocyte dependent. *Diabetes* **36**, 535–538.

Wraith, D. C., Smilek, D. E., Michell, D. J., Steinman, L. & McDevitt, H. O. (1989). Antigen recognition in autoimmune encephalomyelitis and the potential for peptides mediated immunotherapy. *Cell* **59**, 247–255.

Chapter 13
Anti-MHC class II antibodies

Christian Boitard

Introduction

The major histocompatibility complex (MHC) is a critical genetic region which controls various immunological functions. Class I MHC antigens play a central role in cellular interactions between $CD8^+$ T cells and most nucleated cells, including non-lymphoid cells. Antigens that are synthesized within cells, including constitutive self proteins and viral antigens in infected cells, are presented to $CD8^+$ T cells through their association with class I molecules. Class II antigens, which are encoded by I-region H-2 genes in the mouse, D-region genes within the human leucocyte antigen (HLA) system in the human, play a major role in cellular interactions between $CD4^+$ T cells and other lymphoid cells, including B lymphocytes and antigen-presenting cells (APC). Class II MHC antigens are directly involved in antigen presentation to $CD4^+$ T cells *in vitro* and *in vivo*. Exogenous antigens processed by APCs, including soluble and particulate antigens, are presented in the form of peptides in association with class II antigens. Class II genes are referred to as immune response (Ir) genes which determine the response to T-cell-dependent antigens as exemplified by the immune response to synthetic copolymers. Beyond their role in antigen presentation, MHC antigens expressed by resident or migrant cells present within the thymus are crucial to the central selection of the T-cell repertoire. Genetic studies have demonstrated a polygenic basis for susceptibility to autoimmunity. In most experimental models, at least one major susceptibility component maps within the MHC, as exemplified by genetic studies following crosses of animal models of autoimmune diseases

270

with conventional laboratory strains. A strong association has been evidenced between most human autoimmune diseases and definite class II MHC alleles (Todd *et al.*, 1988).

Polyclonal sera and monoclonal antibodies directed against class II MHC antigens have been shown to block antigen presentation to T cells, as well as primary or secondary antibody responses *in vitro* (Shevach *et al.*, 1974; Frelinger *et al.*, 1975; Schwartz *et al.*, 1976; Berzofsky & Richman, 1981). Beyond their role in presenting processed peptides to CD4$^+$ T cells (Rudensky *et al.*, 1991), class II MHC antigens can directly mediate transduction signal on cells on which they are expressed, as shown in case of B lymphocytes and monocytes (Cambier *et al.*, 1987; Chen *et al.*, 1987; Mooney *et al.*, 1989; Brick-Ghannam *et al.*, 1991). *In vivo* treatment with anti-class II monoclonal antibodies interferes with CD4$^+$ T-cell function (Sprent, 1980), antigen presentation (Kruisbeek *et al.*, 1985b,c; Aberer *et al.*, 1986) antibody production to branched multichain synthetic polypeptide antigens in the mouse (Rosenbaum *et al.*, 1981), the clonal deletion of developing T cells within the thymus both *in vivo* (Cosgrove *et al.*, 1991) and *in vitro* (DeLuca, 1986), and with the differentiation of class II-restricted T cells in the neonatal period (Kruisbeek *et al.*, 1983, 1985a,b; Kimoto & Kishimoto, 1986). The suppression of humoral immune responses *in vivo* in adult H-2^{k,b} F1 mice, treated with monoclonal anti-class II antibodies is haplotype specific, since the only response inhibited by anti-I-A^k is that against (HG)-AL which is under I-A^k control while (TG)-AL which is under I-A^b control is unaffected. Such haplotype specificity is observed in cases of immunization with antigen in aqueous solution but not in complete Freund's adjuvant (Rosenbaum *et al.*, 1981). By contrast, no inhibition of B-cell responses to thymo-independent antigens is observed following *in vivo* treatment with anti-class II monoclonal antibodies (Fultz *et al.*, 1989). Treatment of mouse neonates with anti-I-A^k monoclonal antibodies for 3 weeks following birth induce a depletion of class II-expressing cells within the spleen, abrogate alloantigen and trinitrophenyl-specific T-lymphocyte responses, helper function for the generation of cytotoxic T cells, reduce I-A antigen expression in the thymus and induce defective class II-bearing accessory cell in the spleen (Kruisbeek *et al.*, 1983). Such treatment deplete CD8$^-$ CD4$^+$ thymic T cells and is followed by an absence of peripheral CD4$^+$ T cells which is reversible upon cessation of treatment. The absence of recruitment of CD4$^+$ T cells in this model correlates with the absence of thymic-antigen presenting cell function in treated animals (Kruisbeek *et al.*, 1985b).

In vivo treatment with anti-class II polyclonal sera and monoclonal antibodies has further been shown to inhibit delayed-type hypersensitivity reactions against tumoral antigens in the mouse (Perry & Greene, 1982) through the induction of protective T cells which can transfer antigen-specific protection to syngeneic recipients (Perry *et al.*, 1979). T cells which are responsible for transferring protection in this last model are sensitive to low-dose cyclophosphamide. Interestingly, in the case of delayed-type hypersensitivity reactions following infection of H-2^b mice with *Listeria monocytogenes*, *in vivo* treatment of infected animals with an anti-I-A^b monoclonal antibody markedly inhibited antigen-induced proliferation of *Listeria*-dependent T cells *in vitro*, and I-A expression on spleen cells, and protected treated animals with otherwise lethal concentrations of *Listeria* (Kurlander & Jones, 1987). *Listeria* dissemination was reduced in treated animals, suggesting a possible increase in macrophage bactericidal activity. A differential effect of anti-I-E and anti-I-A antibodies has been further reported in this same model (Blackwell & Roberts, 1987). Anti-class II treatment *in vivo* has also been shown to decrease azobenzene arsonate-induced splenic and nodal trapping at the site of hapten injection under mouse ear skin (Carroll & Greene, 1987). Finally, protection against allograft rejection (Perry & Williams, 1985) and graft-versus-host disease (Prud'homme *et al.*, 1979) has been obtained using anti-class II mono-clonal antibody treatment in the mouse. Pre-treatment of allogeneic islets of Langerhans, thyroid tissue or bone marrow cells with anti-class II monoclonal antibodies *in vitro* has been shown to deplete the graft of class II-expressing cells and significantly prolongs allograft survival in un-treated recipients (Lacy *et al.*, 1979, 1980, 1982; Faustman *et al.*, 1981; Szer *et al.*, 1985; Kaufman *et al.*, 1988; Iwai *et al.*, 1989). Moreover, *ex vivo* treatment of grafts with anti-class II monoclonal antibodies prolongs kidney and liver allograft survival (Jablonski *et al.*, 1989; Kurozumi *et al.*, 1991). Anti-class II-toxin conjugates have been used to deplete lymphoid cell preparations of class II-expressing cells *in vitro* (Nakahara *et al.*, 1985).

The aims of treating autoimmune diseases with anti-class II mono-clonal antibodies are at least twofold. The first is to block antigen presentation to autoreactive T cells, precluding the first activation step of the autoimmune reaction within the T-cell-regulatory cascade traces back to the antigen presentation level. The second is to modulate the activation of autoreactive T cells by blocking their interaction with antigen-present-ing cells and thereby induce long-term tolerance states. *In vivo* treatment with anti-class II monoclonal antibodies has so far been restricted to experimental models of autoimmune diseases in animals, but they ob-viously open new perspectives in human immunotherapy. This therapeutic approach provides several advantages in comparison with conventional immunosuppressive agents. One but not least relates with the expression on cell membranes of different class II antigens encoded at separate loci within the MHC region, allowing the possibility of isotype-specific im-munosuppression. In the mouse, class II antigens are encoded by Aα, Aβ and Eα genes within the I-A region and an Eβ gene within the I-E region (Flavell *et al.*, 1986). In the rat, two different class II antigens are respectively encoded within the B and the D region of the RT1 complex (Gill *et al.*, 1987). Monoclonal antibodies specific for alleles encoded within the I-A and the I-E regions or their equivalent (respectively the B and the D regions in the rat) have been used *in vivo* in experimental models of autoimmune diseases. Although polyclonal antisera specific for I-J region of the H-2 complex in the mouse have been used *in vivo*, they will not be considered in this review. The biochemistry of I-J antigens has remained elusive, casting serious questions regarding the existence of I-J genes within the H-2 MHC of the mouse.

Prevention of experimental autoimmune diseases by anti-class II antibodies

Successful prevention of autoimmune phenomena has been obtained in different experimental models by injecting monoclonal antibodies directed against I-A and, in one case, I-E gene products into the mouse. The largest set of data has been obtained in experimental allergic encephalomyelitis (EAE) which is induced following immunization against myelin, myelin-basic protein or myelin basic protein-derived peptides in complete Freund's adjuvant (CFA). Beyond the prevention of EAE by treatment of SJL/L (H-2^s) mice with anti-I-A^s monoclonal antibodies (Steinman *et al.*, 1981, 1983), efficient reversal of on-going EAE has been obtained in this model using anti-class II monoclonal antibodies (Sriram & Steinman, 1983). Decreased accumulation of radiolabelled lymph node cells in the central nervous system has been demonstrated in anti-class II-treated mice. It has further been shown that the prevention of EAE in (SJL/J × BALB/c)F1 mice combining the SJL/J (H-2^s) high-responder strain to the BALBL/c (H-2^d) low-responder strain is haplotype specific, since suppression of EAE was only seen in F1 mice immunized with antigen in CFA and injected with anti-I-A^s monoclonal antibody. The disease was only partially prevented in this last model by injecting an anti-I-A^s monoclonal antibody. Antibody to the low-responder allele was ineffective in preventing passive transfer of myelin-basic protein-sensitized lymphocytes (Sriram *et al.*, 1987).

Similar prevention has been reported using an anti-I-A^s monoclonal antibody in experimental myasthenia gravis induced in SJL mice following immunization with purified acetylcholine receptor preparations (Waldor *et al.*, 1983, 1987), anti-I-A antibodies of various specificities in experimental allergic thyroiditis (EAT) induced by immunization of AKR (H-2^k) or SJL (H-2^s) mice against thyroglobulin in CFA (Vladutiu & Steinman, 1987; Stull *et al.*, 1990), anti-I-A antibodies in collagen-induced arthritis induced in B10Q and B1O.RIII mice following immunization against collagen type II in CFA (Wooley *et al.*, 1985; Cooper *et al.*, 1988) and finally antibodies directed against B-locus gene products of the RT1

complex in experimental allergic uveitis induced in Lewis rats by immunization against purified S-antigen in CFA (Wetzig *et al.*, 1988; Rao *et al.*,
1989). In the case of EAT, anti-class II treatment was effective when given
shortly before or at the time of antigen administration in a dose-dependent
manner, it also decreased disease severity evaluated in terms of both anti-
thyroglobulin antibodies and thyroid infiltration when given after the
antigenic challenge. Interestingly, the development of EAT requires a first
injection plus a booster injection of thyroglobulin in CFA. The thyroid
disease was prevented by anti-I-A treatment around the first antigenic
challenge although not the booster injection suggesting that the anti-I-A
effect covered the secondary immune response (Vladutiu & Steinman,
1987). In the case of collagen-induced arthritis, the administration of anti-
I-A antibody at the time of antigen administration, (but not 2 weeks after),
significantly decreased the incidence and delayed the onset of arthritis.
Antibody titres and proliferative responses to collagen type II remained
unmodified. In antigen-induced arthritis in mice, flare-up reactions induced by intravenous injection of methylated bovine serum albumin was
suppressed by anti-I-A^b or anti-I-A^k monoclonal antibody treatment. In
C57Bl 10 mice, anti-class II treatment was shown to suppress delayed-type
hypersensitivity but not to reverse the passive Arthus reaction to methylated bovine serum albumin (van den Broek *et al.*, 1986). In the EAT
model, various anti-class II monoclonal antibodies with the same allelic
specificities (Vladutiu & Steinman, 1987) were shown to have different
effects on the development of thyroiditis. Affinity or isotype differences
may explain the different effects of these monoclonal antibodies. In
collagen-induced arthritis, an anti-I-E monoclonal antibody was shown to
be detrimental whereas anti-I-A prevented disease development (Wooley
et al., 1985). However, in other instances such as EAT, anti-I-E monoclonal
antibodies showed the same efficiency as anti-I-A in preventing autoimmunity (Stull *et al.*, 1990). In a model of diabetes induced in the mouse by
low-dose streptozotocin, a toxic agent endowed with highly specific
cytotoxic activity against insulin-secreting cells, partial prevention of
diabetes was obtained using polyclonal H-2 alloantisera (Bonnevie-
Nielsen & Lernmark, 1986) or anti-class II monoclonal antibodies (Kiesel
& Kolb, 1983; Kiesel *et al.*, 1989). The protection against diabetes
development was obtained in C3H mice upon anti-I-A^k or anti-I-E^k
treatment although it was not improved by combining anti-I-A and anti-I-
E. Anti-I-A treatment was only effective when applied at time of streptozotocin injections (Kiesel *et al.*, 1989).

Prevention of spontaneous autoimmune diseases by anti-class II antibodies

Besides the prevention of experimentally-induced autoimmune diseases,
evidence has been obtained indicating that *in vivo* treatment with anti-

class II monoclonal antibodies can prevent the development of spontaneous autoimmune diseases in animals. It was first shown that long-term
treatment with anti-I-A^s monoclonal antibodies prolongs survival and
prevents clinical nephritis in (NZB × NZW)F1 mice (Adelman *et al.*,
1983; Klinman *et al.*, 1986). Using cell-transfer experiments, *in vivo*
treatment with an anti-I-A antibody of either autoimmune NZB donors or
NZB xid recipients significantly reduced the number of B cells secreting
anti-DNA antibodies in the absence of detectable suppressor-cell activation, suggesting a direct effect on autoantibody producing B cells (Klinman *et al.*, 1986).

The same therapeutic approach has been applied to the diabetes-
prone BB rat. The BB rat was developed from an outbred colony of Wistar
rats, the trait being secondarily inbred by sister–brother mating. Metabolic and morphological characteristics of the hyperglycaemic syndrome
in this model show many similarities to human insulin-dependent diabetes
mellitus (IDDM), including islet infiltration by lymphoid cells and the
presence of anti-islet cell antibodies. Clinical diabetes mostly occurs after
60 days of age in diabetes-prone lines with identical prevalence in male and
female animals. It is noteworthy that diabetes-prone BB rats show a
profound T-cell lymphopenia which is not seen in human diabetes.
Genetic susceptibility has been assigned to two independent genetic
regions, one being localized within the rat RT1 MHC region. The BB rat
disease is characterized by the association of diabetes with other autoimmune phenomena, mainly thyroiditis. In this model, the prevention of
diabetes was achieved by *in vivo* treatment with a monoclonal antibody to
I-E equivalent (D-encoded) class II antigens of the rat RT1 complex. No
prevention was obtained in BB rats treated with a monoclonal antibody to
I-A equivalent (B-encoded) class II antigens, indicating that the effect of
anti-class II monoclonal antibody treatment was isotype (locus)-specific.
Thyroiditis was prevented by injecting the anti-I-E monoclonal antibody
preventing IDDM, while treatment with the anti-I-A monoclonal antibody had no such effect. Although genetic susceptibility to thyroiditis has
not been studied in the BB rat model, these data indicate that either similar
genetic background or immunological effector mechanisms are likely to be
involved in both the thyroid and the islet β cell disease (Boitard *et al.*,
1985; Boitard & McDevitt, 1986). In both the (NZB × NZW)F1 mouse
and the BB model, the prevention of spontaneous autoimmunity has been
prevented by long-term treatment with anti-class II monoclonal antibodies.

A second model of autoimmune IDDM has recently been developed
in the non-obese diabetic (NOD) mouse. The spontaneous disease is
predominantly observed in female mice from 10 to 12 weeks of age. Earlier
disease can be induced in females as well as males by two injections of
150–200 mg/kg of cyclophosphamide at a 2-week interval. The role of

autoimmunity in the islet β cell destruction is clearly demonstrated by the prevention of diabetes by neonatal thymectomy, and treatment with anti-CD4 or anti-T cell receptor monoclonal antibodies, or cyclosporin A (CsA). The clinical disease is preceded by an early infiltration of the islets of Langerhans of the pancreas by mononuclear cells, mostly CD4$^+$ T cells. Adoptive transfer of overt diabetes has been obtained by injecting splenic T cells, including CD4$^+$ and CD8$^+$ cells, from diabetic NOD mice into naive NOD neonates, pre-irradiated adult 8-week-old male recipients, or B-cell deprived neonatal recipients. Susceptibility to IDDM in this model has a polygenic basis. A major genetic component maps to the MHC, while other components to chromosomes 3 and 1. The NOD mouse exclusively expresses I-A antigens which show a unique pattern character-ized by five consecutive nucleotide changes on the I-A β chain leading to two amino acid substitutions in positions 56 and 57. The serine at position 57 differs from the aspartic acid present in all non-diabetic inbred strains studied so far, including the non-obese normal (NON) strain. The NOD strain does not express I-E antigens. Expression of I-E antigens in (C57BL/6 $\times$ NOD)F1, in which the parent C57BL/6 expresses an Eα^d transgene, prevents the development of insulitis. Similarly, resistance to diabetes has been reported in transgenic NOD mice expressing Aβ^{nod} with a proline instead of an histidine in position 56, Aβ^k, or Eα transgenes (Boitard & Bach, 1991).

We have found evidence that spontaneous IDDM was prevented in the NOD mouse by injecting 1.2 mg/week of purified anti-I-A^{nod} mono-clonal antibodies, starting treatment at either 3 weeks of age or at birth, providing that continuous treatment was maintained up to the end of experiments. No prevention of insulitis was seen in protected animals. This observation provides a new example of the prevention of a spontaneously occurring autoimmune disease by anti-class II monoclonal antibody treatment (Boitard et al., 1988). In order to study further the mechanisms of protection confered by anti-class II treatment, we attempted to deter-mine whether anti-class II antibodies could protect against diabetes transfer into syngeneic recipients. Evidence was obtained indicating that treatment of neonatal recipients with anti-class II monoclonal antibody did indeed protect against the transfer of diabetes by spleen cells from diabetic mice. By contrast, treatment of recipient male NOD mice with an anti-class II antibody from birth did not confer protection against diabetes transfer performed at 8 weeks, despite maintenance of anti-class II treatment after the transfer. It was thus hypothesized that anti-class II monoclonal antibody treatment could only provide protection if admin-istered to immunocompetent hosts (i.e. non-irradiated recipients), suggest-ing that irradiation abrogated the protection induced by anti-class II monoclonal antibody injections (Boitard et al., 1988).

Mechanisms of protection conferred by anti-class II treatment

The mechanisms of protection observed following anti-class II mono-clonal antibody treatment remain elusive (Vladutiu, 1991). A direct action of anti-class II monoclonal antibodies on T cells is unlikely in the mouse, although it cannot be excluded in other species such as the human or the rat in which activated T cells express class II antigens. A direct action on antigen-presenting cells, e.g. functional impairment or blockade of antigen presentation, is more likely to occur as a general mechanism of action of anti-class II monoclonal antibody treatment, including in the mouse.

A direct action of anti-class II antibodies on target cells of immune reactions must also be considered with regard to the reported expression of class II antigens on target cells such as thyroid epithelial cells at the site of the autoimmune reaction (Hanafusa *et al.*, 1983). However, the signifi-cance of 'aberrant' class II expression on target cells is still a matter of debate. *De novo* expression of class II antigens has been induced by interferon γ on thyroid epithelial cells and by interferon γ plus tumour necrosis factor on pancreatic islet cells (Pujol-Borrell *et al.*, 1987). Class II-expressing thyroid cells have been shown to present viral peptides to specific T-cell clones. However, class II transgene expression on islet β cells in the mouse is not followed by the immune destruction of β cells (Böhme *et al.*, 1989) and the transplantation of islets expressing an I-E class II transgene on β cells in I-E-negative mice induces a tolerance state in recipients (Markmann *et al.*, 1988).

Action of anti-class II *in vitro*

There is overwhelming evidence that anti-class II polyclonal or mono-clonal antibodies block antigen presentation *in vitro* by acting directly on antigen-presenting cells (Frelinger *et al.*, 1975; Schwartz *et al.*, 1976; Berzofsky & Richman, 1981). Beyond the blockade of antigen presenta-tion, anti-class II antibodies have been attributed with other biological effects. Monoclonal antibodies to class II antigens have been shown to partially block lymphocyte interaction with high endothelial venules *in vitro* (Manolios *et al.*, 1988), and thus possibly affect homing processes at inflammation sites (Sriram & Carroll, 1991). There is also evidence that class II MHC antigens can act as signal-transducing molecules on B lymphocytes, by stimulating rapid translocation of cytosolic protein kinase C to the nucleus (Cambier *et al.*, 1987; Mooney *et al.*, 1989; Brick-Ghannam *et al.*, 1991). Some anti-class II antibodies have been further attributed with a direct role in providing a growth signal to B cells. Antibodies to I-A, as well as to I-E, have been shown to enhance anti-μ-

induced B-cell proliferation in the absence of T cells or adherent cells. B-cell responses to lipopolysaccharide or T-cell-derived lymphokines are inhibited by anti-I-A or anti-I-E monoclonal antibodies (Forsgren et al., 1987; Takahama et al., 1989). Finally, the induction of suppressor T cells has been evidenced following treatment with anti-class II antibodies in vitro.

Action of anti-class II on lymphoid cell subsets in vivo

Major modifications of circulating lymphocytes have been evidenced upon in vivo treatment with anti-class II monoclonal antibodies during the first 3 weeks of life in mice (Fultz et al., 1982; Kruisbeek et al., 1983, 1985a,b,c; Fultz et al., 1984; Waldor et al., 1984; Williams et al., 1988). A major decrease in B lymphocyte numbers was first evidenced in anti-class II-treated animals. Both the thymus and the spleen of anti-class II-treated mice have shown a reduction of $CD4^+$ $CD8^-$ T cells as well as antigen presentation by class II-expressing thymic antigen-presenting cells (Kruisbeek et al., 1983, 1985b). These effects are transient upon cessation of anti-class II-treatment. In vivo treatment with anti-I-A was shown to decrease both I-A and I-E expression by 75–90% in spleen-cell populations as well as I-A expression (but not I-E expression) in thymic antigen-presenting cells. Anti-class II treatment during embryonal life in the mouse has been shown to alter the selection of self-class II reactive T cells. The action of anti-class II monoclonal antibodies injected at birth on B and $CD4^+$ T-cell population has not been observed to the same extent in adult animals. In the NOD model, we observed a transient depletion of B cells following treatment of 3-week-old animals by anti-class II antibodies but lymphocyte populations recovered their normal distribution within weeks despite the maintenance of the anti-class II treatment (unpublished data). The mechanisms of action of anti-class II treatment is unlikely to depend on B cells in this diabetes model which is largely, if not exclusively, dependent on the activation of the T-cell compartment (Boitard & Bach, 1991).

Induction of suppressor T cells by anti-class II treatment in vivo

The induction of suppressor T cells may mediate the action of anti-class II treatment in vivo (Perry & Greene, 1982; Williams & Perry, 1985; Aoki et al., 1987; Adelman et al., 1988). Evidence has been obtained in vitro that a direct effect on antigen-presenting cells may indeed be the first step in the subsequent induction of suppressor T cells, as in the case of T cells primed to sperm-whale myoglobin (Broder et al., 1980; Lamb et al., 1982). Since anti-class II conferred no protection against diabetes transfer to pre-irradiated adult recipients, we evaluated radiation-sensitive mechanisms mediating anti-class II monoclonal antibody-induced protection. Irradiated 8-week-old male recipients were reconstituted with spleen cells from anti-class II monoclonal antibody-treated NOD donors prior to the transfer of spleen cells from diabetic NOD mice (Boitard & Bach, 1988; Boitard et al., 1988; Boitard et al., 1991). Restoration of irradiated male recipients with spleen cells from 8-week-old NOD mice treated from birth or from 3–8 weeks of age with an anti-I-A^{nod} monoclonal antibody, (but not an irrelevant anti-class II antibody of same isotype), 24 h prior to the transfer of spleen cells from diabetic mice afforded effective protection of recipients against the ultimate development of diabetes. By contrast, spleen cells from mice treated for only 7 days prior to transfer were not protective. T cells were responsible for restoring anti-class II-induced protection in irradiated adult recipients and were further characterized as CD4$^+$ cells. Present evidence for the induction of suppressor T cells upon treatment with anti-class II monoclonal antibodies must be considered in the light of previous observations based on in vitro assays in models of active immunization against viral or allogeneic antigens. One should also recall that inhibition of DTH reactions against tumoral antigens by anti-class II antibody treatment has been transferred in vivo by spleen cells obtained from anti-class II antibody-treated mice. The transfer of protection in this last model is abrogated by T-cell depletion and is sensitive to low-dose cyclophosphamide (Perry & Green, 1982). In all the previously mentioned models, including the NOD mouse, the molecular characterization of suppressor T cells elicited by anti-class II monoclonal antibody treatment is still lacking. Histological analysis of the pancreases of animals transferred with anti-class-II-induced CD4$^+$ protective T cells or non-protective control T cells (obtained from NOD animals treated with an irrelevant anti-class-II-antibody-prior to the injection of spleen cells from diabetic NOD mice was followed, in both cases, by the homing of transferred cells around the islets of Langerhans (periinsulitis). No destructive insulitis was seen in animals which received spleen cells from anti-I-A^{nod}-treated animals in contrast with animals which received nonprotective control spleen cells. These data bring histological evidence that non-specific homing of CD4$^+$ T cells is not sufficient to protect against the development of diabetes upon injection of spleen cells from diabetic animals.

Modulation of autoreactive T cells

Beyond the induction of suppressor T cells by anti-class II treatment, other and non-exclusive protection mechanisms are likely to be at play in the protection observed. The blockade of autoreactive T cell homing to the site of target cells is one possibility. There is experimental evidence that anti-class II treatment inhibits the homing of myelin-basic protein-sensitized T cells in a passive transfer model of EAE in the mouse (Sriram & Carroll, 1991). In the NOD mouse, transferred suppressor T cells were only evidenced if anti-class II treatment was maintained in recipients (Boitard *et al.*, 1988). In this last model, transient treatment with anti-I-A^{nod} antibody prevented the development of IDDM, provided that anti-class II treatment was applied early in the natural history of the disease (Jonker *et al.*, 1988; Boitard *et al.*, 1991). The long-term effect of transient anti-class II treatment was not observed in cases of anti-class I, anti-CD8 or a depleting anti-CD4 monoclonal antibody treatment applied within the same early therapeutic window. It is thus possible that induction of suppressor T cells summarizes one aspect of anti-class II induced protection but that other mechanisms are at play following *in vivo* treatment. The long-term effect of transient anti-class II treatment will need further evaluation as for the mechanism of long-term inactivation of autoreactive T cells.

Conclusion

Although large-scale use of anti-class II monoclonal antibodies in human therapeutics is premature given the large number of unanswered questions, e.g. the mechanisms of protection at play *in vivo*, this therapeutic approach has been evaluated in the EAE primate model (Broder *et al.*, 1980) and has been reported in rheumatoid arthritis (Abderrazi *et al.*, 1990). Major issues to be addressed in the perspective of human therapy will need further insight into the mechanisms of action of anti-class II monoclonal antibodies. The choice between antibodies directed against public and private class II epitopes or between depleting versus non-depleting antibodies, and the role of isotype or affinity of antibodies, have not been fully evaluated in experimental models. The possibility that anti-class II antibodies modulate autoreactive T cells by blocking a crucial activation pathway and thereby confer long-term protection in autoimmune animals requires further clarification. Nevertheless, the possibility of locus and/or haplotype-specific protection when targeting class II antigens and the possibility of prolonged protection following transient treatment in animals open new perspectives in the treatment of human autoimmune diseases.

References

Abderrazik, M., Moynier, M., Eliaou, J. F., Levy-Biau, D., Combe, B., Sany, J., Clot, J. & Brochier, J. (1990). Anti-F(ab′)2 antibody response to the injection of anti-class II HLA alloantibodies in patients with rheumatoid arthritis. *Journal of Rheumatology* **17**, 758–763.

Aberer, W., Kruisbeek, A. M., Shimada, S. & Katz, S. I. (1986). *In vivo* treatment with anti-I-A antibodies: differential effects on Ia antigens and antigen-presenting cell function of spleen cells and epidermal Langerhans cells. *Journal of Immunology* **136**, 830–836.

Adelman, N. E., Watling, D. L. & McDevitt, H. O. (1983). Treatment of (NZB × NZW)F1 disease with anti-I-A monoclonal antibodies. *Journal of Experimental Medicine* **158**, 1350–1355.

Adelman, N. E., Watling, D. & McDevitt, H. O. (1988). *In vivo* effects of antibodies to immune response gene products. II. Suppression of humoral immune responses with monoclonal anti-I-A is due to suppressor cells. *International Reviews of Immunology* **3**, 333–344.

Aoki, I., Ishii, N., Minami, M., Nagashima, Y., Misugi, K. & Okuda, K. (1987). Induction of suppressor T cells by intravenous administration of monoclonal anti-I-A antibody. *Transplantation* **44**, 421–425.

Berzofsky, J. A. & Richman, L. K. (1981). Genetic control of the immune response to myoglobins. IV. Inhibition of determinant-specific Ir gene-controlled antigen presentation and induction of suppression by pretreatment of presenting cells with anti-Ia antibodies. *Journal of Immunology* **126**, 1898–1904.

Blackwell, J. M. & Roberts, M. B. (1987). Immunomodulation of murine visceral leishmaniasis by administration of monoclonal anti-Ia antibodies: differential effects of anti-I-A vs. anti-I-E antibodies. *European Journal of Immunology* **17**, 1669–1672.

Bohme, J., Haskins, K., Stecha, P., van Ewijk, W., Le Meur, M., Gerlinger, P., Benoist, C. & Mathis, D. (1989). Transgenic mice with I-A on islet cells are normoglycemic but immunologically intolerant. *Science* **224**, 1179–1183.

Boitard, C. & Bach, J. F. (1988). Therapy of autoimmune diseases with monoclonal antibodies to class II major histocompatibility complex antigens: the role of T lymphocytes. *Journal of Autoimmunity* **1**, 663–671.

Boitard, C. & Bach, J. F. (1991). Insulin-dependent diabetes mellitus: an autoimmune disease. In Talal, N. (ed) *Molecular Autoimmunity* pp. 273–318. Academic Press, London.

Boitard, C., Bendelac, A., Richard, M. F., Carnaud, C. & Bach, J. F. (1988). Prevention of diabetes in nonobese diabetic mice by anti-I-A monoclonal antibodies: transfer of protection by splenic T cells. *Proceedings of the National Academy of Sciences USA* **85**, 9719–9723.

Boitard, C. & McDevitt, H. O. (1986). Prevention of polyendocrine autoimmune disease by antibodies to class II major histocompatibility complex antigens in the rat. In Brochier, J. Clot, J. & Sany, J. (eds) *Anti-Ia Antibodies in the Treatment of Autoimmune Disease* Vol. 2, pp. 129–134. Academic Press, London.

Boitard, C., Michie, S., Serrurier, P., Butcher, G. W., Larkins, A. P. & McDevitt, H. O. (1985). *In vivo* prevention of thyroid and pancreatic autoimmunity in the BB rat by antibody to class II major histocompatibility complex gene products. *Proceedings of the National Academy of Sciences USA* **82**, 6627–6631.

Boitard, C., Sempé, P., Villa, M. C., Becourt, C., Richard, M. F., Timsit, J. & Bach, J. F. (1991). Monoclonal antibodies: probes for studying experimental autoimmunity in animals. *Research in Immunology* **142**, 495–503.

Bonnevie-Nielsen, V. & Lernmark, A. (1986). An H-2 allo-antiserum preserves β-cell function in mice made diabetic by low-dose streptozocin. *Diabetes* **35**, 570–573.

Brick-Ghannam, C., Mooney, N. & Charron, D. (1991). Signal transduction in B lymphocytes. *Human Immunology* **30**, 202–207.

Broder, S., Mann, D. L. & Waldmann, T. A. (1980). Participation of suppressor T cells in the immunosuppressive activity of a heteroantiserum to human Ia-like antigens (p23, 30). *Journal of Experimental Medicine* **151**, 257–262.

Cambier, J. C., Newell, M. K., Justement, L. B., McGuire, J. C., Leach, K. L. & Chen, Z. Z. (1987). Ia binding ligands and cAMP stimulate nuclear translocation of PKC in B lymphocytes. *Nature* **327**, 629–632.

Carroll, A. M. & Greene, M. I. (1987). Anti-I-A antibody modulation of lymphocyte traffic in hapten-stimulated inbred mice. *Immunology* **62**, 471–475.

Chen, Z. Z., McGuire, J. C., Leach, K. L. & Cambier, J. C. (1987). Transmembrane signaling through B cell MHC class II molecules: anti-Ia antibodies induce protein kinase C translocation to the nuclear fraction. *Journal of Immunology* **138**, 2345–2352.

Cooper, S. M., Sriram, S. & Ranges, G. E. (1988). Suppression of murine collagen-induced arthritis with monoclonal anti-Ia antibodies and augmentation with IFNγ. *Journal of Immunology* **141**, 1958–1962.

DeLuca, D. (1986). Ia-positive nonlymphoid cells and T cell development in murine fetal thymus organ cultures: monoclonal anti-Ia antibodies inhibit the development of T cells. *Journal of Immunology* **136**, 430–9.

Faustman, D., Hauptfeld, V., Lacy, P. & Davie, J. (1981). Prolongation of murine islet allograft survival by pretreatment of islets with antibody directed to Ia determinants. *Proceedings of the National Academy of Sciences USA* **78**, 5156–5159.

Flavell, R. A., Allen, H., Burkly, L. C., Sherman, D. H., Waneck, G. L. & Widera, G. (1986). Molecular biology of the H-2 histocompatibility complex. *Science* **233**, 437–443.

Forsgren, S., Martinez, A. C. & Coutinho, A. (1987). The role of I-A/E molecules in B-lymphocyte activation. II. Mechanism of inhibition of the response to lipopolysaccharide by anti-I-A/E antibodies. *Scandinavian Journal of Immunology* **25**, 225–234.

Frelinger, J. A., Niederhuber, J. E. & Shreffler, D. C. (1975). Inhibition of immune responses in vitro by specific antiserums to Ia antigens. *Science* **188**, 268–270.

Fultz, M., Carman, J., Finkelman, F. D. & Mond, J. J. (1989). Neonatal suppression with anti-Ia antibody. III. In vivo responses to the type 2 antigen TNP-Ficoll. *Journal of Immunology* **143**, 403–406.

Fultz, M., Finkelman, F. D. & Mond, J. J. (1984). *In vivo* administration of anti-I-A antibody induces the internalization of B-cell surface I-A and I-E without affecting the expression of surface immunoglobulin. *Journal of Immunology* **133**, 91–97.

Fultz, M. J., Scher, I., Finkelman, F. D., Kincade, P. & Mond, J. J. (1982). Neonatal suppression with anti-Ia antibody. I. Suppression of murine B lymphocyte development. *Journal of Immunology* **129**, 992–995.

Gill III, T. J., Kunz, H. W., Misra, D. N. & Hassett, A. L. C. (1987). The major histocompatibility complex of the rat. *Transplantation* **43**, 773–785.

Gosgrove, D., Gray, D., Dierich, A., Kaufman, J., Lemeur, M., Benoist, C. & Mathis, D. (1991). Mice lacking MHC class II molecules. *Cell* **66**, 1051–1066.

Hanafusa, T., Pujol-Borrell, R., Chiovato, L., Russell, R. C. G., Doniach, D. & Bottazzo, G. F. (1983). Aberrant expression of HLA-DR antigen on thyrocytes in Graves' disease: relevance for autoimmunity. *Lancet* **ii**, 1111–1115.

Iwai, H., Kuma, S., Inaba, M. M., Good, R. A., Yamashita, T., Kumazawa, T. & Ikehara, S. (1989). Acceptance of murine thyroid allografts by pretreatment of anti-Ia antibody or anti-dendritic cell antibody *in vitro*. *Transplantation* **47**, 45–49.

Jablonski, P., Kraft, N., Howden, B. O., Thomson, N. M., Atkins, R. C. & Marshall, V. C. (1989). Transplantation of rat kidneys following perfusion with anti-Ia monoclonal antibody. *Transplantation Proceedings* **21**, 1123–1124.

Jonker, M., van Lambalgen, R., Mitchell, D. J., Durham, S. K. & Steinman, L. (1988). Successfull treatment of EAE in Rhesus monkeys with MHC class II specific monoclonal antibodies. *Autoimmunity* **1**, 399–414.

Kaufman, D. S., Kong, C. S., Shizuru, J. A., Gregory, A. K. & Fathman, C. G. (1988). Use of anti-L3T4 and anti-Ia treatments for prolongation of xenogeneic islet tranplants. *Transplantation* **46**, 210–215.

Kiesel, U. & Kolb, H. (1983). Suppressive effect of antibodies to immune response gene products on the development of low-dose streptozotocin-induced diabetes. *Diabetes* **32**, 869–871.

Kiesel, U., Oschilewski, M., Taniguchi, M. & Kolb, H. (1989). Modulation of low-dose streptozotocin-induced diabetes in mice by administration of antibodies to I-A, I-E and I-J determinants. *Diabetologia* **32**, 173–176.

Kimoto, M. & Kishimoto, S. (1986). Alteration of the T cell self-specificity repertoire by treatment with anti-Ia antibody during embryonic life. *European Journal of Immunology* **16**, 835–839.

Klinman, D. M., Lefkowitz, M. D., Raveche, E. S. & Steinberg, A. D. (1986). Effect of anti-Ia treatment on the production of anti-DNA antibody by NZB mice. *European Journal of Immunology* **16**, 939–944.

Kruisbeek, A. M., Bridges, S., Carmen, J., Longo, D. L. & Mond, J. J. (1985a). *In vivo* treatment of neonatal mice with anti-I-A antibodies interferes with the development of the class I, class II, and Mls-reactive proliferating T cell subset. *Journal of Immunology* **134**, 3597–3604.

Kruisbeek, A. M., Fultz, M. J., Sharrow, S. O., Singer, A. & Mond, J. J. (1983). Early development of the T cell repertoire. *In vivo* treatment of neonatal mice with anti-Ia antibodies interferes with differentiation of I-restricted T cells but not K/D-restricted T cells. *Journal of Experimental Medicine* **157**, 1932–1946.

Kruisbeek, A. M., Mond, J. J., Fowlkes, B. J., Carmen, J. A., Bridges, S. & Longo, D. L. (1985b). Absence of the Lyt-2-, L3T4 + lineage of T cells in mice treated neonatally with anti-I-A correlates with absence of intrathymic I-A-bearing antigen-presenting cell function. *Journal of Experimental Medicine* **161**, 1029–1047.

Kruisbeek, A. M., Titus, J. A., Stephany, D. A., Gause, B. L. & Longo, D. L. (1985c). *In vivo* treatment with monoclonal anti-I-A antibodies: disappearance of splenic antigen-presenting cell function concomitant with modulation of splenic cell surface I-A and I-E antigens. *Journal of Immunology* **134**, 3605–3614.

Kurlander, R. J. & Jones, F. (1987). The effects of an anti-I-Ab antibody on murine host resistance to *Listeria monocytogenes. Journal of Immunology* **138**, 2679–2686.

Kurozumi, Y., Sakagami, K., Takasu, S., Haisa, M., Oiwa, T., Hasuoka, H., Yagi, T., Saito, S., Inagaki, M., Niguma, T., Miyoshi, K., Kobayashi, N., Fuziwara, T., Kusaka, S., Matuoka, J. & Orika, K. (1991). The effect of *ex vivo* perfusion of the liver with anti-class II antibody on acute rejection in canine liver transplantation. *Transplantation* **52**, 170–172.

Lacy, P. E., Davie, J. M. & Finke, E. H. (1979). Prolongation of islet allograft survival following *in vitro* culture (24°C) and a single injection of ALS. *Science* **204**, 312–313.

Lacy, P. E., Davie, J. M. & Finke, E. H. (1980). Prolongation of islet xenograft survival without continuous immunosuppression. *Science* **209**, 283–285.

Lacy, P. E., Finke, E. H., Janney, C. G. & Davie, J. M. (1982). Prolongation of islet xenograft survival by *in vitro* culture of rat megaislets in 95% O_2. *Transplantation* **33**, 588–592.

Lamb, J. R., Eckels, D. D., Ketterer, E. A., Sell, T. W. & Woody, J. N. (1982). Antigen-specific human T lymphocyte clones: mechanisms of inhibition of proliferative responses by xenoantiserum to human nonpolymorphic HLA-DR antigens. *Journal of Immunology* **129**, 1085–1090.

Manolios, N., Geczy, C. & Schrieber, L. (1988). Anti-Ia monoclonal antibody (10-2.16) inhibits lymphocyte-high endothelial venule (HEV) interaction. *Cellular Immunology* **117**, 152–164.

Markmann, J., Lo, D., Naji, A., Palmiter, R. D., Brinster, R. L. & Heber-Katz, E. (1988). Antigen presenting function of class II MHC expressing pancreatic beta cells. *Nature* **336**, 476–479.

Mooney, N., Hivroz, C., Ziai-Talebian, S., Grillot-Courvalin, C. & Charron, D. (1989). Signal transduction via MHC class II antigens on B lymphocytes. *Journal of Immunogenetics* **16**, 273–281.

Nakahara, K., Kaplan, D., Bjorn, M. & Fathman,C. G. (1985). The effectiveness of anti-Ia-immunotoxins in the suppression of MLR. *Transplantation* **40**, 62–67.

Perry, L. L., Dorf, M. E., Benecerraf, B. & Greene, M. I. (1979). Regulation of immune response to tumor antigen: interference with syngeneic tumor immunity by anti-IA alloantisera. *Proceedings of the National Academy of Sciences USA* **76**, 920–924.

Perry, L. L. & Greene, M. I. (1982). Conversion of immunity to suppression by *in vivo* administration of I-A subregion-specific antibodies. *Journal of Experimental Medicine* **156**, 480–491.

Perry, L. L. & Williams, I. R. (1985). Regulation of transplantation immunity *in vivo* by monoclonal antibodies recognizing host class II restriction elements. I. Genetics and specificity of anti-Ia immunotherapy in murine skin allograft recipients. *Journal of Immunology* **134**, 2935–2941.

Prud'homme, G. J., Sohn, U. & Delovitch, T. L. (1979). The role of H-2 and Ia antigens in graft-versus-host reactions (GVHR): presence of host alloantigens on donor cells after GVHR and suppression of GVHR with an anti-Ia antiserum against host Ia antigens. *Journal of Experimental Medicine* **149**, 137–149.

Pujol-Borrell, R., Todd, I., Doshi, M., Bottazzo, G. F., Sutton, R., Gray, D., Adolf, G. R. & Feldmann, M. (1987). HLA-class II induction in human islet cells by interferon-gamma plus tumour necrosis factor or lymphotoxin. *Nature* **326**, 304–306.

Rao, N. A., Atalla, L., Linker-Israeli, M., Chen, F. Y., George, F. W., Martin, W. J. & Steinman, L. (1989). Suppression of experimental uveitis in rats by anti-I-A antibodies. *Investigative Ophthalmology and Visual Science* **30**, 2348–2355.

Rosenbaum, J. T., Adelman, N. E. & McDevitt, H. O. (1981). *In vitro* effects of antibodies to immune response gene products. I. Haplotype-specific suppression of humoral immune responses with a monoclonal anti-I-A. *Journal of Experimental Medicine* **154**, 1694–1702.

Rudensky, A. Yu., Preston-Hurlburt, P., Hong, S-C., Barlow, A & Janeway, Jr, C. A. (1991). Sequence analysis of peptides bound to MHC class II molecules. *Nature* **353**, 622–627.

Schwartz, R. H., David, C. S., Sachs, D. H. & Paul, W. E. (1976). T lymphocyte-enriched murine peritoneal exudate cells. III. Inhibition of antigen-induced T lymphocyte proliferation with anti-Ia antisera. *Journal of Immunology* **117**, 531–540.

Shevach, E. M., Green, I. & Paul, W. E. (1974). Alloantiserum-induced inhibition of immune response gene product function. II. Genetic analysis of target antigens. *Journal of Experimental Medicine* **139**, 679–695.

Singh, B., Dillon, T., Fraga, E. & Lauzon, J. (1990). Role of the first external domain of I-Aβ chain in immune responses and diabetes in on-obese diabetic (NOD) mice. *Journal of Autoimmunity* **3**, 507–521.

Sprent, J. (1980). Effect of blocking helper T cell induction *in vivo* with anti-Ia antibodies: possible role of I-A/E hybrid molecules as restriction elements. *Journal of Experimental Medicine* **152**, 996–1010.

Sriram, S. & Carroll, L. (1991). Haplotype-specific inhibition of homing of radiolabeled lymphocytes in experimental allergic encephalomyelitis following treatment with anti-IA antibodies. *Cellular Immunology* **135**, 222–231.

Sriram, S. & Steinman, L. (1983). Anti-I-A antibody suppresses active encephalomyelitis: treatment model for diseases linked to Ir genes. *Journal of Experimental Medicine* **158**, 1362–1367.

Sriram, S., Topham, D. J. & Caroll, L. (1987). Haplotype-specific suppression of experimental allergic encephelomyelitis with anti-IA antibodies. *Journal of Immunology* **139**, 1485–1489.

Steinman, L., Rosenbaum, J. T., Sriram, S. & McDevitt, H. O. (1981). *In vivo* effects of antibodies to immune response gene products: Prevention of experimental allergic encephalitis. *Proceedings of the National Academy of Sciences USA* **78**, 7111–7114.

Steinman, L., Solomon, D., Lim, M., Zamvil, S. & Sriram, S. (1983). Prevention of experimental allergic encephalitis with in vivo administration of anti-I-A antibody. Decreased accumulation of radiolabelled lymph node cells in the central nervous system. *Journal of Neuroimmunology* **5**, 91–97.

Stull, S. J., Kyriakos, M., Sharp, G. C., Bickel, J. T. & Braley-Mullen, H. (1990). Effects of anti-I-A and anti-I-E monoclonal antibodies on the induction and expression of experimental autoimmune thyroiditis in mice. *Autoimmunity* **6**, 23–36.

Szer, J., Deeg, H. J., Appelbaum, F. R. & Storb, R. (1985). Failure of autologous marrow reconstitution after cytolytic treatment of marrow with anti-Ia monoclonal antibody. *Blood* **65**, 819–822.

Takahama, Y., Ono, S., Ishihara, K., Muramatsu, M. & Hamaoka, T. (1989). Disparate functions of I-A and I-E molecules on B cells as evidenced by the inhibition with anti-I-A and anti-I-E antibodies of polyclonal B cell activation. *European Journal of Immunology* **19**, 2227–2235.

Todd, J. A., Acha-Orbea, H., Bell, J. I., Chao, N., Fronek, Z., Jacob, C. O., McDermott, M., Sinha, A. A., Timmerman, L., Steinman, L. & McDevitt, H. O. (1988). A molecular basis for MHC class II-associated autoimmunity. *Science* **240**, 1003–1009.

Van den Broek, M. F., Van der Berg, W. B. & Van de Putte, L. B. (1986). Monoclonal anti-Ia antibodies suppress the flare up reaction of antigen induced arthritis in mice. *Clinical and Experimental Immunology* **66**, 320–330.

Vladutiu, A. O. (1991). Treatment of autoimmune diseases with antibodies to class II major histocompatibility complex antigens. *Clinical Immunology and Immunopathology* **61**, 1–17.

Vladutiu, A. O. & Steinman, L. (1987). Inhibition of experimental autoimmune thyroiditis in mice by anti-I-A antibodies. *Cellular Immunology* **109**, 169–180.

Waldor, M. K., Hardy, R. R., Hayakawa, K., Steinman, L., Herzenberg, L. A. & Herzenberg, L. A. (1984). Disappearance and reapparance of B cells after *in vivo* treatment with monoclonal anti-I-A antibodies. *Proceedings of the National Academy of Sciences USA* **81**, 2855–2858.

Waldor, M. K., O'Hearn, M., Sriram, S. & Steinman, L. (1987). Treatment of experimental autoimmune myasthenia gravis with monoclonal antibodies to immune response gene products. *Annals of the New York Academy of Sciences* **505**, 655–668.

Waldor, M. K., Sriram, S., McDevitt, H. O. & Steinman, L. (1983). *In vivo* therapy with monoclonal anti-I-A antibody suppresses immune responses to acetylcholine receptor. *Proceedings of the National Academy of Sciences USA* **80**, 2713–2717.

Wetzig, R., Hooks, J. J., Percopo, C. M., Nussenblatt, R., Chan, C. C. & Detrick, B. (1988). Anti-Ia antibody diminishes ocular inflammation in experimental autoimmune uveitis. *Current Eye Research* **7**, 809–818.

Williams, W. W., Falo, L. D. Jr., Lu, C. Y., Benacerraf, B. & Sy, M. S. (1988). Effects of *in vivo* monoclonal anti-I-A antibody treatment in neonatal mice on intrathymic and peripheral class II antigen expression. *Cellular Immunology* **111**, 126–138.

Williams, I. R. & Perry, L. L. (1985). Regulation of transplantation immunity in vivo by monoclonal antibodies recognizing host class II restriction elements. II. Effects of anti-Ia immunotherapy on host T-cell responses to graft alloantigens. *Journal of Immunology* **134**, 2942–2947.

Wooley, P. H., Luthra, H. S., Lafuse, W. P., Huse, A., Stuart, J. M. & David, C. S. (1985). Type II collagen-induced arthritis in mice. III. Suppression of arthritis by using monoclonal and polyclonal anti-Ia antisera. *Journal of Immunology* **134**, 2366–2374.

Chapter 14
Use of MHC antagonists to prevent and treat autoimmune disease in animal models

Jonathan B. Rothbard & Hugh O. McDevitt

Introduction

The dramatic increase in the understanding of antigen-specific T-cell recognition has led to the exploration of novel immunotherapeutic approaches to treat a variety of autoimmune syndromes. The logical basis of these strategies is to interfere with the activation of $CD4^+$ T lymphocytes, known to be essential in the generation of the inflammatory responses inherent in many autoimmune diseases. If drugs can be designed that specifically inhibit the expansions of this population of cells they might represent the first effective therapy for this large class of diseases. These therapeutics are envisioned to be radically different from the current drugs on the market, which only modulate the symptoms of these diseases and are not directed at the fundamental causes of the syndromes.

One strategy for immunomodulation that several groups are exploring is to develop small molecular weight antagonists for major histocompatibility complex (MHC) class II proteins. These polymorphic membrane proteins have evolved to bind, transport and display on the surface of antigen-presenting cells proteolytic fragments of proteins. The MHC–peptide complexes are recognized by the antigen-specific receptor of T lymphocytes. In the case of autoimmunity, T cells believed to be central to the aetiology of the disease are activated by the engagement of specific fragments of either the autoantigen bound by MHC class II proteins. If the concentration of the complexes can be reduced sufficiently, then the antigen-specific T-cell response should be inhibited, which in turn should result in the reduction of the symptoms of the disease. At the present time, this logic has not been explicitly proved. If feasible, and the antagonist was bound by one, or a limited number, of MHC class II alleles, this strategy would be more selective than more broadly based immuno-suppressive approaches such as the use of cyclosporin, FK 506, or antibodies that would interfere with T-cell recognition by inhibiting cell adhesion. Because an effective MHC antagonist would inhibit all T cells restricted by the particular MHC allele, this approach would not be as specific as strategies aimed at inhibiting specific subpopulations of T cells.

In vitro inhibition experiments

The initial experiments demonstrating that T-cell activation could be blocked by competing at the level of antigen presentation were performed by Werdelin, Banceraff and Goodman. Each of these three groups separately demonstrated that structurally related, as well as distinct, antigens could compete for T-cell recognition by interfering with antigen presentation (Werdelin, 1982; Rock & Benacerrat, 1983; Godfrey *et al.*, 1984).

Guillet *et al.* (1986) were able to inhibit the proliferative response of a class-II restricted hybridoma specific for a bacteriophage peptide sequence with a staphylococcal nuclease peptide previously shown to bind the same MHC allele. This series of experiments was also the first demonstration that there was a single peptide combining site on class II proteins and that each complex was not the result of a unique association, but that MHC molecules were a general receptor for peptides.

Competition between peptides for binding MHC class II proteins was unequivocally demonstrated using purified, detergent solubilized proteins soon after peptides were shown to bind specifically to the receptors (Babbitt, *et al.*, 1986; Buus *et al.*, 1987). These studies were extended by Adorin *et al.* (1988) who demonstrated a direct correlation between the apparent affinity with which peptide was bound by a class II protein and its ability to inhibit T cells restricted by the same MHC molecule. A key aspect of these early experiments, which was not emphasized at the time, was that only a small percentage of the purified MHC molecules were able to bind added ligand. Consequently, only a small subpopulation of the protein was involved in the competition experiments. This was particularly important to consider in the context of those experiments that added the agonist and the antagonist simultaneously. In these cases successful competition *in vitro* might not be easily extrapolated to the more complex situation *in vivo*. At the present time the molecular basis for the limited binding is poorly understood, with two possibilities being equally likely. The first is based on the presence of endogenous peptides in the site, while the second invokes conformational changes either on behalf of the receptor or the peptide.

Several groups have isolated and sequenced the most highly repre-sented of the endogenous peptides from murine and human class II proteins (Rudensky *et al.*, 1991; Hunt *et al.*, 1992; Chicz *et al.*, 1992; Cammeron *et al.*, personal communication). The vast majority are derived from either membrane proteins that recycle into the lysosome, or proteins existing in high concentrations in serum. Their affinity for class II proteins is in the same range as peptides previously shown to bind (between 5 and 500 nM), and therefore the basis for their relatively high occupancy appears to be high local concentration in the lysosome and not unusually high affinity.

Inhibition of peptide binding on cell surfaces appears to be significantly more difficult to observe than in assays using purified MHC proteins. The observed inhibition still involves the same small percentage of the MHC class II protein that binds exogenous peptide. Consequently, if little peptide exchange occurs on the cell surface, then the endogenous peptides only can be effectively replaced if the antagonist is present in the cellular location where MHC–peptide complexes are formed.

The biosynthetic pathway of MHC class II proteins is reasonably well understood. The α and β chains of MHC class II proteins are bound by a 33 kDa invariant chain as they are translated in the rough endoplasmic reticulum. The invariant chain serves three separate functions: (i) it facilitates the formation of the heterodime, in the same manner than Bip interacts the heavy and light chains of immunoglobulins; (ii) it contains the appropriate intracellular trafficking signal which results in the transport of the complex to lysosomes; and (iii) it prevents peptides present in the biosynthetic pathway from associating with the class II protein until it reaches the lysosome. In the lysosome the invariant chain is cleaved, and the peptide–class II complexes are formed that eventually will be displayed on the cell surface.

The experiments by Lorenz *et al.* (1990) demonstrated that normal serum proteins compete for the processing and presentation of exogenously added proteins. The competition could have occurred at any of three levels: (i) uptake of the protein by antigen-presenting cells; (ii) at the level of proteolytic cleavage in the lysosome; or (iii) the binding of the fragment to MHC class II proteins. In these studies the authors could not detect any competition at the level of uptake or processing, however, inhibition was observed when the amount of peptide–MHC complexes was assayed as measured by T-cell recognition. However, this competition could be overcome by increased uptake of the antigen by modifying the antigen with mannan, which enabled the protein to be more rapidly incorporated by macrophages by receptor-mediated endocytosis.

In vivo inhibition experiments

Soluble peptides were first shown to be effective inhibitors of the priming of class II restricted proliferative T-cell responses by Muller *et al.* (1991).

In this study, mice were immunized with a peptide immunogen, either alone or with a competitor, injected at a different anatomical site. As in earlier studies, the competitive peptides inhibited only those T-cell responses restricted by the allele or isotype they were known to bind. The observed inhibition was dose dependent and correlated with the known affinities between the peptide and the MHC protein. Peptides emulsified in complete Freund's adjuvant were approximately four times more potent than when the peptides were delivered in phosphate buffered saline. These differences were sufficiently small that they could be compensated for by an increase in dosage. The most effective method of delivery was mini-pumps implanted subcutaneously.

An important and interesting detail was that there were no detectable T-cell responses to the competitors when they were administered in a soluble form. Clearly, for them to be effective competitors the local concentration of the peptides in the lymph nodes must be considerable. The authors tried to minimize the immunogenicity of the competitors by using relatively short analogues. However, even these analogues elicit an immune response. This is an important issue because as valuable as these studies were, they do not prove that the inhibition in the T-cell response was due to reduction in the number of peptide–MHC complexes displayed on the surface of antigen-presenting cells. One of several alternative explanations of the phenomenon was that the competitors were sufficiently immunogenic to indirectly reduce the response to the agonist peptides. Obviously, if the competitive peptides were not immunogenic this concern need not be considered.

To investigate these issues more directly Guery et al. (1992) established an ex vivo system to detect peptide–MHC complexes generated in vivo. The authors assembled a set of T-cell hybridomas specific for each of four lysozyme peptides and restricted by either I-A^k, I-E^d, or I-E^k. Each of the hybridomas were shown to be stimulated by popliteal lymph node cells from mice immunized either with intact lysozyme or synthetic peptides corresponding to the T-cell determinants. A direct relationship was demonstrated between the dose of the antigen injected and the degree of T-cell-hybridoma activation induced by the lymph node cells. The ability of the lymph nodes to present peptide was detected between 6 and 12 days after immunization, but was maximal after 8 days.

The T-cell responses elicited by these antigen-presenting cells were shown to arise from recognition of peptide-MHC complexes formed in vivo and not to a small amount of intact lysozyme isolated in the cell preparation. Treatment of lymph node cells from unimmunized mice with chloroquine prior to exposure to intact lysozyme completely prevented proliferation of the hybridomas. Similar treatment of lymph node cells from immunized mice did not have any affect on T-cell recognition, consistent with the hybridomas recognizing preformed complexes on the surface of the dissected lymph node cells. Coinjection of a T-cell determinant of one of the hybridomas with a second peptide known to bind the same MHC protein resulted in a reduction in the ability of the lymph node cells to stimulate the cell line *in vitro*. The most convincing experiments used a murine lysozyme peptide, known to bind I-A^k, to prevent priming to intact chicken lysozyme. The lymph node cell from these mice were unable to restimulate a chicken lysozyme-specific hybridoma restricted by I-A^k, but were very effective in stimulating hybridoma restricted by I-E^k. This experiment verified many of the key attributes of a perceived MHC antagonists: (i) it was not immunogenic, being a murine peptide; (ii) it was effective at reducing peptide-class II complexes on the surface of antigen presenting cells; and (iii) it was selective for a single allele of I-A, being unable to bind either to I-A^d or I-E^k.

Finally, the authors confirmed that the antigen-presenting ability in the lymph node cells did not involve T cells by treating the cells with anti-Thy 1 antibodies and complement. Cells treated in this manner acted similarly to untreated cells from mice given the immunogen alone or in the presence of inhibitory peptides. These experiments allowed them to conclude that a subset of T cells, such as suppressor T cells, were not responsible for this phenomenon. Finally because the peptides used to inhibit the T-cell responses in this study were structurally unrelated, mechanisms of antigen specific modulation, such as tolerance induction or the modification in the spectrum of cytokines produced (Evavold & Allen, 1991), do not need to be considered. A major issue not addressed by this study was the ability of exogenously added antagonists being effective against endogenously generated peptide-MHC complexes.

Two groups have investigated the inhibition of endogenous peptide-class II complexes by the addition of exogenous antagonists. In addition to the previously mentioned study by Allen and coworkers reducing the amount of murine haemoglobin complexes in mice (Rudensky *et al.*, 1991), Adornie *et al.* (1991) have created a useful system. They transfected a fusion protein composed of the first 80 residues of chicken lysozyme attached to the transmembrane and cytoplasmic portions of a murine MHC class I protein into a B-cell hybridoma expressing both I-A^k and I-E^k. This cell was shown to process and present lysozyme peptides by its ability to stimulate murine T-cell hybridomas specific for determinants in the first 80 amino acids. As expected, this cell line did not stimulate a hybridoma specific for residues 112–129 of lysozyme. As in their earlier studies they used a peptide from murine lysozyme (residues 46–64) as an inhibitor of I-A^k-restricted responses. Incubation of living transfected cells with the peptide antagonist resulted in a dose-dependent inhibition of stimulation of a lysozyme-specific T-cell hybridoma. No effect was seen on presentation of a lysozyme peptide to an I-E^k-restricted hybridoma, consistent with the inhibition arising from reduction of I-A^k-peptide complexes. The competition for the presentation of the engodenous antigen depended on the number of lysozyme transfected cells used in the experiment. A tenfold increase in the number of these cells resulted in a proportional increase in cytokine production.

These experiments provide strong support for the feasibility of the approach. However, a cautionary remark is important. In each cited investigation, the authors purposely selected agonists and antagonists that most effectively demonstrated the principle they wanted to establish. Consequently, the long-term efficacy of this approach in a specific autoimmune disease will depend on both the concentration and affinity the autoantigenic peptides appears to be attainable only at the level of newly synthesized MHC. Consequently any prospective antagonist must be able to maintain a high local concentration in the biosynthetic pathway where peptide–MHC complexes are formed. The design of an effective antagonist necessarily includes the problem of targeting to particular cells and cellular compartments. In the context of MHC class II proteins this corresponds to the lysosomal–endosomal network.

Animal models

Experimental allergic encephalomyelitis

Experimental allergic encephalomyelitis (EAE) is an autoimmune, T-cell mediated demyelinating disease which can be induced in many species of experimental animals by immunization with spinal cord, crude myelin, purified myelin basic protein or synthetic peptide epitopes of myelin basic protein emulsified in complete Freund's adjuvant, often with the help of additional adjuvants such as pertussis bacilli. EAE can also be induced with proteolipid protein, and in most instances is an abrupt onset, short duration, self-limited autoimmune disease in which it is difficult to induce a second episode in those animals which survive the first episode. Susceptibility is linked to both MHC and non-MHC linked genes (Williams & Moore, 1973; McFarlin et al., 1975; Fritz et al., 1985), and each susceptible MHC allele presents a characteristic myelin basic protein peptide epitope to induce disease causing T-cell-immune responses. In H-2^u mice, the immunodominant peptide presented by I-A^u is MBP Ac1-11, while the major epitope presented by I-E^u is MBP 35–47. MBP Ac1-11 is by far the strongest peptide epitope in H-2^u mice and the majority of T cells are restricted to I-A^u and specific for Ac1-11. In addition, in PL/J mice and to a lesser extent in (PL × SJL) F1 mice, many of these T cells express T-cell receptor molecules utilizing V$_{\alpha 8.2}$ and V$_{\beta 2,4}$. In H-2^s mice (SJL) there are several major peptide epitopes included within residues 89–101, including 89–101, 89–100, and a third not yet fully characterized epitope (Zamvil *et al.*, 1986; Sakai *et al.*, 1988). The proteolipid protein peptide 139–151 is major peptide epitope presented by I-A^s in SJL mice (Tuohy *et al.*, 1989).

Prevention of EAE with MHC binding peptides

Induction of EAE has been prevented through the use of Ac1-11 analogues, as well as peptides of unrelated sequence, when these are added in a 3–30-fold molar excess in the immunizing complete Freund's adjuvant mixture. Table 14.1 gives a summary of results obtained in several laboratories using a variety of blocking peptides and proteins.

Induction of EAE by MBP Ac1-11, PLP 139-151, and whole MBP has been prevented by using MBP Ac1-11 analogues of related and sometimes longer sequence as well as unrelated peptides, unrelated proteins, synthetic amino acid polymers, and unrelated non-immunogenic peptides. Lamont *et al.* (1990) used a peptide (KM core) related to ovalbumin 323–339 with high affinity to I-A^s to block EAE induced in SJL mice by PLP 139–151. This was one of the first examples of the prevention of EAE by a peptide with a high affinity for the relevant I-A allele but of a sequence unrelated to the immunizing peptide. However, this peptide was also highly immunogenic in these mice. Subsequently, Gautam and Glynn (1990) showed that Ova 323-339 is non-immunogenic in (PL × SJL)F1 mice, binds to I-A^u, and is effective in preventing EAE induced in this strain by MBP Ac1-11. This is the first example of prevention of an autoimmune disease by an MHC-binding peptide which is unrelated to the immunizing peptide and is itself non-immunogenic. This peptide thus fulfills all of the criteria, in this strain, for an ideal MHC competitor peptide.

As indicated in Table 14.1, a peptide analogue of MBP Ac1-11, namely Ac1-11 with alanine replacing lysine at position 4, is capable of preventing EAE in (PL × SJL)F1 mice. This peptide has several unusual properties. First, it is heteroclitic for disease-inducing T cells, and second, it has a much higher binding affinity for I-A^u than does Ac1-11 (Wraith *et al.*, 1989). These findings suggested that AC1-11[4A] would be a very strong immunogen. Paradoxically, this peptide induces a very poor immune response in (PL × SJL)F1 mice, despite the fact that it is heteroclitic for T cells specific for Ac1-11. When mixed in a three–sixfold molar excess with Ac1-11 in complete Freund's adjuvant, Ac1-11[4A] causes a striking reduction in the incidence and severity of EAE. There are several paradoxes in this result. Because Ac1-11[4A] is a poor immunogen but binds with higher affinity to I-A^u, it could block induction of EAE by competitively binding to I-A^u. However, Ac1-11[4A] is also a heteroclitic agonist for Ac1-11-specific T cells and therefore might anergize these T cells or stimulate them in the periphery, which could prevent them from

Table 14.1. Peptides and polypeptides used for disease prevention in EAE

Disease-inducing agent	Sequence	Disease-preventing molecule	Sequence	Animal	Reference
1. MBP analogues					
MBP Ac1–11	AcASQKRPSQRHG	Ac1–11[4A]	AcASQARPSQRHG	(PL/J × SJL)F1	Wraith et al., 1989
MBP Ac1–11	AcASQKRPSQRHG	N1–20	ASQKRQPSQRHGSKYLATAST	Mouse	Hunt et al., 1992
MBP Ac1–11	AcASQKRPSQRHG	AcN9–20	AcRHGSKYLATAST	Mouse	Zaki et al., 1989
2. Unrelated peptides					
PLP 139–151	HSLGKWLGHPDKF			SJL mouse	Lamont et al., 1990
KM core exten.	KMKMVHAAAHAKMKM				
3. Unrelated proteins and synthetic polymers					
Whole MBP	—	Whole ovalbumin		Lewis rat	Gautam & Glynn, 1990
Whole MBP	—	Cop 1	Random copolymer A:E:K:Y	(SJL × BALB/C)F1	Lando et al., 1979
4. Unrelated, non-immunogenic peptides					
MBP Ac1–11	AcASQKRPSQRHG	Ovalbumin 323–339	ISQAVHAAHAEINEAGR	(PL × SJL)F1 Mouse	Gautam et al., 1992

inducing disease in the central nervous system (CNS). (It should be noted that this mechanism is distinct from the mechanism recently demonstrated by De Magistris *et al.* (1992). In that study, greater competition was seen with a peptide analogue of the immunizing peptide than with a peptide of equal affinity but unrelated sequence implying that MHC plus peptide analogue is a competitive antagonist for the T-cell receptor.) A number of studies (Smilek & McDevitt, unpublished observations) have failed to demonstrate the induction of anergy, suppression, or other mechanism which might explain the unique properties of Ac1-11[4A].

However, further studies with Ac1-11[4A] and Ac1-11 have shown that both peptides are capable of preventing induction of EAE if they are injected in incomplete Freund's adjuvant 5–10 days prior to immunization with Ac1-11 in complete Freund's adjuvant (Smilek *et al.*, 1991). This result is similar to numerous earlier demonstrations that pre-immunization of animals with whole myelin basic protein or its peptides in aqueous solution, or in incomplete Freund's adjuvant prevented subsequent induction of EAE. The mechanism of this prevention is unknown. Nonetheless, there is an apparent dissociation in the effects of Ac1-11 and Ac1-11[4A] in *treating* EAE once the disease has been induced and the animals are showing early neurological symptoms. In this setting, with onset of disease at day 9–11 following immunization, injection of large doses of Ac1-11 in incomplete Freund's adjuvant failed to affect the course of disease when compared to untreated control animals. In contrast, injection of similar doses of Ac1-11[4A] in incomplete Freund's adjuvant resulted in a striking reduction in symptoms and signs of EAE and a marked shortening of disease duration to a period of 1–3 days.

Once again, there is no evidence for T-cell anergy induced by Ac1-11[4A] in these animals. This peptide might stimulate Ac1-11 specific T cells in the peripheral lymphoid system where they remain, and are thus prevented from migrating to the CNS. This possibility as well as several others require further investigation before the mechanism by which AC1-11[4A] is successful in treating EAE can be elucidated. Such studies are of considerable importance because they raise the possibility that an immunodominant peptide epitope which is itself the target of the autoimmune process could be used in the treatment of a particular autoimmune disease. In addition to this possibility, the results in Table 14.1, particularly sections 2 and 4 indicate that MHC-binding peptides of related and unrelated sequence (to the autoantigen) can function effectively as competitive inhibitors for the induction of an autoimmune disease and may in future be used to treat already established autoimmune disease processes.

Type 1 insulin-dependent diabetes mellitus in the non-obese diabetic mouse

As an autoimmune disease model for peptide immunotherapy, EAE has several limitations. The disease is of abrupt onset, explosive in nature in most immunization regimens, of short duration and difficult to reinduce once the animals have recovered from an episode of EAE. This makes it particularly difficult to study peptides which might be used to *treat* an already established autoimmune process. The non-obese diabetic (NOD) mouse model on the other hand, offers the advantage that it is a spontaneous autoimmune disease with close similarity to its human counterpart, develops slowly over a period of months, has a specific target organ and is well characterized in terms of the T-cell-immune response and the autoantibodies produced, and the histological changes which are progressively seen in the islets of Langerhans. However, insulin-dependent diabetes mellitus (IDDM) in the NOD mouse suffers from the drawback that the molecular target autoantigen is as yet unknown, although several candidates have been identified recently.

NOD mice manifest a progressive autoimmune insulitis with lymphocytic accumulation in the islets of Langerhans beginning at 4–6 weeks of age and ending in diabetes in 60–80% of females by 8–9 months of age (Makino *et al.*, 1980; Rossini *et al.*, 1985). The disease is T-cell mediated and a number of laboratories have devised an adoptive transfer system which demonstrates that disease transfer required both $CD4^+$ and $CD8^+$ T cells (Wicker *et al.*, 1986; Thivolet *et al.*, 1991). IDDM in the NOD mouse can be prevented with antibodies to the $I\text{-}A^{NOD}$ class II molecules (Boitard *et al.*, 1988), anti-CD4 (Koike *et al.*, 1987; Wang *et al.*, 1987; Shizuru *et al.*, 1988), thymectomy (Ogawa *et al.*, 1985), and cyclosporin (Wang *et al.*, 1988). Since the NOD mouse is I-E negative and expressed only $I\text{-}A^{NOD}$ at the cell surface and since introduction of a site specific mutated $I\text{-}A^{NOD}$ β chain can greatly reduce the incidence of diabetes in NOD mice, there is every reason to believe that the MHC-linked gene responsible for susceptibility to IDDM in this strain is the $I\text{-}A^{NOD}$ molecule itself (Shizuru *et al.*, 1988).

The α chain of $I\text{-}A^{NOD}$ is identical in sequence to $I\text{-}A_a{}^d$. The β chain in $I\text{-}A^{NOD}$ is different from all other inbred murine haplotypes in that it carries histidine at position 56 and serine at position 57, in contrast to proline at 56 and aspartic acid at 57 in other murine strains (Lund *et al.*, 1990). This is similar to the finding that the presence of a non-charged amino acid at position 57 in the $DQ\beta$ chain is strongly associated with susceptibility to IDDM in man (Acha-Orbea & McDevitt, 1987; Todd, 1990). Peptides which bind strongly to $I\text{-}A^{NOD}$ should be affective competitors for the putative autoantigenic peptide being presented by $I\text{-}A^{NOD}$ in the lymph nodes draining the pancreas. Experiments by McDevitt *et al.* (1991) have identified five different peptides which are antigenic in NOD mice and which are capable of binding to $I\text{-}A^{NOD}$. Other peptides have been identified which are non-immunogenic in NOD mice but are also incapable of competing for T-cell stimulation using spleen cells from immunized NOD mice, implying that these peptides do not bind to $I\text{-}A^{NOD}$.

Utilizing a standard method for transfer of IDDM, Lock has shown that peptides which bind to I-A^{NOD} can prevent transfer of disease, while non-binding control peptides are unable to do so. The disease transfer model is one in which 10^7 spleen cells from recently diabetic NOD females are injected into 650 rad irradiated young NOD males and females, and the recipients are followed by type I IDDM. Diabetes develops in 80-90% of the recipients with 20-30 days and this incidence can be reduced to 20% or less by the injection of 1-2 mg of a blocking peptide in incomplete Freund's adjuvant at the time of cell transfer. These experimental results, while encouraging, suffer from the drawback that all of the binding peptides identified so far are immunogenic in the NOD mouse. Experiments are currently underway to identify peptides which bind to I-A^{NOD}, are unrelated to the sequences of known islet cell specific proteins such as glutamic acid decarboxylas 1 and 2, and which are non-immunogenic in the NOD mouse. Such a peptide would be an ideal candidate for attempts to prevent transfer of IDDM, and for immunotherapy of spontaneous IDDM in normal, unmanipulated NOD mice.

Conclusion

The results obtained to date with a variety of competitive antagonists of peptide binding to MHC class II proteins collectively support the premise that reducing the density or number of MHC autoantigenic peptide complexes *in vivo* will result in a reduction in the severity of the autoimmune disease. In addition to identifying MHC antagonists, the success of this approach will require solution of several complex problems. These include the stability, metabolism and targeting of the antagonist to the endosomal-lysosomal compartments in antigen-presenting cells. Furthermore, the local concentration and affinity of the antagonist must exceed that of the autoantigenic peptide(s), which will differ in each disease. While MHC antagonists have been shown to be effective in preventing the induction of autoimmune disease, they have yet to be shown to be therapeutically useful in an ongoing autoimmune process. Clearly, the major challenge at the present time is to design MHC antagonists which are non-immunogenic and capable of achieving sufficient concentration in antigen-presenting cells to permit them to be effective therapeutic agents.

References

Acha-Orbea, H. & McDevitt, H. O. (1987). The first domain of the nonobese diabetic mouse class II I-Ab-chain is unique. *Proceedings of the National Academy of Sciences USA* **84**, 2435-2439.

Adorini, L., Moreno, J., Momburg, F., Hammerling, G., Guery, J.-C., Valli, A. & Fuchs, S. (1991). Exogenous peptides compete for the presentation of endogenous antigens to major histocompatibility complex class II restricted T cells. *Journal of Experimental Medicine* **174**, 945–948.

Adorini, L., Sette, A., Buus, S., Grey, H., Darsley, M., Lehmann, P., Doria, G., Nagy, Z. & Appella, E. (1988). Interaction of an immunodominant epitope with Ia molecule in T cell activation. *Proceedings of the National Academy of Sciences USA* **85**, 5181.

Babbitt, B., Matsueda, G., Haber, E., Unanue, E. & Allen, P. (1986). Antigenic competition at the level of peptide-Ia molecules. *Proceedings of the National Academy of Sciences USA* **83**, 4509.

Boitard, C., Bendelac, A., Richard, M. F., Carnaud, C. & Bach, J. F. (1988). Prevention of diabetes in nonobese diabetic mice by anti-Ia monoclonal antibodies: transfer of protection by splenic T cells. *Proceedings of the National Academy of Sciences USA* **85**, 9719–9723.

Buus, S., Sette, A., Colon, S., Miles, C. & Grey, H. (1987). The relation between major histocompatibility complex restriction and the capacity of Ia to bind immunogenic peptides. *Science* **235**, 1353.

Chicz, R., Urban, R., Gorga, J., Lane, W., Stern, L., Vignali, D. & Strominger, J. (1992). The predominant naturally processed peptides bound to HLA-DR1 are derived from MHC related molecules and are heterogeneous in size. (Submitted).

DeMagistris, D., Alexander, J., Coggeshall, M., Altman, A., Gaeta, F. C. A., Grey, H. M. & Sette, A. (1992). Antigen analog-major histocompatibility complexes act as antagonist of the T cell receptor. *Cell* **68**, 625–629.

Evavold, B. & Allen, P. (1991). Separation of IL-4 production from Th cell proliferation by an altered T cell receptor ligand. *Science* **252**, 1308.

Fritz, R. B., Skeen, M. J., Jen Chou, C.-H., Garcia, M. & Egorov, I. K. (1985). Major histocompatibility complex-linked control of the murine immune response to myelin basic protein. *Journal of Immunology* **134**, 3238–2332.

Gautam, A. M. & Glynn, P. (1990). Competition between foreign and self proteins in antigen presentation. Ovalbumin can inhibit activation of myelin basic protein-specific T cells. *Journal of Immunology* **144**, 1177–1180.

Gautam, A. M., Pearson, C. I., Sinha, A. A., Smilek, D. E., Stiman, L. & McDevitt, H. O. (1992). Inhibition of experimental autoimmune encephalomyelitis by a nonmimmunogenic non-self peptide that binds to I-A^u. *Journal of Immunology* **148**, 3049–3055.

Godfrey, W., Lewis, G. & Goodman, J. (1984). The anatomy of an antigen molecule: functional subregions of L-tyrosine-p-azobenzenearsonate. *Molecular Immunology* **21**, 969–978.

Guery, J.-C., Sette, A., Leighton, J., Dragomir, A. & Adorini, L. (1992). Selective immunosuppression by administration of major complex (MHC) class II binding peptides. *Journal of Experimental Medicine* **175**, 1345–1352.

Guillet, J., Lai, M., Briner, T., Smith, J. & Gefter, M. (1986). Interaction of peptide antigens and class-II major histocompatibility complex antigens. *Nature* **324**, 260–263.

Hunt, D., Michel, H., Dickinson, T., Shabanowitz, J., Cox, A., Sakaguchi, K., Appella, E., Grey, H. & Sette, A. (1992). Peptides presented to the immune system by the murine class II molecule, I-A^d. *Science* (in press).

Koike, T., Itoh, Y., Ishi, Ito, I., Takabayashi, K., Maruyama, N., Tomioka, H. & Yoshida, S. (1987). Preventative effect of monoclonal anti-L3T4 antibody on development of diabetes in NOD mice. *Diabetes* **36**, 539–541.

Lamont, A. G., Sette, A., Fujinami, R., Colon, S. M., Miles, C. & Grey, H. M. (1990). Inhibition of experimental autoimmune encephalomyelitis induction in SJL/J mice by using a peptide with high affinity for IA^s molecules. *Journal of Immunology* **145**, 1687–1693.

Lando, Z., Teitelbaum, D. & Arnon, R. (1979). Effect of cyclophosphamide on suppressor cell activity in mice unresponsive to EAE. *Journal of Immunology* **123**, 2156–2160.

Lorenz, R., Blum, J. & Allen, P. (1990). Constitutive competition by self proteins for antigen presentation can be overcome by receptor enhanced uptake. *Journal of Immunology* **144**, 1660–1606.

Lund, T., O'Reilly, L., Hutchings, P., Kanagawa, O., Simpson, E., Gravely, R., Chandler, P., Dyson, J., Picard, J. K., Edwards, A., Kioussis, D. & Cooke, A. (1990). Prevention of insulin-dependent diabetes mellitus in non-obese diabetic mice by transgenes encoding modified I-Ab-chain or normal I-Ea chain. *Nature* **345**, 727–729.

Makino, S., Kunimoto, D., Muraoka, Y., Mizushima, Y., Katagiri, K. & Tochino, Y. (1980). Breeding of non-obese, diabetic strain of mice. *Experimental Animals* **29**, 1–13.

McDevitt, H. O., Lock, C. & Vaysburd, M. (1991). Analysis of the role of MHC class II molecules in autoimmune disease. *Diabetes Research and Clinical Practice*, Vol 14, p. S35, 11th International Diabetes Workshop Nagasaki, Japan.

McFarlin, D., Hsu, S. C., Selemenda, S. B., Chou, F. C. & Kibler, R. (1975). The immune response against myelin basic protein in two strains of rat with different genetic capacity to develop experimental allergic encephalomyelitis. *Journal of Experimental Medicine* **141**, 72–81.

Muller, S., Adorini, L., Juretic, A. & Nagy, Z. (1991). Selective *in vivo* inhibition of T cell activation by class II MHC binding peptides administered in soluble form. *Journal of Immunology* **145**, 4006–4011.

Ogawa, M., Maruyama, T., Hasegawa, T., Kanaya, T., Kobayashi, F., Tochino, Y. & Uta, H. (1985). The inhibitory effect of neonatal thymectomy on the incidence of insulitis in non-obese diabetes (NOD) mice. *Biomedical Research* **6**, 103–105.

Rock, K. L. & Benacerraf, B. (1983). Inhibition of antigen specific T lymphocyte activation by structurally related Ir gene controlled polymers. Evidence of specific competition for accessory cell antigen presentation. *Journal of Experimental Medicine* **157**, 1618–1634.

Rossini, A. A., Morders, J. P. & Like, A. A. (1985). Immunology of insulin-dependent diabetes mellitus. *Annual Review of Immunology* **3**, 289–320.

Rudensky, A., Preston-Hurlburt, P., Hong, S., Barlow, A. & Janeway, C. (1991). Sequence analysis of peptides bound to MHC class II molecules. *Nature* **353**, 622–627.

Sakai, K., Zamvil, S. S., Mitchell, D. J., Lim, M., Rothbard, J. B. & Steinman, L. (1988). Characterization of a major encephalitogenic T cell epitope in SJL/J mice with synthetic oligopeptides of myelin basic protein. *Journal of Neuroimmunology* **19**, 21–31.

Shizuru, J. A., Taylor-Edwards, C., Banks, B. A., Gregory, A. K. & Fathman, C. G. (1988). Immunotherapy of the nonobese diabetic mouse: treatment with an antibody to T helped lymphocytes. *Science* **240**, 659–662.

Smilek, D., Wraith, D. C., Hodgkinson, S., Dwivedy, S., Steinman, L. & McDevitt, H. O. (1991). A single amino acid change in a myelin basic protein peptide confers the capacity to prevent rather than induce experimental autoimmune encephalomyetis. *Proceedings of the National Academy of Sciences USA* **88**, 9633–9637.

Thivolet, C., Benelac, A., Bedossa, P., Bach, J.-F. & Carnaud, C. (1991). CD8[+] T cell homing to the pancreas in the non-obese diabetic (NOD) mouse is CD4[+] T cell dependent. *Journal of Immunology* **146**, 85–88.

Todd, J. A. (1990). Genetic control of autoimmunity in type I diabetes. *Immunology Today* **11**, 122–129.

Tuohy, V. K., Lu, Z., Sobel, R. A., Laursen, R. A. & Lees, M. B. (1989). Identification of an encephalitogenic determinant of myelin proteolipid for SJL mice. *Journal of Immunology* **142**, 1523–1527.

Wang, Y., Hao, L., Gill, R. G., Lafferty, K. J. (1987). Autoimmune diabetes in NOD mouse is L3T4 T lymphocyte dependent. *Diabetes* **36**, 535–538.

Wang, Y., McDuffie, M., Nomikos, I. N., Hao, L. & Lafferty, K. J. (1988). Effect of cyclosporine on immunologically mediated diabetes in nonobese diabetic mice. *Transplantation* **46**, 101s–106s.

Werdelin, O. (1982). Chemically related antigens compete for presentation by accessory cells to T cells. *Journal of Immunology* **129**, 1883–1891.

Wicker, L. S., Miller, B. J. & Mullen, Y. (1986). Transfer of autoimmune, diabetes mellitus with splenocytes from nonobese diabetic (NOD) mice. *Diabetes* **35**, 855–860.

Williams, R. M. & Moore, M. J. (1973). Linkage of susceptibility to experimental allergic encephalomyelitis to the major histocompatibility locus in the rat. *Journal of Experimental Medicine* **138**, 775–783.

Wraith, D. C., Smilek, D. E., Mitchell, D. J., Steinman, L. & McDevitt, H. O. (1989). Antigen recognition in autoimmune encephalomyelitis and the potential for peptide-mediated immunotherapy. *Cell* **59**, 247–255.

Zakai, K., Zamvil, S. S., Mitchell, D. J., Hodgkinson,S., Rothbard, J. B. & Steinman, L. (1989). Prevention of experimental encephalomyelitis with peptides that block interaction of T cells with major histocompatibility complex proteins. *Proceedings of the National Academy of Sciences USA* **86**, 9470–9474.

Zamvil, S. S., Mitchell, D. J., Moore, A. C., Kitamura, K., Steinman, L. & Rothbard, J. B. (1986). T cell epitope of the autoantigen myelin basic protein that induces encephalomyelitis. *Nature* **324**, 258–260.

Index